Disability Studies and Disability Evaluation

Disability Studies and Disability Evaluation

Guest Editors

Debra Harley
Siyi Chao

MDPI

Basel • Beijing • Wuhan • Barcelona • Belgrade • Novi Sad • Cluj • Manchester

Guest Editors
Debra Harley
Department of Early Childhood, Special Education, & Counselor Education
University of Kentucky
Lexington
USA

Siyi Chao
Department of Early Childhood, Special Education, & Counselor Education
University of Kentucky
Lexington
USA

Editorial Office
MDPI AG
Grosspeteranlage 5
4052 Basel, Switzerland

This is a reprint of the Special Issue, published open access by the journal *Healthcare* (ISSN 2227-9032), freely accessible at: https://www.mdpi.com/journal/healthcare/special_issues/DAVZ8RZ7VF.

For citation purposes, cite each article independently as indicated on the article page online and as indicated below:

Lastname, A.A.; Lastname, B.B. Article Title. *Journal Name* **Year**, *Volume Number*, Page Range.

ISBN 978-3-7258-7887-1 (Hbk)
ISBN 978-3-7258-7888-8 (PDF)
https://doi.org/10.3390/books978-3-7258-7888-8

Contents

About the Editors

Debra Harley

Debra Harley is a professor and a coordinator of the Counselor Education and Supervision Doctoral Program at the University of Kentucky. Her main research interests include disability and mental health concerns of diverse populations, intersectionality, substance use disorder, and ethics. She has published 100 peer-reviewed articles, 91 book chapters and six books on disability-related topics. Recently, she was a recipient of the Distinguished Career in Rehabilitation Award from the Association for Rehabilitation, Research, Policy and Education.

Siyi Chao

Siyi Chao is an assistant professor in the Counselor Education Program at University of Kentucky. Her research focuses on social identity and intersectionality among people with disabilities, with an emphasis on disability identity development, discrimination, career development, mental health, and multicultural counseling competencies. Her work also addresses career development for school-age populations, community-based rehabilitation, and the training of supervisors and human service professionals. She has published fifteen peer-reviewed articles, three edited books, one translated book, and seven book chapters.

Preface

Disabilities studies focuses on the lived experiences and knowledges of disabled individuals. Recognizing the vast diversity in health and function in people with chronic illness and disability, this Reprint aims to call attention to disparities in healthcare for disabled people. It is important to understand the factors that influence the health outcomes of disabled people in order to improve them.

Debra Harley and Siyi Chao
Guest Editors

healthcare

MDPI

Editorial

Disability Studies and Disability Evaluation in Healthcare—Themes and Challenges Moving Forward

Debra A. Harley * and Si-Yi Chao

Department of Early Childhood, Special Education, and Counselor Education, University of Kentucky, 229 Taylor Education Building, 597 S Upper St, Lexington, KY 40506-0001, USA; siyichao7185@uky.edu
* Correspondence: debra.harley@uky.edu

1. Introduction

Persons with disabilities experience significant barriers to accessing healthcare, yet the gap between disability studies and healthcare service delivery remains a persistent structural problem. The number of individuals living with disabilities is growing, which is attributed to factors such as population increase, aging, and medical advances that increase survival rates and prolong life; this has increased the demand for health services [1]. However, demand alone does not translate into access. Persons with disabilities and their families experience significant barriers to accessing inclusive healthcare on a global scale [2]. Building health systems that genuinely respond to the complexity of disability-related needs requires a deliberate, coordinated effort across research, policy, and practice [3].

Among the most immediate human consequences of inadequate systemic support is the burden carried by family caregivers. Caregivers of persons with disabilities, especially those supporting children with intellectual and developmental disabilities (IDD), bear substantial burden and stress in managing the demands of daily care [4]. Having a child with special health and care needs creates multiple challenges for families as a unit, for this individual child, and for the parents and/or caregivers. These children require levels of medical care and daily assistance that exceed those of children without disabilities, placing demands on families that adversely affect their work–life balance [5]. Social support is related to better long-term care planning for a child or adult with IDD, but fewer than 40% of caregivers report having the social support they need [6].

The challenges do not diminish as individuals with disabilities age and, in many respects, they intensify with time. People with IDD are living longer and experiencing life transitions, such as retirement, that the existing service and policy frameworks were not designed to address [7]. Functional aging among people with IDD accelerates relative to the general population, and the mismatch between chronological age and functional capacity exposes a structural inadequacy in how care systems categorize and respond to needs. Although the importance of interdisciplinary collaboration in developing planning, pathways, and the integration of disability within the broader healthcare services is recognized, the extent to which disability studies and disability evaluation research examine disability inclusion in healthcare and from an interdisciplinary perspective is limited. Building on efforts to create a more inclusive healthcare and recognizing that a variety of people with chronic illnesses and disabilities exist along a spectrum of health and function, Gulley et al. [8] argue that the existing frameworks for addressing the health of persons with chronic conditions and disabilities require fundamental evaluation and reform, particularly for those whose care needs are ongoing or elevated. This Special Issue enters this broader discourse precisely when the consequences of inadequate response—for caregivers, aging adults with disabilities, and marginalized communities worldwide—remain profound and pressing.

2. An Overview of Published Articles in This Special Issue

The aim of this Special Issue, "Disability Studies and Disability Evaluation", is to evaluate how disability studies impacts service delivery and the health and social outcomes of people with disability through an examination of disability awareness, perceptions of healthcare providers, and the influence of social factors on quality of life. Emphasis is placed on the implications of individual, psychosocial, and organizational elements of improving health and mental health outcomes among people with chronic illness and disability. The articles included in this Special Issue address a broad spectrum of topics within this framework and reflect perspectives including caregiver burden in families; interdisciplinary research between critical disability studies and healthcare; person-centered management in disability services; age disparities between disability types; intersecting identities in college students across ethnicities; enhancing social, financial and health service inclusivity; the support of workers with intellectual and developmental disabilities transitioning into retirement; disability-inclusive approaches within neglected tropical disease programming; and the structural evolution of inclusive healthcare systems for children with disabilities. The nine articles trace a path from family caregiving and research epistemology through systemic inequities in service delivery, workforce participation, and global health infrastructure.

Caregivers of children with disabilities carry a disproportionate burden, with diminished support and reduced coping capacity. Garcia-Grau et al. [Contributor 1] present a fuzzy-set qualitative comparative analysis of causal configurations of psychosocial conditions associated with both high and low levels of caregiver burden in families of children receiving early intervention services. Low family confidence emerges as the central driver of elevated burden, while parental self-efficacy and social support retain protective value regardless of a child's functional level [Contributor 1]. Toman et al. [Contributor 2] raise critical questions for researchers when conducting disability research and challenges the oppositional training of professionals in disability studies and the healthcare and medical research fields, highlighting that continued non-collaboration inflicts measurable harm on the populations that both fields claim to serve and that repositioning disabled individuals as active research partners is an ethical requirement, rather than a programmatic aspiration. Disability services are recognized as being person-centered approaches to promote positive outcomes for individuals with disabilities, of which adequate allocation of resources is required to meet the planned services [Contributor 2]. Bianchi et al. [Contributor 3] investigate how individual and contextual factors shape resource use in individualized support planning of those with intellectual and developmental disabilities (IDD) who receive services in residential, family, or independent living. As individuals with developmental disabilities grow older, the effects of their functional age are accelerated compared to their non-IDD counterparts [Contributor 3]. Jeong [Contributor 4] measures the disparity in functional ability and chronic illness prevalence between adults with developmental disabilities and other disabilities, finding activity limitations that current policy frameworks are inadequate to respond to and for which function-based care models are urgently needed [Contributor 4].

Structural disadvantage extends beyond care and service systems. Students with disabilities are underrepresented in college and face compounded disadvantages in career-related factors. Chao and Wilson [Contributor 5] explore the influence of intersecting disabilities and ethnic identities on career decision self-efficacy, career outcome expectations, perceived career barriers, and support among college students with disabilities from diverse

https://doi.org/10.3390/healthcare14081016

racial and ethnic backgrounds, indicating that students from underrepresented ethnic groups face markedly greater career-related barriers than their European American peers and that culturally responsive interventions affirming multiple identities are structurally necessary [Contributor 5]. Access to social support and financial means can influence the inclusion of persons with disabilities in service utilization. Alturif et al. [Contributor 6] explore caregivers' perspectives on awareness, perceived barriers, and accessibility of social and financial services for people with disabilities in Saudi Arabia, documenting that over 70% of caregivers remain unaware of available supports, a gap deepened by technological barriers, administrative complexity, and the near-absence of decentralized outreach in rural areas [Contributor 6]. The effects of disability across the lifespan elicit different adjustments. Sanchez et al. [Contributor 7] focus on needs of aging workers with IDD who experience a declining work ability because of aging and disability and who transition to retirement, underscoring that flexible workplace accommodations and individualized planning across families, employers, and professionals are critical for dignified aging [Contributor 7]. The most marginalized populations are disproportionately faced with disease and illness that are further perpetuated by structural, social, and political attributes of exclusion. Juma et al. [Contributor 8] examine the concept of inclusion within neglected tropical disease (NTD) programming, with a particular focus on intersecting forms of marginalization, including poverty, gender, disability, and displacement. The authors contend that disability-inclusive strategies and community empowerment must be embedded throughout health systems, rather than treated as peripheral concerns [Contributor 8]. Children with disabilities continue to face systemic challenges in healthcare. Gulgosteren et al. [Contributor 9] employ bibliometric methods and analyze the structure and evolution of the scientific literature on inclusive healthcare systems for children with disabilities, identifying growing academic attention to neurodevelopmental disorders and family-centered care since 2015. Still, the dominance of high-income countries in the literature remains a structural barrier to equitable, community-based care globally [Contributor 9].

3. Conclusions

Collectively, the contributors in this Special Issue call attention to the current state of evaluation or measurement of disabilities, as well as a need for coordinated interdisciplinary research between disability studies and healthcare. Several themes emerged from the contribution in this Special Issue:

- The healthcare needs of children and adults with intellectual and developmental disabilities;
- Support for caregivers of persons with disabilities;
- The intersectionality of disability and demographic characteristics;
- The social determinants of inclusion of persons with disabilities in healthcare service utilization;
- Life transitions of people with disabilities.

Disability is extraordinarily diverse, yet across different national contexts and population groups, people with disabilities experience remarkably consistent barriers when seeking healthcare, including exclusion, lack of autonomy in decision-making about their health, healthcare costs, poor availability of services, and physical and systematic inaccessibility [3]. The gap in disability studies and evaluation in healthcare causes consideration for a comprehensive, inclusive approach that accounts for people with disabilities as active participants, integrates family members and informal supports, aligns planned services with real-world needs, and attends to the full range of transitions across the lifespan. Movement from policy to practice is a foundational requirement of any comprehensive disability healthcare approach. The present Special Issue addresses this gap through building de-

https://doi.org/10.3390/healthcare14081016

terminants of enablement that can lead to better management of healthcare services for people with disabilities and their families.

Moving forward, to better address the interplay between disability and healthcare, future research should be collaborative across disability studies and healthcare disciplines, and structurally integrated in design, methodology, and dissemination, rather than parallel or nominally interdisciplinary. A lifespan perspective is essential because the sequence and progression of many types of disabilities are expected to continue indefinitely, and frameworks that only address discrete life stages will remain inadequate to the realities that people with disabilities actually face. Persons with disabilities continue to encounter considerable barriers when accessing healthcare services, which negatively affects their chances of achieving their highest attainable standard of living and might contribute to their shorter life expectancy and poorer health outcomes than people without disabilities [8]. Sustained commitment to collaborative, lifespan-oriented, and structurally integrated research remains the most defensible means of achieving the equitable healthcare outcomes that people with disabilities deserve.

Author Contributions: D.A.H. and S.-Y.C. contributed equally to the conceptualization, curation, and writing of this editorial. All authors have read and agreed to the published version of the manuscript.

Conflicts of Interest: The authors declare no conflicts of interest.

List of Contributions:

1. García-Grau, P.; Argente-Tormo, J.; Gabriel Martínez-Rico, G.; Rómulo González-García, R.J. Caregiver Burden in Early Intervention: A Fuzzy-Set Qualitative Comparative Analysis of Causal Configurations. *Healthcare* **2025**, *13*, 3026. https://doi.org/10.3390/healthcare13233026.
2. Toman, M.; Atanasio, M.; Teaster, P.B. The Questions, Challenges, and Possibilities When Joining Critical Disabilities Studies and Healthcare Research. *Healthcare* **2025**, *13*, 2925. https://doi.org/10.3390/healthcare13222925.
3. Bianchi, P.; Lombardi, M.; Croce, L.; Caserta, A.; Speziale, R. The Impact of Support Intensity Needs on Person-Centered Case Management. *Healthcare* **2025**, *13*, 2697. https://doi.org/10.3390/healthcare13212697.
4. Jeong, J.U. Aging Unequally: Functional Age Disparities Between Developmental and Non-Developmental Disabilities. *Healthcare* **2025**, *13*, 2412. https://doi.org/10.3390/healthcare13192412.
5. Chao, S.Y.; Wilson, K.B. Intersecting Identities and Career-Related Factors Among College Students with Disabilities Across Ethnic Groups. *Healthcare* **2025**, *13*, 2119. https://doi.org/10.3390/healthcare13172119.
6. Alturif, G.; Saleh, W.; Alsanad, H.; Ababio-Donkor, A. Enhancing Inclusive Social, Financial, and Health Services for People with Disabilities in Saudi Arabia: Insights from Caregivers. *Healthcare* **2025**, *13*, 1901. https://doi.org/10.3390/healthcare13151901.
7. Sánchez, B.; de Borja Jordán de Urríes, F.; Verdugo, M.A.; de Jesús Abena, C.; Sanblás, V. Strategies to Prevent Work Ability Decline and Support Retirement Transition in Workers with Intellectual and Developmental Disabilities. *Healthcare* **2025**, *13*, 1766. https://doi.org/10.3390/healthcare13141766.
8. Juma, I.Z.; Oguntoye, O.; Sankar, G.; Weber, J.; Qureshi, B.; Amanyi-Enegela, J. Inclusion in Neglected Tropical Disease Programmes: A Review of Inclusive Approaches for Control and Elimination. *Healthcare* **2026**, *14*, 27. https://doi.org/10.3390/healthcare14010027.
9. Gulgosteren, E.; Onturk, Y.; Cuhadar, A.; Zahiu, M.; Stanescu, M.; Stanescu, R. Inclusive Healthcare Systems for Children with Disabilities: A Bibliometric Analysis and Visualization. *Healthcare* **2025**, *13*, 2106. https://doi.org/10.3390/healthcare13172106.

References

1. Galvin, A.E.; Friedman, D.B.; Hebert, J.R. Focus on disability-free life expectancy: Implications for health-related quality of life. *Qual. Life Res.* **2021**, *30*, 2187–2195. [CrossRef] [PubMed]
2. Global Disability Summit. Global Disability Inclusion Report: Accelerating Disability Inclusion in a Changing and Diverse World. Available online: http://www.globaldisabilitysummit.org/resource/global-disability-inclusion-report (accessed on 5 April 2025).
3. Kuper, H.; Aziztunnisa, L.; Gatta, D.R.; Rotenberg, S.; Banks, L.M.; Smythe, T.; Heydt, P. Building disability-inclusive health systems. *Lancet* **2024**, *9*, E316–E325. [CrossRef] [PubMed]
4. Lahije, S.T.A.; Lujikx, J.; Waninge, A.; van der Putten, A.A.J. Family resilience affecting well-being of families with a child with profound intellectual and multiple disabilities. *Intellect. Dev. Disabil.* **2024**, *62*, 101–113. [CrossRef] [PubMed]
5. Stevns, E.K.; Aziz, S.; Wuensch, K.L.; Walcott, C. Caregivers of children with special healthcare needs: A quantitative examination of work-family culture, caregiver burden, and work-life balance. *J. Child Fam. Stud.* **2024**, *33*, 1365–1377. [CrossRef]
6. Santos, T.; Steinway, C.; Mastrogiannis, A.; Chen, J.; Woodward, J.; Riddle, I.; Spicer, B.; Berens, J.; Davis, T.; Cornacchia, M.; et al. Caregiver support, burden, and long-term planning among caregiver support, burden, and long-term planning among caregivers of individuals with intellectual and developmental disabilities: A cross-sectional study. *J. Appl. Res. Intellect. Disabil.* **2023**, *36*, 1229–1240. [CrossRef] [PubMed]
7. Anderson, L.L.; Hall, S.; Kramme, J.E.D.; Stancliffe, R. Transition to retirement: The lived experiences of adults with intellectual disabilities. *J. Appl. Res. Intellect. Disabil.* **2023**, *36*, 547–557. [CrossRef] [PubMed]
8. Gulley, S.P.; Rasch, E.K.; Bethell, C.D.; Carle, A.C.; Druss, B.G.; Houtrow, A.J.; Reichard, A.; Chan, L. At the intersection of chronic disease, disability and health services research: A scoping literature review. *Disabil. Health J.* **2018**, *11*, 192–203. [CrossRef] [PubMed]

https://doi.org/10.3390/healthcare14081016

healthcare

MDPI

Article

Intersecting Identities and Career-Related Factors Among College Students with Disabilities Across Ethnic Groups

Si-Yi Chao * and Keith B. Wilson

Early Childhood, Special Education & Counselor Education Department, University of Kentucky, Lexington, KY 40506, USA; keithbwilson@uky.edu
* Correspondence: siyichao7185@uky.edu

Abstract

This study explores how intersecting disabilities and ethnic identities influence key career-related factors, including career decision self-efficacy, career outcome expectations, perceived career barriers, and social support, among college students with disabilities from diverse racial and ethnic backgrounds. **Background/Objectives:** Applying social cognitive career theory (SCCT) and intersectionality frameworks, this research addresses a critical gap in understanding the unique challenges and strengths experienced by underrepresented students with disabilities in postsecondary education. **Method:** Quantitative data were collected from approximately 306 participants representing various ethnic groups, including African American, Asian American, Hispanic, and other ethnic backgrounds, alongside European American peers. **Results:** Findings revealed that underrepresented students with disabilities reported significantly stronger ethnic identity affirmation but also perceived greater career-related barriers compared to their European American counterparts. These results demonstrate the need for culturally responsive career development practices and inclusive campus environments that affirm students' multiple identities. **Conclusions:** Implications are discussed for higher education professionals, rehabilitation counselors, disability service providers, and career counselors seeking to promote equitable career outcomes and identity-conscious support systems.

Keywords: disability identity; ethnicity identity; intersectionality; college students with disabilities; perceived career barriers; social support

1. Introduction

In recent years, social justice debates have increasingly focused on making higher education institutions more accessible to historically marginalized groups of students, such as students of color, LGBTQ+ students, women in science, technology, engineering, and math (STEM) fields, students from low-income families, and most critically, students with disabilities. Colleges and universities today enroll more students with disabilities than ever before [1]. The growth in college students with disabilities from different backgrounds is a broader trend toward greater diversity on campuses throughout the nation.

National data reports a growing trend that more students with disabilities are enrolled in college and represent a wide range of racial and ethnic backgrounds. The percentage of undergraduates reporting a disability has increased significantly, rising from 10.8% in the 2007–2008 academic year to 20.5% in the 2019–2020 academic year [2,3]. This increase is due to better awareness and access to disability services at colleges. Furthermore, the characteristics of students with disabilities have changed, becoming more racially and ethnically diverse over the past two decades. The percentage of students who identified as two or more races and had a disability was highest in 2019–2020, at 25.4%. They were followed by American Indian/Alaska Native students at 23.7%, Pacific Islander students at 22.1%, Hispanic students at 21.3%, White students at 21.1%, Black students at 18.0%, and Asian students at 13.9%. These numbers reflect a clear shift from the year 2016, when the population of students with disabilities in higher education was both smaller and less diverse [2]. The proportion of Hispanic and Black students with disabilities has increased with their college attendance. At large, these trends highlight the significance of inclusive and culturally responsive services that address the unique needs of college students of color with disabilities at the postsecondary level.

The campus environment, which is increasingly multicultural but still subject to predominant cultural pressures, typically reveals larger societal dynamics through the lens of a disability and ethnic minority college student. For underrepresented students, coping with predominantly European American institutional demands is stressful and frustrating. Decision-making, interests, goals, and engagement in career tasks are all influenced by intersection of disability and racial/ethnic identity [4]. College students of color with disabilities face unique and multifaceted career development challenges rooted in systemic racism, ableism, and a lack of culturally responsive support services. The students often experience issues such as a shortage of diverse role models, career counseling that is insufficiently inclusive, and limited participation in internships and employment-based learning experiences. The structural barriers impede a minority college student with a disability in following through and retaining high career aspirations through significantly damaging self-confidence, lowering motivation, and negatively impacting career outcome expectations [5,6]. Identity development can be challenging for students with multiple marginalized identities as they navigate higher education in the complex sociocultural environment, which is characterized by power disparities, social inequalities, and intersecting forms of privilege and oppression. Multiple marginalized students might struggle to build and evolve complex selves despite constant processes of surveillance and negotiation [7]. Intersectional racial/ethnic and disability identity affirmation and the pursuit of academic and professional fulfillment require ongoing observation, constant self-reflection, and assessment of one's own self-efficacy [6]. Moreover, social support from families, peers, mentors, and the campus is crucial in fostering resilience and perseverance, particularly when students experience discrimination or inadequate representation in mainstream career services [8,9].

Despite these challenges, few empirical studies have explored the complex perspectives of college students with disabilities from racially and ethnically diverse backgrounds. Research on the different perceptions between intersecting identities and important career-related factors is desperately needed. Implications for career counselors, disability service professionals, academic advisers, and postsecondary institutions are provided. Developing culturally responsive, identity-conscious career development programs and fostering inclusive campus climates should be emphasized to effectively address the specific needs and barriers for underrepresented college students of color with disabilities.

1.1. Career Decision Self-Efficacy and Outcome Expectations

The social cognitive career theory (SCCT) [10] offers a comprehensive framework for understanding the career development of individuals, especially of those with intersecting marginalized identities, such as race/ethnicity, and disability. The two main concepts that SCCT focuses on are career decision self-efficacy, which is defined as one's belief in and confidence about their abilities to successfully make career-related decisions, and career outcome expectations, which are defined as one's beliefs about their ability to achieve successful academic and vocational outcomes, engage in competitive employment, and progress in their career trajectory [11]. Lent et al. [10] highlighted that career self-efficacy plays a foundational role in shaping an individual's career outcome expectations. These constructs are shaped by personal characteristics, learning experiences, and sociocultural contexts.

According to the SCCT framework, Ochs and Roessler [12] discovered that adolescents with disabilities reported much lower levels of career skills self-efficacy and career outcome expectations in comparison to their peers without disabilities. These disparities have aligned with previous studies showing that career choices, decisions, goals, and outcome expectations are more likely to differ for women, people with disabilities, and racial/ethnic minorities than the majority of White, non-disabled men in the workforce [13–15]. For racially/ethnically diverse college students with disabilities, the development of career decision self-efficacy and positive outcome expectations is typically undermined by multiple intersecting barriers. These may include systemic racism, ableism, limited access to role models, and a lack of culturally responsive institutional support [16,17]. Research consistently shows that underrepresented students, particularly those with intersecting marginalized identities, report lower career decision self-efficacy due to experiences of discrimination and reduced access to affirming environments [18,19]. Thus, college students with disabilities need to evaluate disability conditions in academia and career development, identify self-identity status involving the environment, and finally, believe in one's abilities, and persist through achievement. Career decision self-efficacy is an essential ability of a college student with disabilities to make decisions and develop one's career path.

Despite the theoretical linkage of SCCT, relatively few empirical studies have simultaneously examined both constructs, career decision self-efficacy and career outcome expectations, in the context of college students of color with disabilities. Most of the existing literature focuses on either career decision self-efficacy or outcome expectations separately, thereby overlooking the role of self-efficacy beliefs and decisions on minoritized college students with disabilities' perceptions of their future career success. Additionally, the gap restricts our understanding of how these beliefs are intertwined with the development and the affirmation of their intersectional identities.

1.2. Intersectionality of Disability and Ethnic Identities

In recent years, an increasing number of researchers in vocational psychology and career development have begun to report on the experiences of individuals with intersecting social identities related to race, ethnicity, gender, disability, and sexual orientation [20,21]. Mpofu and Harley [4] pointed out that identity is a key factor in career development. The way that the students understood their disability and racial/ethnic identity played a role in their understanding of strengths, career goals, and challenges, and the way that they viewed or responded to career barriers. Building on the foundational constructs of SCCT, it is essential to examine how these theoretical principles manifest in the lived experiences of individuals with intersecting marginalized identities. In particular, understanding how disability intersects with racial and ethnic identities offers critical insight into the career development processes of underrepresented college students with disabilities.

Intersectionality, first conceptualized by Crenshaw [22], refers to how two or more identities overlap and how individuals experience compounded effects of marginalization based on dominant power structures. These intersecting identities range from race, ethnicity, gender, disability, sexual orientation, and socioeconomic status, among many others. Intersectionality entails two important implications. First, intersectionality acknowledges that social identities are jointly constructed and inseparable nature [23]. A Hispanic American with a disability that impacts mental health is an example of the intersection of ethnic and disability identities. Second, intersectionality highlights the consequences of overlapping identity, including compounded discrimination or social exclusion. As noted by Alvarado and Hurtado [24], one's sociocultural context greatly determines how one identifies. For example, a Hispanic American with a mental health issue may be marginalized based on ethnicity and disability, respectively, while situated in the United States. However, should a Hispanic American migrate to Colombia, while potential marginalization for disability may persist, the marginalization of ethnicity may be obscured. In this situation, the Hispanic American may face new issues requiring consideration of marginalization based on gender, language, or citizenship, reflecting new potential default identifications. These affordances demonstrate the person–environment interaction central to the theory of intersectionality [23,25]. That is, identity is fluid, as shaped by place, time, and culture.

While the theoretical foundation of intersectionality continues to grow, many fields within human services and disability studies continue to view client identities as separate and distinct, rather than as connected and interacting [26]. In a systematic review of 41 peer-reviewed articles on disability identity, Forber-Pratt et al. [21] noted an average of only 24% of studies integrated or recognized intersectionality in the disability research field. In addition, half of the studies did not even report participant race. Among the remaining studies, 70% of the participants were European American; only 9.4% were African American, 8.8% Latino/a, and 11.8% in another racial/ethnic group. Very few studies examined how intersectional identities impact the psychosocial development, academic success, career pathways, or community involvement of underrepresented communities. Therefore, people with disabilities from various cultural backgrounds (e.g., people of color, women, and LGBTQ+) have their own unique needs and expectations that deserve greater attention in research and practice.

Indeed, during formative years like college, when identity development is particularly salient, the intersection of disability with race and ethnicity may significantly impact self-concept, self-esteem, and self-efficacy. Foster and Kinuthia [27] explored multicultural identity development among 33 deaf college students from underrepresented racial/ethnic backgrounds, including African American, Asian American, and Hispanic students. Their study emphasized the role that self-reflection, K–12 educational experiences, and family upbringing played in the development of disability identities. Notably, participants described identity as fluid and context-dependent, often shifting based on life transitions, peer interactions, and institutional messaging. After speaking with a college disability support provider who explained the difference, one student in the study who had previously identified as hard of hearing changed their identity to deaf. Others shared experiences when they prioritized their deaf identity over their racial identity, or the reverse, depending on the context. These narratives of participants present that identity is not just a static label but a biographical process, like a story students construct and reconstruct while they navigate different environments and evolving social expectations.

Mejia-Smith and Gushue [19] found that for Latina/o college students, ethnic identity pride was associated with greater awareness of career barriers. However, students who held stronger ethnic identity also reported higher career decision self-efficacy, which in turn was negatively associated with perceived barriers. The findings suggest that identity can be a source of both challenge and resilience. Similarly, Bounds [28] reported that among African American high school students, academic self-concept and ethnic identity were positively linked to career decision self-efficacy. The role of both cultural affirmation and academic confidence are emphasized in supporting vocational development [28]. For college students with disabilities, especially those from racial and ethnic minority backgrounds, the intersecting marginalized identities significantly influence their career development, decision-making confidence, and career outcome expectations [19,27]. Foster and Kinuthia's [27] findings challenge practitioners to recognize that intersecting identities are not additive but dynamic and deeply contextual. They serve as lenses through which individuals experience the world, seek support, and shape their sense of self. Understanding how students of color with disabilities navigate their identities can offer valuable insight into their help-seeking behaviors, community involvement, and career pathways.

Lastly, Chao et al. [29] investigated the factors comprising ethnic identity, disability identity, perceived career barriers, and social support that influence career decision self-efficacy and outcome expectations among 312 college students with disabilities. The study found that 30.1% of the variability in career decision self-efficacy was explained by social support, ethnic identity, and disability identity. Furthermore, 56.1% of the variance in career outcome expectations was explained by career decision self-efficacy, ethnic identity, and perceived career barriers. While ethnic identity significantly predicted both career decision self-efficacy and outcome expectations, disability identity contributed to the model for self-efficacy but did not show a significant relationship with outcome expectations. However, the study did not explore whether perceptions of intersectional identities differed across ethnic groups among college students with disabilities, leaving this important dimension unaddressed. This gap signals the need to further examine how perceptions of intersecting identities and career barriers vary across ethnic groups among college students with disabilities in pursuing their career goals.

1.3. Career Barriers

The intersection of disability and racial/ethnic identities creates complex challenges for students' career aspirations, career decision-making self-efficacy, and outcome expectations. While these identities contribute to professional development, they simultaneously expose students to multifaceted structural and cultural barriers that extend beyond single identity experiences [29,30]. The growing diversity in higher education brings both opportunities and challenges for students' academic and career trajectories, particularly affecting those navigating multiple marginalized identities. College students with disabilities from racially and ethnically diverse backgrounds encounter more intricate challenges in pursuing their career goals than their European American peers. These students must navigate disability-related obstacles while simultaneously managing ethnic identity development and confronting others' perceptions about their intersectional status. The compounded effects of marginalization create additional barriers that influence their career choices, goals, and perceived barriers [16]. Furthermore, students positioned at the intersection of disability and racial/ethnic minority status face multilayered difficulties including disability-related barriers, systemic racism, cultural stigma, and underrepresentation in academic spaces [1].

The literature reveals that ableism and racism operate differently when experienced simultaneously rather than in isolation. For example, ableism manifests differently for a Black college student with a disability compared to a White student with a disability. A Black student using a wheelchair encounters physical inaccessibility and disability-related stereotypes, but the Black student additionally experiences race-based profiling on campus, adding another layer of scrutiny from peers and faculty [31,32]. Likewise, consider a Black student with Autism Spectrum Disorder (ASD) requesting extended exam time. While White peers with similar accommodations are viewed as "hardworking individuals overcoming challenges," the Black student might face skepticism about seeking "unfair advantages" and questions about academic belonging based on intersecting racial and ableist assumptions. Conversely, racism is experienced differently by students with disabilities than by non-disabled peers from the same racial/ethnic background. For instance, while a non-disabled Black student might face assumptions about academic preparation, A Black student with ASD encounters compounded stereotypes which are attributed to both racial assumptions about the education and learning opportunities they had before college and disability-related assumptions about cognitive ability, creating intensified perceptions of academic incapability [9,33]. These overlapping biases exacerbate exclusion from academic opportunities and career networks, demonstrating that ableism and racism are not merely additive but mutually reinforcing forces [22,34].

Research has shown that college students with intersectional identities, such as disability and race/ethnicity, manage college expectations while attempting to navigate and explore spaces that do not necessarily recognize, understand, or support their complex individual identity experiences. Additionally, perceived stigma, cultural expectations, and stereotypes about discrimination in the labor market negatively impact education and career paths [19,35]. Although the previous literature has not explicitly focused on students with disabilities, the research indicates that developing an intersectional identity [36] during the college years is an important factor in shaping career self-efficacy and outcome expectations for underrepresented students with disabilities [4,21]. Transferring from a local high school to a college or university, which often functions as a more diverse environment like a small society. For racially and ethnically diverse students with disabilities, this shift often required them to re-evaluate their sense of identity and determine where they belong and how they position themselves within the new environment [24,37]. This identity renegotiation process occurs alongside academic adjustment and career exploration, creating multiple developmental demands simultaneously.

To fully acknowledge the challenges faced by these marginalized students, it is essential to examine the varying levels of perceived career-related barriers experienced by college students with disabilities from different racial and ethnic backgrounds, both within educational institutions and across broader sociocultural systems [5,30]. This research foundation supports the critical need for appropriate career counseling and career-related development in postsecondary education. Effective career services could assist underrepresented college students with disabilities to build identity-affirming confidence, develop beliefs about their competencies for career decisions and outcomes, and eliminate perceptions of career barriers related to their intersecting identities [38–40].

1.4. Social Support

Social support is essential for the career success and well-being of college students with disabilities and those who manage intersecting disability and racial/ethnic identities. Students with disabilities are more likely to face unique challenges, including physical barriers, stigma, and the need to request accommodation [41,42]. Family, peer support, affinity groups, culturally sensitive instructors, and disability services are examples of supportive networks that can offer emotional validation, a sense of community, and guidance in navigating social and academic settings [43,44]. Students feel valued and empowered when their instructors and program faculty are understanding and accommodating [42,43]. Peer support through mentoring programs or student organizations can reduce feelings of isolation, build resilience, and foster a sense of belonging [41,44]. Positive campus climates supported by institutes provide easily accessible resources and encourage inclusive practices [41,43]. Research shows that minority students with disabilities living with strong support networks and inclusive campus climate report higher self-efficacy confidence, mental well-being, and academic engagement [43,44]. A study by Dutta et al. [45] examined career interests and goal persistence in STEM (science, technology, engineering, and mathematics) among 115 college students with disabilities, of whom 82 (71%) identified as African American and 33 (29%) as Hispanic. The study investigated several SCCT-related factors, including barriers to coping efficacy, academic self-efficacy, career outcome expectations, and social support. Their findings revealed that social support had a direct effect on STEM goal persistence and an indirect effect on academic self-efficacy. In contrast, barriers to coping self-efficacy were negatively associated with academic self-efficacy and indirectly reduced students' interest in STEM careers. Moreover, positive career outcome expectations strongly predicted both STEM interest and goal persistence [45]. Additionally, Chao et al. [29] indicated that the intersection of social identities, the presence of adequate social support, perceptions of barriers related to social identity, and higher levels of career decision self-efficacy are crucial factors in promoting positive career outcomes among college students with disabilities. These results underscore the pivotal role that social support plays, especially for students who report low academic and career self-efficacy. Enhancing academic self-efficacy may not only boost career interest and persistence but also buffer the negative effects of identity-related barriers. Strengthening a support system and creating inclusive and affirming spaces where intersectional identities and cultural backgrounds are both acknowledged are crucial to ensuring equity and success for college students of color with disabilities in higher education [41]. Hence, there is a need to understand how college students with disabilities from diverse racial/ethnic groups perceive social support in relation to their dual identities, career development factors, and barriers they face.

1.5. Purpose and Significance of the Study

Despite the increasing focus on equity and inclusion in higher education, there remains limited research on how college students with disabilities navigate career development through their intersecting identities, particularly in relation to disability and race/ethnicity, and other factors. Building on the work of Chao et al. [29], they found that social support was the strongest predictor of career decision self-efficacy, followed by ethnic identity and disability identity. Additionally, career decision self-efficacy, ethnic identity, and perceived career barriers were significantly associated with career outcome expectations. The present study seeks to address how perceptions of disability identity, ethnic identity, perceived career barriers, social support, career decision self-efficacy, and career outcome expectations differ among college students with disabilities from diverse racial and ethnic backgrounds. Determination of such differences is important as the population of students with disabilities in higher education continues to become more diverse.

This study foregrounds the voices and life experiences of students with intersectional marginalized identities, therefore contributing to initiatives towards creating more inclusive and supportive learning environments. The results are expected to inform culturally responsive practice in the disability support industry, career counseling, academic advising, and school policy development. The study highlights the critical need for educators, counselors, rehabilitation and human services professionals, and disability support specialists to advance multicultural competence. It is imperative that multicultural competence be developed to make sure that all students, particularly those who are experiencing the intersection of disability, race, and ethnicity, obtain the validation, resources, and support they require to thrive in their academic and professional success.

1.6. Research Question

To explore these concerns, this study examines the following research question: are there significant differences among racial/ethnic groups of college students with disabilities regarding disability identity, ethnic identity, perceived career barriers, social support, career decision self-efficacy, and career outcome expectations?

2. Method

2.1. Participants and Sampling

The target population for this study was college students with disabilities enrolled in postsecondary education in the United States. Eligibility criteria included (1) current or prior enrollment in a college or university, (2) being 18 years of age or older, and (3) self-identification as having a physical or mental impairment that substantially limits one or more major life activities, as defined by the Americans with Disabilities Act (ADA). A cross-sectional survey design using a non-probability convenience sampling method was employed at two four-year public universities, one located in the midwestern region and the other in the southeastern region of the United States. This sampling method was selected due to the researchers' prior affiliation with both institutions, which provided them with access and familiarity that facilitated participant recruitment and data collection. The total number of college students with disabilities enrolled at the two universities during the 2018–2019 academic year was approximately 2900, including about 500 students at the midwestern university and about 2400 students at the southeastern university. Eligible students were invited to participate in the study via email distributed by the Directors of Disability Support Services at each institution. A total of 306 valid participants who completed the entire questionnaire were included in the final analysis.

Among the 306 participants, 225 (73.5%) identified themselves as White/European Americans, 19 (6.2%) identified themselves as Black/African Americans, 21 (6.9%) identified themselves as Hispanics, 17 (5.6%) identified themselves as Asian Americans, and 24 (7.9%) responded other ethnicities, including multiethnicities, American Indian/Alaska Native, Arab, Hebrew, Appalachian, Pakistani, and Jewish. Among 306 participants, there were
94 male participants (30.7%), 208 female participants (68%), and 4 transgender participants (1.3%). Regarding disability onset type, 67 (21.9%) reported themselves as congenital disabilities, 87 (28.4%) reported as acquired disabilities, 123 (40.2%) reported they were not sure about their disability onset type, and 29 (9.5%) reported that they preferred not to answer. Regarding age, the majority of participants (n = 264, 86.3%) ranged 18–24 years and 13 participants (4.2%) were 25–34 years. Regarding education class, 103 (33.7%) participants reported as freshman, 75 (24.5%) as sophomores, 49 (16.0%) as juniors, 40 (13.1%) as seniors, 18 (5.9%) as master's students, and 6 (2.0%) as doctoral students. In terms of disability type, 16 participants (5.2%) reported having physical disability, 88 (28.8%) having a mental illness and psychiatric disability, 50 (16.3%) having Attention Deficit/Hyperactivity Disorder (ADD/ADHD), 9 (2.9%) having Autism Spectrum Disorder (ASD), 23 (7.5%) having learning disabilities, 35 (11.4%) having chronic disorders, 8 (2.6%) reported having low vision or blindness, 3 (1.0%) being hard of hearing or having deafness, and 4 (1.3%) having intellectual or developmental disability (Table 1).

Table 1. Demographic data of participants.

			n		Valid Percent
Race/Ethnicity		306		100%	
	White/European		225		73.5%
	Black/African		19		6.2%
	Hispanic		21		6.9%
	Asian		17		5.6%
	Others		24		7.9%
Gender		306		100%	
	Female		208		68.0%
	Male		94		30.7%
	Transgender		4		1.3%

Table 1. *Cont.*

		n		Valid Percent
Disability Onset	277		100%	
Congenital		67		21.9%
Acquired		87		28.4%
Not sure		123		40.2%
Age	295		100%	
18–24		264		86.3%
25–34		13		4.2%
35–44		9		2.9%
45–54		3		1.0%
55 or older		6		2.0%
Class	291		100%	
Freshman		103		34.8%
Sophomore		76		25.7%
Junior		49		16.6%
Senior		41		13.9%
Master		19		6.4%
PhD		8		2.7%
Disability Type	260		100%	
Physical Disability		16		5.2%
Mental Health Issues/Emotional Disability/Psychiatric Disability		88		28.8%
Attention Deficit/Hyperactivity Disorder (ADD/ADHD)		50		16.3%
Autism Spectrum Disorder		9		2.9%
Learning Disability		23		7.5%
Chronic Disorders (e.g., Rare Diseases, Diabetes, Sickle Cell Disease, etc.)		35		11.4%
Low Vision/ Blindness		8		2.6%
Hard of Hearing/ Deafness		3		1.0%
Brain Injury		6		2.0%
Temporary Disability		15		4.9%
Epilepsy		3		1.0%
Intellectual/Developmental Disability		4		1.3%

2.2. Independent Variable

The independent variable in this study was the self-reported race/ethnicity of college students with disabilities. Participants were categorized into five groups:

1. White/European American;
2. Black/African American;
3. Hispanic/Latino(a);
4. Asian/Asian American;
5. Other ethnicities, which include college students with disabilities identified themselves as Jewish, Irish, Pakistan, Arabic, and multi-races/ethnicities.

2.3. Dependent Variables

The six dependent variables as below were examined as the perceptions and the experiences of college students with disabilities.

1. Disability Identity;
2. Ethnic Identity;
3. Perceived Career Barriers;
4. Social Support;
5. Career Decision Self-Efficacy;

6. Career Outcome Expectations.

2.4. Instruments

Six dependent variables were assessed using validated instruments designed for diverse populations, with prior studies reporting reliability coefficients ranging from acceptable to high internal consistency. Each instrument was selected based on its relevance to the constructions examined in this study, which comprise disability identity, ethnic identity, perceived career barriers, social support, career decision self-efficacy, and career outcome expectations. The following sections provide a brief description of each instrument, including purpose, structure, scaling, and reliability evidence.

Personal Disability Identity Scale (PDI). Disability identity was measured using the PDI, developed by Hahn and Belt [46]. The PDI is an eight-item instrument that measures two dimensions, including *disability affirmation* and *disability denial*. Items are rated on a 5-point Likert scale (1 = strongly disagree to 5 = strongly agree), with reverse scoring applied to denial items. Average scores range from 1 to 5, with higher scores indicating stronger disability identity. Sample items include "I feel proud to be a person with a disability" (affirmation) and "My disability sometimes makes me feel ashamed" (denial). Previous studies reported Cronbach's α ranging from 0.43 to 0.81 for affirmation and 0.50 to 0.79 for denial. The Cronbach's α was 0.84 in this study, reflecting good reliability.

Multigroup Ethnic Identity Measure—Revised (MEIM-R). The MEIM-R adapted from Phinney [47], is a twelve-item scale assessing two dimensions: (1) ethnic identity search, which evaluates a developmental and cognitive component and (2) affirmation, belonging, and commitment, which reflects an affective component [48]. Responses use a 4-point Likert scale (1 = strongly disagree to 4 = strongly agree). No items require reverse scoring. Mean scores range from 1 to 4, with higher scores indicating stronger ethnic identity. The MEIM-R consistently shows good reliability ($\alpha > 0.80$) across diverse groups [49]. The Cronbach's α was 0.93 in this study, reflecting excellent reliability.

Perception of Barriers Scale (POB). Originally developed by McWhirter [50], the POB was adapted in this study to assess disability-related barriers alongside racial and ethnic barriers. A total of 13 items were used: four items measuring perceived ethnic discrimination, five items for disability-related barriers (modified from original gender items), and four items for general career barrier. Items are scored on a 5-point Likert scale (1 = strongly disagree to 5 = strongly agree), with one reverse-coded item. Higher mean scores indicate greater perceived barriers. Previous studies reported a Cronbach's α of 0.87 for the POB [50]. The Cronbach's α was 0.91 in this study, confirming excellent internal consistency.

College Students with Disabilities Campus Climate Survey (CSDCC). The CSDCC, developed by Lombardi et al. [51], assesses perceptions of social support and campus climate. In this research, 22 items were taken from five subscales, including peer support (4 items), family support (4 items), disability services (4 items), campus climate (5 items, with an additional item on ethnicity), and faculty support (5 items, taken from teaching practices and accommodation categories). Items are rated on a 6-point Likert scale (1 = never true to 6 = always true). Higher mean scores reflect higher perceived social support. Prior studies report subscale reliabilities ranging from $\alpha = 0.62$ to 0.88 [51]. Convergent validity was demonstrated through correlations with GPA, self-efficacy, and campus belonging. Cronbach's α in this study was 0.85, confirming good internal consistency.

Career Decision Self-Efficacy Scale—Short Form (CDSE-SF). The CDSE-SF is a 25-item scale that measures a person's self-perceived confidence in career decision-making [52]. The CDSE-SF consists of five subscales: self-appraisal, occupational information, goal selection, planning, and problem-solving. Each subscale has five items. The participants rate their responses on a 5-point Likert scale, from 1 (no confidence at all) to 5 (complete confidence). High mean scores reflect a greater level of career decision self-efficacy. The CDSE-SF is widely validated and has demonstrated excellent internal consistency ($\alpha = 0.94$) [53]. The Cronbach's α was 0.96 in this study, reflecting excellent reliability.

Vocational Outcome Expectations (VOE) Scale. The VOE developed by McWhirter et al. [54], is a 12-item scale assessing expectations about future career success. This study used 10 items, omitting two that were unrelated to career goals. Responses are rated on a 4-point Likert scale (1 = strongly disagree to 4 = strongly agree), and the mean score of all items is used for scoring. Higher mean scores reflect more positive career outcome expectations. McWhirter et al. [54] reported Cronbach's $\alpha = 0.83$, and concurrent validity was supported through correlations with CDSE [36]. The Cronbach's α was 0.94 in this study, reflecting excellent internal consistency.

2.5. Research Procedure

This study was approved by the Institutional Review Board (IRB) at two four-year public universities to ensure that participants' rights and procedures complied with ethical research standards. Prior to recruitment, formal permission was obtained from the Directors of Disability Support Services at both universities. Data was collected using an online survey administered via Qualtrics. The survey was restricted to students with self-identified disabilities to ensure the appropriateness of responses. An email invitation outlined the purpose of the study, the survey link, the approximate time required to complete the survey (about 20 min), anonymous participation, assurances of confidentiality, and academic use of data. The initial email invitation and the survey link were distributed by the Directors to all students with disabilities registered with the Offices of Disability Support Services, inviting their voluntary participation. To encourage participation, the researchers requested that the Directors send two follow-up recruitment emails to the same population. The first follow-up was sent 14 days after the initial invitation, and the second follow-up was sent 14 days after the first follow-up. Participants were offered the opportunity to enter a drawing for a $5 gift card [55]. The data were collected from 15 September 2019 to 15 December 2019.

2.6. Data Analysis

All data were analyzed using IBM SPSS Statistics Version 28. Descriptive statistics, including frequency and percentage distributions, were used to summarize demographic characteristics such as race/ethnicity, gender, and education level. A one-way Multivariate Analysis of Variance (MANOVA) was conducted to examine whether students' racial/ethnic backgrounds were significantly associated with differences across the six dependent variables. MANOVA was chosen due to its ability to assess multiple dependent variables simultaneously while controlling for Type I error [56,57]. Assumptions for normality, linearity, homogeneity of variance–covariance matrices, independence of observations, and multicollinearity were evaluated prior to conducting the analysis. There was no linearity, normality, multicollinearity, and homoscedasticity assumption violations in the study. Wilks' Lambda (Λ) was used as the multivariate test statistic. Smaller Λ values indicate stronger group effects. If Box's M test indicated a violation of the homogeneity of covariance matrices ($p < 0.001$), Pillai's Trace was used as a more robust alternative [56]. In the event of a statistically significant MANOVA, follow-up univariate ANOVAs and post hoc tests (e.g., Scheffé test) were conducted to explore group differences.

3. Results

According to the analysis principles of MANOVA, the correlation values of dependent variables were 0.3 to 0.8. Because of variables somehow correlated with each other, it is appropriate to put all dependent variables in a complex for the MANOVA analysis. Before running the MANOVA, the assumptions were examined, including normal distribution, linearity, homogeneity of variances and covariances, and multicollinearity. Additionally, the assumptions of homogeneity of variance and covariance were tested for all dependent variables by using Box's M test and the Levene's test.

3.1. Box's M Test and Levene's F Test

The test yielded a value of Box's $M = 126.80$, $F(84, 13{,}666.94) = 1.33$, $p = 0.024$. Since the p value of 0.024 is greater than the alpha level of 0.001, the result is not statistically significant. Therefore, the assumption of homogeneity of covariance matrices was met. The observed covariance matrices of the dependent variables in the study were equal across ethnicity groups, including European Americans, African Americans, Hispanics, Asian Americans, and other ethnicities in college students with disabilities.

In the study, the probability (p) value of Levene's test of five dependent variables including ethnicity identity, perceived career barriers, social support, career self-efficacy, and career outcome expectation were larger than 0.05. Namely, these five dependent variables followed the homogeneity of error variance across different ethnicity groups. However, the disability identity variable was not homogenous across error variances in Levene's test, $F(4, 301) = 2.90$, $p = 0.012$. Although the assumption of homogeneity of variance for the disability identity variable was violated, further examination showed that the largest standard deviation was not four times greater than the smallest, meeting the robustness guideline suggested by Mertler and Reinhart [56]. Therefore, the univariate analysis was considered robust and appropriate for use. Consequently, the MANOVA was conducted using Wilks' Λ as multivariate test statistic to evaluate overall group differences.

3.2. Multivariate Analysis

A one-way MANOVA was conducted to examine whether there were significant mean differences across ethnicity groups of college students with disabilities on six dependent variables, consisting of disability identity, ethnic identity, perceived career barriers, social support, career decision self-efficacy, and career outcome expectations. The analysis revealed a statistically significant multivariate effect of ethnicity, Wilk's $\Lambda = 0.75$, $F(24, 1033.83) = 3.73$, $p < 0.001$, partial $\eta^2 = 0.070$ (see Table 2). Partial eta squared (η^2), similarly to R^2 in regression, indicates the proportion of variance explained by the independent variable. According to Tabachnick and Fidell [57], a value of 0.02 represents a small effect size, 0.13 a medium effect, and 0.26 a large effect. Therefore, ethnicity accounted for 7% of the variance across the six dependent variables, indicating a small to moderate effect size.

3.3. Univariate Analysis

A series of one-way analysis of variance on six dependent variables were conducted following the multivariate analysis to examine which specific variable had statistically significant difference across ethnicity groups. The results showed that there was a significant difference in European Americans, African Americans, Hispanics, Asian Americans, and other ethnicities in college students with disabilities on ethnic identity, $F(4, 301) = 7.88$, $p < 0.001$, partial $\eta^2 = 0.095$ (Table 3). Hence, 9.5% of the variability of the difference in ethnicity identity can be explained by college students with disabilities with different ethnicities, which had a small to medium effect size.

Table 2. Multivariate tests [a] of variance table on ethnicity groups.

	Effect	Value	F	Hypothesis df	Error df	p	Partial η^2
Intercept	Pillai's Trace	0.98	2065.39 [b]	6.00	296.00	0.000	0.98
	Wilks' Lambda	0.02	2065.39 [b]	6.00	296.00	0.000	0.98
	Hotelling's Trace	41.87	2065.39 [b]	6.00	296.00	0.000	0.98
	Roy's Largest Root	41.87	2065.39 [b]	6.00	296.00	0.000	0.98
Ethnicity	Pillai's Trace	0.26	3.51 ***	24.00	1196.00	0.000	0.07
	Wilks' Lambda	0.75	3.73 ***	24.00	1033.83	0.000	0.07
	Hotelling's Trace	0.32	3.94 ***	24.00	1178.00	0.000	0.07
	Roy's Largest Root	0.27	13.42 [c]***	6.00	299.00	0.000	0.21

[a] Design: Intercept + Ethnicity. [b] Exact statistics. [c] The statistic is an upper bound on F that yields a lower bound on the significance level. *** $p < 0.001$.

Table 3. Tests of between-subjects effects on ethnicity groups.

Source	Dependent Variable	Type III SS	df	MS	F	p	Partial η^2
Corrected Model	Disability Identity	2.70	4	0.68	1.15	0.332	0.015
	Ethnicity Identity	11.13	4	2.78	7.87 ***	0.000	0.095
	Perceived Career Barrier	25.31	4	6.33	11.26 ***	0.000	0.130
	Social Support	2.90	4	0.73	1.44	0.221	0.019
	Career Decision Self-Efficacy	1.94	4	0.48	0.97	0.425	0.013
	Career Outcome Expectation	1.51	4	0.38	1.54	0.189	0.020
Error	Disability Identity	176.60	301	0.59			
	Ethnicity Identity	106.37	301	0.35			
	Perceived Career Barrier	169.18	301	0.56			
	Social Support	151.73	301	0.50			
	Career Decision Self-Efficacy	150.39	301	0.50			
	Career Outcome Expectation	73.41	301	0.24			
Corrected Total	Disability Identity	3156.66	306				
	Ethnicity Identity	2459.67	306				
	Perceived Career Barrier	2391.87	306				
	Social Support	5340.25	306				
	Career Decision Self-Efficacy	4607.37	306				
	Career Outcome Expectation	3299.25	306				

*** $p < 0.001$.

Due to the unequal sample size of five ethnicity categories investigated in the study, Scheffé test post hoc pairwise comparison is adequate for the unequal sample size of each ethnicity group in the study [57]. The results indicated statistically significant differences in the average scores of ethnic identity among college students with disabilities. Specifically, European American students (M = 2.66, SD = 0.57) reported significantly lower ethnic identity compared to Hispanic students (M = 3.18, SD = 0.62), mean difference = −0.52, SE = 0.14, $p = 0.006$; Black/African American students (M = 3.12, SD = 0.62), mean difference = −0.46, SE = 0.14, $p = 0.035$; and students from other ethnicities (M = 3.09, SD = 0.56), mean difference = −0.43, SE = 0.13, $p = 0.026$ (see Table 4). No significant difference was found between European American and Asian American students (M = 2.83, SD= 0.82), mean difference = −0.17, SE = 0.15, $p = 0.85$. These findings suggest that, on average, Black/African American, Hispanic, and students from other ethnic backgrounds reported higher levels of ethnic identity than their European American counterparts.

Table 4. Scheffé post hoc comparison table in ethnic identity of ethnicity groups.

(I) Ethnicity	(J) Ethnicity	ΔMean (I-J)	*SE*	*p*	95% Confidence Interval (CI)
White/European	Black/African	−0.46 *	0.14	0.035	[−0.90, −0.02]
	Hispanic	−0.52 **	0.14	0.006	[−0.94, −0.10]
	Asian	−0.17	0.15	0.851	[−0.64, 0.29]
	Other ethnicities	−0.43 *	0.13	0.026	[−0.82, −0.03]
Black/African	White/European	0.46 *	0.14	0.035	[0.01, 0.90]
	Hispanic	−0.06	0.19	0.998	[−0.65, 0.52]
	Asian	0.29	0.20	0.724	[−0.33, 0.90]
	Other ethnicities	0.03	0.18	1.000	[−0.53, 0.60]
Hispanic	White/European	0.52 **	0.14	0.006	[0.10, 0.94]
	Black/African	0.06	0.19	0.998	[−0.52, 0.65]
	Asian	0.35	0.19	0.519	[−0.25, 0.95]
	Other ethnicities	0.10	0.18	0.990	[−0.45, 0.65]
Asian	White/European	0.17	0.15	0.851	[−0.29, 0.64]
	Black/African	−0.29	0.20	0.724	[−0.90, 0.33]
	Hispanic	−0.35	0.19	0.519	[−0.95, 0.25]
	Other ethnicities	−0.25	0.19	0.771	[−0.84, 0.33]
Other ethnicities	White/European	0.43 *	0.13	0.026	[−0.03, 0.82]
	Black/African	−0.03	0.18	1.000	[−0.60, 0.53]
	Hispanic	−0.10	0.18	0.990	[−0.65, 0.45]
	Asian	0.25	0.19	0.771	[−0.33, 0.84]

Note. Based on observed means. The error term is Mean Square (Error) = 0.244. * $p < 0.05$. ** $p < 0.01$.

In addition, a statistically significant difference in perceived career barriers was found across ethnic groups of college students with disabilities: European American, African American, Hispanic, Asian American, and other ethnicities, $F(4, 301) = 25.31$, $p < 0.001$, partial $\eta^2 = 0.13$. This indicates that approximately 13% of the variance in perceived career barriers can be explained by students' ethnicity, representing a medium effect size (Table 3). Scheffé post hoc analyses revealed statistically significant differences between European American students ($M = 2.66$, $SD = 0.57$) and the following groups: Asian American students ($M = 3.41$, $SD = 0.65$), mean difference = −0.90, $SE = 0.19$, $p < 0.001$; other students ($M = 3.16$, $SD = 0.82$), mean difference = −0.65, $SE = 0.16$, $p = 0.003$; and African American students ($M = 3.12$, $SD = 0.62$), mean difference = −0.60, $SE = 0.18$, $p = 0.025$ (see Table 4). No significant difference was found between European American and Hispanic students ($M = 2.89$, $SD = 0.95$), mean difference = −0.37, $SE = 0.17$, $p = 0.31$ (see Table 5). These findings suggested that African American, Asian American, and other ethnicities college students with disabilities perceived significantly greater career barriers compared to their European American counterparts. By contrast, no significant differences were found across ethnic groups for disability identity, $F(4, 301) = 1.2$, $p = 0.33$, partial $\eta^2 = 0.02$; social support, $F(4, 301) = 1.4$, $p = 0.22$, partial $\eta^2 = 0.02$; career decision self-efficacy, $F(4, 301) = 0.48$, $p = 0.97$, partial $\eta^2 = 0.013$; and career outcome expectation, $F(4, 301) = 1.55$, $p = 0.19$, partial $\eta^2 = 0.02$ (Table 3).

Table 5. Scheffé post hoc comparison table in perceived career barriers of ethnicity groups.

(I) Ethnicity	(J) Ethnicity	ΔMean (I-J)	*SE*	*p*	95% CI
White/European	Black/African	−0.60 *	0.18	0.025	[−1.16, −0.05]
	Hispanic	−0.37	0.17	0.313	[−0.90, 0.16]
	Asian	−0.90 ***	0.19	0.000	[−1.48, −0.31]
	Other ethnicities	−0.65 **	0.16	0.003	[−1.15, −0.15]
Black/African	White/European	0.60 *	0.18	0.025	[0.05, 1.16]
	Hispanic	0.23	0.24	0.922	[−0.51, 0.96]
	Asian	−0.29	0.25	0.847	[−1.07, 0.48]
	Other ethnicities	−0.05	0.23	1.000	[−0.76, 0.67]
Hispanic	White/European	0.37	0.17	0.313	[−0.16, 0.90]
	Black/African	−0.23	0.24	0.922	[−0.96, 0.51]
	Asian	−0.52	0.24	0.339	[−1.28, 0.24]
	Other ethnicities	−0.27	0.22	0.828	[−0.97, 0.42]
Asian	White/European	0.90 ***	0.19	0.000	[0.31, 1.48]
	Black/African	0.29	0.25	0.847	[−0.48, 1.07]
	Hispanic	0.52	0.24	0.339	[−0.24, 1.28]
	Other ethnicities	0.25	0.24	0.895	[−0.49, 0.98]
Other ethnicities	White/European	0.65 **	0.16	0.003	[0.15, 1.15]
	Black/African	0.05	0.23	1.000	[−0.67, 0.76]
	Hispanic	0.27	0.22	0.828	[−0.42, 0.97]
	Asian	−0.25	0.24	0.895	[−0.98, 0.49]

Note. Based on observed means. The error term is Mean Square (Error) = 0.244. * $p < 0.05$. ** $p < 0.01$. *** $p < 0.001$.

4. Discussion

The purpose of this research was to investigate whether there are significant differences among diverse ethnic groups of students with disabilities in higher education across six main constructs: disability identity, ethnic identity, perceived career barriers, social support, career decision self-efficacy, and career outcome expectations. By integrating both the social cognitive career theory [10] and intersectionality theory [22], the results provide insight into how the intersection of disability and ethnicity influences the identity development and career-related experiences of college students with disabilities within the postsecondary education context.

4.1. Discrepancies of Ethnic Identity Among Groups

The first primary finding indicated a significant difference in ethnic identity among students from varying racial and ethnic groups. Specifically, Hispanic, Black/African American, and other marginalized ethnic groups had a higher degree of affirmation, engagement, and commitment of their ethnic identities in comparison with their European American counterparts. As Islam [58] emphasizes, ethnic identity is not simply determined by skin color or understood on a binary basis. Instead, it is contingent upon an individual's cultural heritage, family descent, religious background, and sociocultural values. Disabled and non-disabled adolescents in Islam's study [58] described their ethnic identity as being firmly rooted in intergenerational and cultural traditions.

This finding supports prior research which has demonstrated that for individuals from underrepresented groups, ethnic identity becomes more salient than disability identity when engaged in environments that are predominantly marked by standards, in this case, European American, cisgender, and non-disabled institutions [59]. The salience and dynamic development of ethnic identity among underrepresented college students with disabilities help them navigate dominant cultural contexts in higher education. For European American students, ethnic identity tends to be implicit or concealed since it is part of hegemonic cultural norms. In contrast, college students from marginalized backgrounds must engage in more conscious negotiation and affirmation of both disability and ethnic identities in contexts where such identities are either underrepresented or misunderstood within postsecondary education institutes.

From an intersectionality perspective, the identity development process becomes more complex for college students with disabilities from marginalized racial and ethnic backgrounds. These students are actively navigating identities that are frequently minimized or invisible in institutional settings rather than just confronting isolated forms of marginalization. Individuals experience social systems such as racism, ableism, sexism, and classism as interconnected and compounding systems of oppression rather than as separate forces [22]. Students who live at the intersection of marginalized racial/ethnic identities and disabilities in higher education encounter challenges in defining themselves and accessing opportunities.

This nuanced interplay between social identity and structural oppression is also illuminated by SCCT [10], which conceptualized identity-relevant experiences as part of one's "learning experiences". These experiences shape self-efficacy beliefs, outcome expectations, and ultimately, career decision-making. SCCT emphasizes the dynamic interaction between personal and environmental factors and sheds light on how identity development influences the formation of career decision self-efficacy and outcome expectations. For students navigating multiple marginalized identities, these learning experiences are particularly intricate, as they must simultaneously develop strategies for succeeding within systems that may not fully recognize or value their intersectional identities.

Dual negotiation of ethnic and disability identities is both a reaction to ongoing marginalization and a form of empowerment. Individuals who face persistent discrimination tend to reconstruct and redefine numerous elements of their identities to obtain access to resources, enhance self-esteem, and achieve career satisfaction [30]. Identity negotiation is crucial for determining career development, access to resources, and level of engagement in academic activities for students with disabilities from underrepresented groups. Within the SCCT framework, this negotiation is seen as a protective and adaptive behavior. Students who successfully navigate intersectional identity development in the face of discrimination may build stronger self-efficacy and develop more realistic and hopeful outcome expectations.

Collectively, the findings demonstrate that ethnic and disability identity development plays a fundamental role in framing students' career-related beliefs and experiences. The integration of SCCT and intersectionality frameworks reveals that postsecondary institutions must move beyond one-dimensional diversity initiatives to develop comprehensive approaches that recognize and support the intersectional identity work required by students with multiple marginalized identities. Developing equitable career development outcomes requires an understanding of and a validation of such intersecting identities. Additionally, supporting the ongoing identity negotiation processes enables students to thrive in academic and professional contexts

4.2. Perceived Career Barriers Among Racial/Ethnic Groups

According to the second finding, students with disabilities from non-European backgrounds, including African American and Asian American students, reported greater levels of career-related obstacles in contrast to their European American peers. This pattern of differential barrier perception provides crucial insight into how intersecting marginalized identities shape career development experiences in higher education. The disparities closely align with SCCT, which emphasizes how contextual factors, such as systemic discrimination, exposure to marginalization, and limited access to social capital, contribute to career self-efficacy and outcome expectations among marginalized groups. SCCT positions that both perceived support and barriers are central in constructing individuals' confidence and future-oriented beliefs about their career expectations [10]. For students from marginalized racial and ethnic backgrounds, systemic discrimination, limited access to social capital, and repeated exposure to marginalization create environmental conditions that heighten awareness of career barriers. This perceived barrier is not simply negative thinking; rather, it reflects a valid assessment of real structural challenges that these students encounter in academic and professional contexts.

The relationship between ethnic identity strength and barrier perception introduces an additional dimension to this finding. Research by [19] demonstrated that Latina/o students who had a strong sense of ethnic identity were not only more conscious of systemic discrimination but also more likely to identify structural career barriers. This suggests that ethnic identity development serves a dual function: while it provides cultural grounding and resilience, it also increases sensitivity to social injustice and structural inequities [4]. For students with disabilities from marginalized racial and ethnic backgrounds, this heightened awareness represents both an obstacle and a form of critical consciousness that can inform strategic career planning.

Viewed through an intersectional lens, the finding reflects how racism, ableism, and other systems of oppression intersect in complex ways that uniquely affect the career trajectories of college students with multiple marginalized identities. Supporting the framework of this study, Aquino et al. [60] found that underrepresented students with disabilities, including those identifying as Asian American, African American, Hispanic, multiracial, or LGBTQ+, were more likely to perceive discrimination than European American students with disabilities. These students frequently encountered multiple forms of marginalization, such as ableism, racism, sexism, and homophobia, reinforcing the intersectionality framework that social identities are not experienced in isolation [1]. For students who hold multiple minoritized identities, these barriers are not theoretical but are lived experiences that continuously surface in interactions with institutional systems and throughout career development efforts.

In the present study, Asian, African American, and other racially and ethnically underrepresented college students with disabilities reported significantly more perceived career barriers than their European American counterparts. According to the SCCT framework, non-European college students with disabilities who reported greater perceived career barriers than their European American peers probably lead to lower self-efficacy in making career decisions and lower expectations [29]. As a result, marginalized students may restrict their ability to pursue their goals and succeed in their careers. Also, SCCT draws attention to the mitigating role of contextual support, including affirming relationships and inclusive campus climates, that can help counteract these negative effects. These results provide empirical validation for faculty, disability services staff, diversity and inclusion professionals, and higher education leaders regarding the connection between identity-based stigma and career development challenges. Furthermore, this pattern suggests that traditional career development models, which often assume relatively uniform experiences across student populations, may inadequately address the complex realities facing students at intersectional margins.

Therefore, institutions must consider both the structural barriers and the supportive mechanisms that influence students' career development, particularly for those with multiple marginalized identities. Synthesizing SCCT and intersectionality frameworks offers a comprehensive approach for moving beyond surface-level inclusion efforts toward structurally informed practices that acknowledge and respond to students' complex lived experiences. Effective interventions must simultaneously address the systemic barriers these students face while providing the contextual support necessary for career development success. Culturally responsive, equity-driven interventions are essential to advance access, foster career readiness, and promote long-term success for racially and ethnically diverse college students with disabilities.

5. Implications for Practice: Professional and Institutional Responsibilities

5.1. Fostering Multicultural Counseling Competencies in Rehabilitation and Human Services

For students with disabilities navigating higher education, identity development is a multidimensional process shaped by disability, race, ethnicity, gender, and other sociocultural factors [37]. Nevertheless, disability is still too often viewed through a narrow lens of legal compliance, which is centered on accommodation rather than as a meaningful social and cultural identity [38]. This limited approach marginalizes students whose identities diverge from dominant norms and fails to fully recognize their lived experiences. Professionals in rehabilitation and human services, including disability support staff, rehabilitation counselors, and career counselors, must move beyond procedural frameworks and develop multicultural counseling competencies. These include cultural humility, intersectionality awareness, and the ability to validate students' experiences with ableism, racism, and other systemic barriers [40,61]. Students whose social identities are repeatedly devalued may internalize stigma, experience emotional distress, and face barriers to academic and career engagement [1,62]. Rehabilitation professionals should respond not only as service providers but also as advocates and institutional change agents, supporting underrepresented students' needs and affirming their complex identities to strengthen career decision self-efficacy and outcome expectations.

5.2. Advancing Culturally Responsive Career Development and Identity-Based Support

Culturally diverse students with disabilities frequently encounter systemic barriers to career opportunities, including underdeveloped mentorship networks, culturally insensitive programming, and limited internship representation [19,60]. When students must balance competing expectations in the academic, professional, and cultural domains, these obstacles can cause them to lose confidence in their ability to navigate career paths and impede their ability to achieve their career goals [39].

Career service providers, faculty, and disability support staff must collaborate to design and implement career development programs grounded in cultural responsiveness, systematic barrier navigations, and identity affirmation. This includes accessible and inclusive workshops, internships designed for diverse learners, and mentoring relationships that reflect the cultural and linguistic backgrounds of students. When students are given space to reflect on their intersecting identities and how these shape their aspirations, they are better positioned to develop resilience and career clarity [19]. Programs should also confront the broader institutional norms that discourage full participation. Institutions should recognize the systemic causes of career barriers rather than portraying them as personal constraints. This will give students the language and resources they need to confront and overcome injustices [35,61]. Culturally responsive and collaborative career development programs that affirm identity and address systemic barriers are essential for fostering inclusive participation, empowering students to explore their intersecting identities, and building resilience and career clarity.

5.3. Embedding Disability Culture and Intersectionality Within Institutional Inclusion Framework

Despite progress in diversity, equity, and inclusion (DEI) across higher education, disability remains underrepresented in DEI frameworks. Multicultural centers and diversity initiatives often exclude disability identity, and students are typically referred only to Disability Support Services, where the emphasis remains on documentation and compliance [38]. This practice sidelines the cultural, social, and intersectional dimensions of disability and contributes to feelings of isolation and marginalization.

Disability culture acknowledges disability as a natural and valuable aspect of human diversity and includes the shared history, values, language, artistic expression, and collective identity of individuals with disabilities [63]. As Hopson [64] explains, disability culture fosters a feeling of shared identity and passions that binds PWDs together and aids in developing and maintaining meanings, identities, and the consciousness that propels a political movement. This collective identity encompassing both cultural and sociopolitical dimensions is expressed through narrative and identity pride and is grounded in shared experiences of oppression and resilience [65]. In light of this, incorporating disability culture into campus life, we must go beyond accommodation. We need to acknowledge disability as an identity category that is equal to race, ethnicity, gender, and sexual orientation within DEI frameworks. This involves including disability perspectives in curricula, organizing disability cultural programming, and developing visible spaces that build community and pride.

To create genuinely inclusive environments, institutions must integrate disability culture and intersectionality into their DEI frameworks. Establishing Disability Cultural Centers as spaces that provide integrated wellness, identity development, vocational preparation, and social engagement can provide students with holistic support [62]. These centers should operate in partnership with Disability Resource Center, Offices of Diversity and Inclusion, Student Success, and Career Services to promote interdisciplinary collaboration and integration and dismantle structural impediments. This approach requires developing culturally responsive career services that address intersectional discrimination and mentorship programs connecting students with professionals sharing similar identity experiences.

Theoretically, integrating disability culture aligns with SCCT [10] by enhancing students' self-efficacy, shaping positive outcome expectations, and supporting meaningful academic and career goals. This approach also reinforces intersectionality theory [22] by recognizing how disability intersects with other marginalized identities, influencing access to opportunities and resources and perceiving barriers. Creating environments where disability identity is affirmed increases students' confidence in navigating career barriers, expands perceived career possibilities, and encourages persistence toward goals. Research demonstrates that when students' intersecting ethnic and disability identity is affirmed, they report higher levels of belonging, self-efficacy, and engagement, which are significant predictors of career development outcomes [66]. These recommendations must be considered within the current sociopolitical climate, where DEI initiatives may face institutional and legislative resistance. Disability culture initiatives can be strong and practical ways to sustain inclusive practices while cultivating partnerships across identity groups to prevent marginalization.

Institutional staff, faculty, and administrators should receive training on disability identity, culture, and intersectionality, fostering environments where students with disabilities from all racial and ethnic backgrounds feel valued [38]. Such efforts can reduce microaggressions, improve campus interactions, and promote empathy across groups [1]. Cross-campus collaboration among peers, faculty, families, and campus leaders is essential for building supportive ecosystems where students' identities are affirmed and their strengths acknowledged as fundamental to institutional diversity. These efforts must validate students navigating multiple marginalized identities, fostering climates that advance meaningful access, career readiness, and long-term professional success for all students.

6. Limitations of the Study

The first limitation of the study involves research design. The present study was a cross-sectional data collection. However, perceptions of identities, social support, career barriers, career decision self-efficacy, and outcome expectation among college students with disabilities are more likely dynamic and subject to change over time. The data was collected within a discreet period of time, which can affect the findings and the interpretations. As noted by Johnson and Christensen [67], cross-sectional designs often require large and representative samples for meaningful generalization.

The second limitation concerns the statistical power of subgroup analyses. While 250 participants identified themselves as European American, only 50 participants identified as non-European ethnicities, including African American, Asian American, Hispanic, multiethnic, Irish, and Jewish backgrounds. This distribution broadly reflects recent U.S. census data showing approximately 58% non-Hispanic White and 42% people of color. Hence, the imbalance in sample size aligns with population demographics and is not inherently problematic. That said, the relatively small size of the non-European groups may affect the robustness of statistical comparisons and limit the power to detect significant differences across ethnic groups. Even though conservative and appropriate statistical methods were employed (e.g., Scheffé post hoc analysis), the findings regarding ethnic group differences should be carefully interpreted, especially when making generalized conclusions. Given the increasing diversity of the population, future research should aim for larger and more representative samples to enhance statistical power and better reflect the broader population.

Third, the data were collected from two four-year public universities in the midwestern and southeastern regions of the United States. As a result, the present study findings cannot be generalized to college students with disabilities in all types of nationwide postsecondary education (e.g., community colleges, private universities, or institutes of technology). Future research should seek to replicate this study using more diverse institutional types and geographic regions to enhance external validity.

Fourth, participants' responses might have been impacted by social desirability bias [68]. For instance, participants might understate perceived barriers on campus or exaggerate positive experiences with faculty support. Informed consent and confidentiality measures were taken to reduce social desirability bias, but participants might have been reluctant to express disagreement or reveal unfavorable opinions, which could potentially affect the validity of self-reported data. Researchers should remain cautious in interpreting results that may be influenced by such biases and consider incorporating methods to detect or control for social desirability in future studies.

7. Recommendations for Future Research

The results of this study suggest that more research is necessary to explore the extent to which students' disability identity and ethnic identity inform the career development of college students with disabilities across multiple racial and ethnic groups. Future research also should include larger and more demographically diverse sample sizes of college students with disabilities from historically marginalized racial and ethnic backgrounds. Broader data sets allow for a better understanding of how the intersectionality of identities affects critical constructs like career decision self-efficacy, perceived barriers, social support, and career outcome expectations.

Furthermore, future research should also expand student identity development to other identity dimensions, such as, for instance, gender identity, sexual orientation, socioeconomic status, immigration background, and religious affiliation. Investigating how these constructions of layered identity affect the experience of disability and ethnicity could bring deeper insight. Understanding of identity nuance can emphasize how students experience and contend with structural and cultural barriers in higher education and beyond: for example, how a Black woman with a disability engages in the college, and then how she navigates the intersectionality of disability, ethnicity, and gender identity during the workforce experience.

Additionally, future studies should explore the potential effects of different university attendance modes (in-person vs. e-learning) on students' experiences with identity development and career development. For students with disabilities from diverse ethnic backgrounds, the distinction between in-person and online learning environments may be pertinent because these settings may present unique opportunities and difficulties for identity affirmation and career efficacy and career outcomes [69–72]. In-person learning settings might provide more chances for mentoring and community development, but they might also come with extra challenges because of social isolation, campus climate and physical accessibility. On the other hand, online learning has the potential to improve accessibility and offer flexible accommodations. However, it may limit opportunities for meaningful social connections and access to culturally inclusive and affirming spaces, both of which are fundamental for the development of intersectional identities [70,71]. Promoting more inclusive and efficient support systems that address the individual needs of racially and ethnically diverse students with disabilities across various educational delivery formats is critical. This effort may be facilitated by recognizing how students' perceptions of career barriers and success, social support, and intersectional identity affirmation are influenced by their mode of university attendance.

Lastly, research should not be limited to college experience. Extending research into the workforce may illustrate how identity and intersectionality continue to shape the scope of experience concerning access to career opportunities, perceptions of organizational inclusion in the workplace, and sustainable career satisfaction within the life course of individuals with disabilities. The results of future studies may resonate with rehabilitation professionals, career counselors, and higher education agents and serve to strengthen current efforts to redefine practices supportive of identity development, validate the lived experience, and dismantle systemic inequities.

8. Conclusions

This study illuminates the complex and intersectional influences of disability and ethnic identities on the career-related factors of college students with disabilities across racial/ethnic groups. Two critical patterns were identified. First, students from underrepresented groups reported stronger affirmation and engagement with their ethnic identities than their European American counterparts. Second, they are more likely to perceive career-related barriers compared to those who are European Americans. These patterns highlight the paradox faced by many marginalized students. While ethnic identity can serve as a source of strength, pride, and resilience, it is also associated with a greater awareness of systemic inequities in both educational and career environments.

The findings underscore the need for postsecondary institutions to adopt more nuanced, identity-conscious approaches to career development. One-size-fits-all services fall short in addressing the layered challenges faced by students who navigate the compounded effects of ableism and racism. Instead, career services, academic advising, and campus support systems must be culturally responsive, inclusive, and affirming of students' intersecting identities. This transformation is critical for college students with disabilities from racially and ethnically underrepresented backgrounds. Professionals and institutions need to rethink disability not simply as a category for accommodation but as a dynamic social identity that intersects with race, gender, and culture. Integration of identity-affirming, culturally responsive, and collaborative strategies with career development and student support in institutions helps to reduce barriers and enables students to realize their full academic and professional potential.

Author Contributions: Conceptualization, S.-Y.C.; Methodology, S.-Y.C.; Validation, K.B.W.; Formal analysis, S.-Y.C.; Writing—Ooriginal draft, S.-Y.C.; Writing—review & editing, K.B.W.; Supervision, K.B.W. All authors have read and agreed to the published version of the manuscript.

Funding: This research received no external funding.

Institutional Review Board Statement: The study was conducted in accordance with the Declaration of Helsinki, and approved by the Institutional Review Board of Southern Illinois University Carbondale (protocol code 19177 approved on 5 September 2019) and University of Kentucky (protocol code 54109 approved on 4 November 2019).

Informed Consent Statement: Informed consent was obtained from all subjects involved in the study.

Data Availability Statement: The original contributions presented in this study are included in the article. Further inquiries can be directed to the corresponding author.

Conflicts of Interest: The authors declare no conflicts of interest.

References

1. Harbour, W.S.; Greenberg, D. *Campus Climate and Students with Disabilities*; NCCSD Research Brief; NCCSD: Huntersville, NC, USA, 2017; Volume 1, pp. 1–27.
2. National Center for Education Statistics. *Number and Percentage Distribution of Students Enrolled in Postsecondary Institutions, by Level, Disability Status, and Selected Student Characteristics: Academic Year 2019–2020*; (Table 311.10) [Dataset]; U.S. Department of Education, Institute of Education Sciences: Washington, DA, USA, 2023. Available online: https://nces.ed.gov/programs/digest/d22/tables/dt22_311.10.asp (accessed on 1 August 2025).
3. Snyder, T.D.; Dillow, S.A. *Digest of Education Statistics 2011 (NCES 2012-001)*; National Center for Education Statistics, Institute of Education Sciences, U.S. Department of Education: Washington, DA, USA, 2012. Available online: https://nces.ed.gov/pubs2012/2012001.pdf (accessed on 1 February 2020).
4. Mpofu, E.; Harley, D.A. Racial and disability identity: Implications for the career counseling of African Americans with disabilities. *Rehabil. Couns. Bull.* **2006**, *50*, 14–23. [CrossRef]
5. Isadore, K.M.; Galván, A.; O'Shea, A. Exploring the lived experiences of racially/ethnically minoritized college students with psychiatric disabilities. *J. Postsecond. Educ. Disabil.* **2024**, *37*, 289–305.
6. Pillette, K. *College Students with Disabilities and Employment: Career Development Needs and Models of Support*; NCCSD Research Brief; NCCSD: Huntersville, NC, USA, 2019; Volume 2, pp. 1–17.
7. Ong, M.; Smith, J.M.; Ko, L.T. Counterspaces for women of color in STEM higher education: Marginal and central spaces for persistence and success. *J. Res. Sci. Teach.* **2018**, *55*, 206–245. [CrossRef]
8. Carter, R.T.; Scales, J.E.; Juby, H.L.; Collins, N.M.; Wan, C.M. Seeking Career Services on Campus: Racial Differences in Referral, Process, and Outcome. *J. Career Assess.* **2003**, *11*, 393–404. [CrossRef]
9. Erevelles, N.; Minear, A. Unspeakable offenses: Untangling race and disability in discourses of intersectionality. *J. Lit. Cult. Disabil. Stud.* **2010**, *4*, 127–145. [CrossRef]
10. Lent, R.W.; Brown, S.D.; Hackett, G. Toward a unifying social cognitive theory of career and academic interest, choice, and performance. *J. Vocat. Behav.* **1994**, *45*, 79–122. [CrossRef]
11. Lent, R.W.; Brown, S.D.; Hackett, G. Social cognitive career theory. In *Career Choice and Development*, 4th ed.; Brown, D., Ed.; Jossey-Bass: Hoboken, NJ, USA, 2002; pp. 255–311.
12. Ochs, L.A.; Roessler, R.T. Students with disabilities: How ready are they for the 21st century? *Rehabil. Couns. Bull.* **2001**, *44*, 170–176. [CrossRef]
13. Chan, X.W.; Hutchings, K. Inequalities, barriers, intersectionality, and facilitators of careers of women with disabilities: Themes and future research agenda from a scoping review. *Front. Psychol.* **2023**, *14*, 1104784. [CrossRef]
14. Conyers, L.M.; Szymanski, E.M. Social-cognitive career theory and the career development of African American women. *Rehabil. Couns. Bull.* **1998**, *41*, 198–210.
15. Ozawa, M.N.; Yeo, Y.H. Work status and work performance of people with disabilities: An empirical study. *J. Disabil. Policy Stud.* **2006**, *17*, 180–190. [CrossRef]

16. Kim, Y.H.; Choi, N. Career decision self-efficacy of Asian American students: The role of curiosity and ethnic identity. *Career Dev. Q.* **2019**, *67*, 32–46. [CrossRef]
17. Ma, P.W.W.; Desai, U.; George, L.S.; Filippo, A.A.S.; Varon, S. Managing family conflict over career decisions: The experience of Asian Americans. *J. Career Dev.* **2014**, *41*, 487–506. [CrossRef]
18. Gloria, A.M.; Hird, J.S. Influences of ethnic and nonethnic variables on the career decision-making self-efficacy of college students. *Career Dev. Q.* **1999**, *48*, 157–174. [CrossRef]
19. Mejia-Smith, B.; Gushue, G.V. Latina/o students' perceptions of career barriers: Relations of ethnic identity, acculturation, and self-efficacy. *J. Couns. Psychol.* **2017**, *95*, 145–155. [CrossRef]
20. Brown, S.D.; Lent, R.W. Social cognitive career theory at 25: Progress in studying the domain satisfaction and career self-management models. *J. Career Assess.* **2019**, *27*, 563–578. [CrossRef]
21. Forber-Pratt, A.J.; Lyew, D.A.; Mueller, C.; Samples, L.B. Disability identity development: A systematic review of the literature. *Rehabil. Psychol.* **2017**, *62*, 198–207. [CrossRef]
22. Crenshaw, K. Mapping the margins: Intersectionality, identity politics, and violence against women of color. *Stanf. Law Rev.* **1991**, *43*, 1241–1299. [CrossRef]
23. Shields, S.A. Gender: An intersectionality perspective. *Sex Roles* **2008**, *59*, 301–311. [CrossRef]
24. Ruiz Alvarado, A.; Hurtado, S. Campus Climate, Intersecting Identities, and Institutional Support among Mexican American College Students. In *The Magic Key: The Educational Journey of Mexican Americans from K-12 to College and Beyond*; Ruth Enid Zambrana, R.E., Hurtado, S., Eds.; University of Texas Press: New York, NY, USA, 2015; pp. 168–190. [CrossRef]
25. Prior, S. Gender in schools. In *Intersectionality in Educational Research*; Davis, D.J., Brunn-Bevel, R.J., Olive, J.L., Eds.; Stylus Publishing: Clayton, Australia, 2015; pp. 93–114.
26. Burke, P.J.; Stets, J.E. *Identity Theory*; Oxford University Press: Oxford, UK, 2009.
27. Foster, S.; Kinuthia, W. Deaf persons of Asian American, Hispanic American, and African American backgrounds: A study of intraindividual diversity and identity. *J. Deaf Stud. Deaf Educ.* **2003**, *8*, 271–290. [CrossRef]
28. Bounds, P.S. Contextual factors related to African American adolescent career development. *Career Dev. Q.* **2017**, *65*, 131–144. [CrossRef]
29. Chao, S.Y.; Chen, R.K.; Grizzell, S.T.; Wilson, K.B.; Lewis, T.A. Factors influencing the career decision self-efficacy and outcome expectations of college students with disabilities. *Rehabil. Res. Policy Educ.* **2022**, *36*, 197–212. [CrossRef]
30. Lindsay, S.; Varahra, A.; Ahmed, H.; Abrahamson, S.; Pulver, S.; Primucci, M.; Wong, K. Exploring the relationships between race, ethnicity, and school and work outcomes among youth and young adults with disabilities: A scoping review. *Disabil. Rehabil.* **2022**, *44*, 8110–8129. [CrossRef]
31. Annamma, S.A.; Connor, D.; Ferri, B.A. Dis/ability critical race studies (DisCrit): Theorizing at the intersections of race and dis/ability. *Race Ethn. Educ.* **2013**, *16*, 1–31. [CrossRef]
32. Bell, C.M. *Blackness and Disability: Critical Examinations and Cultural Interventions*; LIT Verlag Münster: Münster, Germany, 2011.
33. Wong, A. *Disability Visibility: First-Person Stories from the Twenty-First Century*; Vintage: Adelaide, Australia, 2020.
34. Purdie-Vaughns, V.; Eibach, R.P. Intersectional invisibility: The distinctive advantages and disadvantages of multiple subordinate-group identities. *Sex Roles* **2008**, *59*, 377–391. [CrossRef]
35. Fabian, E.S.; Ethridge, G.; Beveridge, S. Differences in perceptions of career barriers and supports for people with disabilities by demographic, background and case status factors. *J. Rehabil.* **2009**, *75*, 41–49.
36. Gushue, G.V. The relationship of ethnic identity, career decision-making self-efficacy and outcome expectations among Latino/a high school students. *J. Vocat. Behav.* **2006**, *68*, 85–95. [CrossRef]
37. Jones, S.R.; Abes, E.S. *Identity Development of College Students: Advancing Frameworks for Multiple Dimensions of Identity*; Jossey-Bass: Hoboken, NJ, USA, 2013.
38. Abes, E.S.; Wallace, S.L. "People see me, but they don't see me": An intersectional study of college students with physical disabilities. *J. Coll. Stud. Dev.* **2018**, *59*, 545–562. [CrossRef]
39. Kreider, C.M.; Luna, C.; Lan, M.F.; Wu, C.Y. Disability advocacy messaging and conceptual links to underlying disability identity development among college students with learning disabilities and attention disorders. *Disabil. Health J.* **2020**, *13*, 100827. [CrossRef]
40. Wilson, K.B.; Acklin, C.L.; Chao, S.Y.; Pitt, J.S.; Gines, J.E. The multicultural counseling competencies: An empirical investigation. *Rehabil. Res. Policy Educ.* **2019**, *33*, 260–272. [CrossRef]
41. Kutscher, E.L.; Tuckwiller, E.D. Persistence in higher education for students with disabilities: A mixed systematic review. *J. Divers. High. Educ.* **2019**, *12*, 136–155. [CrossRef]
42. Marshak, L.; Van Wieren, T.; Ferrell, D.R.; Swiss, L.; Dugan, C. Exploring barriers to college student use of disability services and accommodations. *J. Postsecond. Educ. Disabil.* **2010**, *22*, 151–165.
43. Lombardi, A.; Murray, C.; Dallas, B. University faculty attitudes toward disability and inclusive instruction: Comparing two institutions. *J. Postsecond. Educ. Disabil.* **2012**, *25*, 103–117.

44. Test, D.W.; Fowler, C.H.; Wood, W.M.; Brewer, D.M.; Eddy, S. A conceptual framework of self-advocacy for students with disabilities. *Remedial Spec. Educ.* **2009**, *26*, 43–54. [CrossRef]
45. Dutta, A.; Kang, H.J.; Kaya, C.; Benton, S.F.; Sharp, S.E.; Chan, F.; da Silva Cardoso, E.; Kundu, M. Social-Cognitive Career Theory predictors of STEM career interests and goal persistence in minority college students with disabilities: A path analysis. *J. Vocat. Rehabil.* **2015**, *43*, 159–167. [CrossRef]
46. Hahn, H.D.; Belt, T.L. Disability identity and attitudes toward cure in a sample of disabled activists. *J. Health Soc. Behav.* **2004**, *45*, 453–464. [CrossRef]
47. Phinney, J. The Multigroup Ethnic Identity Measure: A new scale for use with adolescents and young adults from diverse groups. *J. Adolesc. Res.* **1992**, *7*, 156–176. [CrossRef]
48. Brown, S.D.; Unger Hu, K.A.; Mevi, A.A.; Hedderson, M.M.; Shan, J.; Quesenberry, C.P.; Ferrara, A. The Multigroup Ethnic Identity Measure—Revised: Measurement invariance across racial and ethnic groups. *J. Couns. Psychol.* **2014**, *61*, 154–161. [CrossRef]
49. Roberts, R.; Phinney, J.; Masse, L.; Chen, Y.; Roberts, C.; Romero, A. The structure of ethnic identity in young adolescents from diverse ethnocultural groups. *J. Early Adolesc.* **1999**, *19*, 301–322. [CrossRef]
50. McWhirter, E.H. Perceived barriers to education and career: Ethnic and gender differences. *J. Vocat. Behav.* **1997**, *50*, 124–140. [CrossRef]
51. Lombardi, A.; Gerdes, H.; Murray, C. Validating an assessment of individual actions, postsecondary, and social supports of college students with disabilities. *J. Stud. Aff. Res. Pract.* **2011**, *48*, 107–126. [CrossRef]
52. Betz, N.E.; Klein, K.L.; Taylor, K.M. Evaluation of a short form of the career decision-making self-efficacy scale. *J. Career Assess.* **1996**, *4*, 47–57. [CrossRef]
53. Betz, N.E.; Taylor, K.M. Manual for the Career Decision Self-Efficacy Scale and CDMSE-Short Form. 2012. Available online: https://www.mindgarden.com/career-decision-self-efficacy-scale/440-cdse-manual.html (accessed on 1 September 2019).
54. McWhirter, E.H.; Crothers, M.; Rasheed, S. The effects of high school career education on social-cognitive variables. *J. Couns. Psychol.* **2000**, *47*, 330–341. [CrossRef]
55. Dillman, D.A.; Smyth, J.D.; Christian, L.M. *Internet, Phone, Mail, and Mixed-Mode Surveys: The Tailored Design Method*, 4th ed.; John Wiley & Sons: Hoboken, NJ, USA, 2014.
56. Mertler, C.A.; Reinhart, R.V. *Advanced and Multivariate Statistical Methods: Practical Application and Interpretation*, 6th ed.; Routledge: London, UK, 2016.
57. Tabachnick, B.G.; Fidell, L.S. *Using Multivariate Statistics*, 7th ed.; Pearson: London, UK, 2018.
58. Islam, Z. Negotiating identities: The lives of Pakistani and Bangladeshi young disabled people. *Disabil. Soc.* **2008**, *23*, 41–52. [CrossRef]
59. Phinney, J.S.; Chavira, V. Parental ethnic socialization and adolescent coping with problems related to ethnicity. *J. Res. Adolesc.* **1995**, *5*, 31–53. [CrossRef]
60. Aquino, K.C.; Alhaddab, T.A.; Kim, E. "Does disability matter?" Students' satisfaction with college experiences. In *Disability as Diversity in Higher Education: Policies and Practices to Enhance Student Success*; Kim, E., Aquino, K.C., Eds.; Routledge: London, UK, 2017; pp. 47–60.
61. Miller, R.A.; Wynn, R.D.; Webb, K.W. Queering disability in higher education: Views from the intersections. In *Disability as Diversity in Higher Education*; Miller, R.A., Wynn, R.D., Webb, K.W., Eds.; Routledge: London, UK, 2017; pp. 31–44.
62. Evans, N.J.; Broido, E.M.; Brown, K.R.; Wilke, A.K. *Disability in Higher Education: A Social Justice Approach*; Jossey-Bass: Hoboken, NJ, USA, 2017.
63. Linton, S. *Claiming Disability: Knowledge and Identity*; New York University Press: New York, NY, USA, 1998.
64. Hopson, J. Disability as Culture. *Sch. Adm. Multicult. Educ. Incl.* **2019**, *27*, 22–24.
65. Saia, T. Embracing disability culture in schools. *Lang. Speech Hear. Serv. Sch.* **2023**, *54*, 794–798. [CrossRef] [PubMed]
66. Vaccaro, A.; Daly-Cano, M.; Newman, B.M. A sense of belonging among college students with disabilities: An emergent theoretical model. *J. Coll. Stud. Dev.* **2015**, *56*, 670–686. [CrossRef]
67. Johnson, R.B.; Christensen, L.B. *Educational Research: Quantitative, Qualitative, and Mixed Approaches*, 3rd ed.; Sage Publications: Thousand Oaks, CA, USA, 2008.
68. Krumpal, I. Determinants of social desirability bias in sensitive surveys: A literature review. *Qual. Quant.* **2013**, *47*, 2025–2047. [CrossRef]
69. Sannipoli, M. UNIversal Inclusion Rights and Opportunities for Students with Disabilities in the Academic Context. 2018, pp. 157–164. Available online: https://research.unipg.it/handle/11391/1576953 (accessed on 22 August 2025).
70. Covelli, V.; Panizza, L.; Trezzi, M.; Zugno, E.; Marelli, A. University Students with Special Educational Needs: An Assessment of Satisfaction and Perceptions of e-Learning and Services Provided. In *International Conference on Higher Education Learning Methodologies and Technologies Online*; Springer Nature: Cham, Switzerland, 2024; pp. 45–58.

71. Kim, S.Y.; Lee, O.E. Examining varying online learning experiences of college students with disabilities by disability type. *Am. J. Distance Educ.* **2024**, *39*, 289–303. [CrossRef]
72. DeRosier, M.E.; McMillen, J.; Davis, N.O.; Kameny, R.; Hoffend, C. Tools to support career advancement of diverse social, behavioral, and mental health researchers: Comparison of in-person and online training delivery modes. *J. Online Learn. Teach.* **2011**, *7*, 43–56.

healthcare

MDPI

Article

Caregiver Burden in Early Intervention: A Fuzzy-Set Qualitative Comparative Analysis of Causal Configurations

Pau García-Grau, Julia Argente-Tormo, Gabriel Martínez-Rico * and Rómulo J. González-García *

Campus Capacitas, Catholic University of Valencia "San Vicente Martir", 46001 Valencia, Spain; pau.garcia@ucv.es (P.G.-G.); julia.argente@ucv.es (J.A.-T.)

* Correspondence: gabi.martinez@ucv.es (G.M.-R.); rj.gonzalez@ucv.es (R.J.G.-G.)

Abstract

Background/Objectives: Caregiver burden is a well-documented phenomenon among families of children with disabilities, particularly within early childhood intervention contexts. Although family-centered practices aim to empower parents and foster collaborative relationships with professionals, the specific contribution of families' psychological and social resources to caregiver burden remains insufficiently understood. This study examined the combinations of psychosocial conditions associated with both high and low levels of caregiver burden in families receiving early intervention services. **Methods:** A total of 117 families of children aged 0–6 years enrolled in an early intervention center in Valencia, Spain, participated in the study. Caregiver burden was assessed using the Zarit Burden Interview. Fuzzy-set qualitative comparative analysis (fsQCA) was applied to identify the combinations of conditions that were necessary and sufficient for the presence or absence of caregiver burden. **Results:** No single condition was necessary for the outcome, but several sufficient combinations were identified. High caregiver burden was associated with configurations involving low resilience, limited perceived social support, and reduced coping capacity, whereas low burden emerged from configurations characterized by stronger psychosocial resources, particularly high family confidence, resilience, and social support. The solutions showed high consistency and coverage, indicating robust explanatory models for both outcomes. **Conclusions:** These findings demonstrate that caregiver burden in early intervention arises not from isolated factors but from specific interactions among psychosocial conditions. Understanding these causal combinations provides a more nuanced perspective on family functioning and highlights the importance of strengthening resilience and social support within early intervention programs to reduce caregiver burden and promote family well-being.

Keywords: caregiver burden; early intervention; psychosocial resources; fsQCA; family-centered practices

1. Introduction

The term "caregiver burden" refers to the physical, psychological, social, and financial difficulties experienced by family members providing care [1,2]. This burden results from caregivers' cognitive appraisal of stressors, influencing their well-being, social functioning, and health [3]. In Early Intervention (EI), burden is particularly relevant because families face prolonged and complex care demands during critical developmental periods, with substantial implications for family quality of life [4].

Parenting a child with disabilities involves multiple responsibilities and varies in satisfaction depending on contextual factors [5]. These responsibilities, often intensified in neurodevelopmental conditions, can generate significant physical, emotional, and financial strain, contributing to parental burden [6]. Although burden has been linked to child-related factors such as age and perceived severity, evidence shows that caregivers' adjustment depends largely on their own resources and skills [7], making empowerment, confidence, and parental competence key factors in managing caregiving demands [8].

1.1. Contextualization of EI Services

The implementation of family-centered practices in EI has been a priority for support services internationally, reflecting a shift from expert-model, deficit-based approaches toward models that highlight environmental and family factors in child development [9–11]. The recommended practices promoted in the United States by the Division for Early Childhood (DEC) contributed to expanding this paradigm globally [12]. In Spain, EI has also evolved following these international influences, although the implementation of family-centered practices is still not fully achieved across services [8,13].

1.2. Capacity-Building Approach to Early Intervention Services

The promotion of child and family functioning is a central priority in EI services [14,15], which requires active collaboration with families throughout assessment, planning, and intervention. Dunst et al., [16] conceptualized help-giving practices as comprising relational and participatory dimensions, both of which have demonstrated positive effects on child and family outcomes [17]. Relational practices refer to respectful, empathetic interactions that recognize family strengths, whereas participatory practices involve shared decision-making and responsiveness to family priorities [17].

Consistent with this evidence, current EI frameworks emphasize strengths-based, collaborative approaches that build family capacity [12], with professionals supporting caregivers in enhancing everyday parenting opportunities and reinforcing parental self-efficacy [18]. Within this paradigm, capacity-building and empowerment are viewed as core outcomes of effective family-centered support [19].

1.3. Family Confidence in EI

Family confidence is one of the consequences of capacity-building and family-centered support services in EI. Family confidence is a component of a person's self-efficacy beliefs [20] that refers to the ability to perform a task competently (for example, the family member's confidence in helping a child participate in a home routine). Therefore, capacity-building practices in EI focus on partnering with caregivers by offering relevant information, guidance, and encouragement, while also fostering the development of their knowledge and skills to address both the child's and the family's needs in a specific context [20]. This approach contributes to improving the caregivers' sense of competence and confidence in their parental role [10].

Previous studies have found that family confidence is a key outcome in attenuating the negative impact that caregiver burden has on family quality of life. In addition, family confidence has also demonstrated to strongly predict better perceptions of family quality of life [4] and decreased parenting burden [21] in the EI field. Furthermore, family confidence can also be understood at the family-system level, encompassing the family's belief in its own ability to manage daily functioning and relational dynamics [22], rather than being limited to confidence in supporting the child's development.

Ref. [13] found that increased confidence contributed to improving child functioning and family quality of life. Families that develop greater confidence in their capabilities are those that more effectively implement intervention strategies in daily life, which translates into greater adherence to the intervention plan and more consistent application of recommended strategies. This effective implementation generates a positive cycle where the child's progress reinforces parental confidence, which in turn facilitates more successful intervention and reduces the perception of family burden.

1.4. Family Confidence and Caregiver Burden in EI

Family-centered EI practices prove to be an effective way to help cope with the perception of burden [9]. These practices aim to promote empowerment, collaboration, and shared decision-making by engaging families as active partners in their child's development through participatory and relational practices [23–25]. Evidence shows that providing support in the form of opportunities for the family to acquire competencies, in turn, has an impact on their children and this affects their parental self-efficacy [9]. Furthermore, in the study by [26], with families of children with ASD, parents obtained a greater sense of parental self-efficacy when they felt more involved in their children's intervention and were more satisfied with the training they received as part of these interventions, which contributes to reducing stress levels associated with burden.

1.5. The Configurational Perspective: fsQCA as a Methodology

Traditionally, research on family burden has employed linear approaches that seek to identify individual predictors through regression analysis. However, these methods may not adequately capture the inherent complexity of family phenomena, where multiple factors interact in non-linear ways to produce diverse outcomes. Qualitative comparative analysis (QCA) based on fuzzy sets (fsQCA) offers an alternative methodological perspective that recognizes equifinality—multiple paths can lead to the same outcome—and configurational causality—outcomes emerge from specific combinations of conditions rather than from independent additive effects [27].

This methodology is particularly appropriate for the study of family burden because it allows for the identification of complex causal configurations, recognizing that different combinations of factors can produce high or low levels of burden. Furthermore, fsQCA is well suited for studying complex social realities because it shows that there can be different combinations of factors leading to the same outcome, and that the absence of the outcome may result from entirely different circumstances [27]. For example, in EI, high family quality of life may emerge from combinations such as high family empowerment and strong social support, while low family quality of life may arise from different configurations, such as low resilience despite high social support.

In the EI context, where families present diversity of resources, needs, and characteristics, this methodological approach can provide more precise and applicable insights for the design of personalized interventions.

Although previous studies have examined the relationships between family confidence, child functioning, and caregiver burden, most have relied on linear approaches that do not capture how these factors operate jointly in Early Intervention. As a result, little is known about the specific combinations of psychosocial and service-related conditions that lead to high or low burden. This gap is particularly relevant in the Spanish EI context, where the implementation of family-centered practices remains uneven. To date, no configurational analyses have explored these interactions, limiting our ability to understand the complexity of caregiver experiences and to tailor supports accordingly.

Given the potential of configurational analysis and the aforementioned influence of family confidence and child functioning on caregiver burden in EI, the present study aimed to: describe the patterns of family confidence and caregiver burden in families receiving EI services in Spain; analyze the relationship between family confidence and caregiver burden scores; and identify the combinations of causal conditions that lead to both high and low levels of burden.

2. Materials and Methods

2.1. Participants

The study included 117 families of children aged 0–6 years receiving Early Intervention (EI) services across four Spanish autonomous communities.

Participating children were predominantly male (n = 42; 35.9%) and had a mean age of 43 months. The concept of family in this study refers to the primary caregiving unit responsible for the daily upbringing and participation of the child in EI activities, which may include biological parents, grandparents, or other legal guardians.

Primary respondents were mainly mothers (58.6%), followed by fathers (17.2%) and grandmothers (3.4%), while 19% of the questionnaires were jointly completed by both parents. Among individual respondents, mothers represented 75.9% (n = 44) and fathers 24.1% (n = 14) of the sample. The mean age of adult respondents was 36.5 years. The duration of EI service receipt ranged from 1 to 48 months (M = 16.6; SD = 12.5).

Regarding caregiving involvement, parents reported the time spent with their children on a 5-point scale (1 = very little to 5 = most of the time), with mothers averaging 4.24 and fathers 3.26. Caregivers rated the perceived severity of their child's disability (M = 1.48; SD = 1.17) and the level of child's functioning level (M = 3.64; SD = 0.88), indicating overall mild to moderate needs within the sample.

The sample size (n = 117) is adequate for fsQCA analyses. Methodological guidelines indicate that fsQCA is particularly suitable for small-to-medium samples, typically ranging from around 50 to 150 cases, as this range provides sufficient empirical diversity to construct meaningful truth tables and identify stable configurational patterns [27,28]. Previous studies in social and health sciences have employed similar sample sizes with robust results, supporting the adequacy of the current dataset for configurational analysis.

2.2. Instruments

Family Quality of Life and Caregiver Burden. Family outcomes were assessed using the Families in Early Intervention Quality of Life Scale (FEIQoL), validated and revised in Spain [29], The scale comprises 39 items rated on a 5-point Likert scale (1 = poor to 5 = excellent) across three dimensions: *Family Relations, Access to Information and Services,* and *Child Functioning*. For this study, the global Family Quality of Life index was used, demonstrating excellent internal consistency (α = 0.98).

Caregiver burden was evaluated using the 12-item Spanish adaptation of the Zarit Burden Interview (ZBI) [30,31]. Although originally designed for caregivers of dependent adults, this reduced version has been widely validated in family caregiving contexts, including parents of children with developmental disabilities. This tool has been widely used and numerous adaptations have emerged in a multitude of fields because it can be easily adapted for different populations. We used the reduced 12-item version because of its length and high internal consistency (α = 0.92) in Spanish [32]. In addition to the applicability of the items to caregivers receiving ECI services in Spain was a key for the instrument selection. Items are rated on a 5-point Likert scale (1 = never to 5 = always), and the overall score in this study demonstrated good reliability (α = 0.87). Its brevity and strong psychometric properties make it suitable for Early Intervention contexts, where participant time is limited.

The Family Confidence in Helping with Child and Family Functioning (Con-Fam) scale [33] was employed to measure parental self-efficacy across two domains: (1) *confidence in supporting the child's participation and independence in daily routines* (20 items), and

(2) *confidence in addressing family functioning aspects* such as informational, emotional, and material support needs (18 items). Responses are scored on a 4-point Likert scale (1 = "I am not quite sure how to help" to 4 = "I have complete confidence"). Reliability was excellent ($\alpha = 0.97$ for child confidence; $\alpha = 0.93$ for family confidence). The instrument demonstrated excellent reliability in the present sample ($\alpha = 0.97$ for child confidence; $\alpha = 0.93$ for family confidence), consistent with previous Spanish studies [13].

Information about the family and the child was collected through an online questionnaire using the same link. Families provided details such as their relationship to the child, caregiver's age, child's age and gender, and the amount of time each adult in the household spent with the child. The child's level of difficulty or severity was assessed through a functional level scale ranging from 1 to 5 (1 = very low functioning, 5 = high functioning), which allowed for a more inclusive description of children with diverse diagnoses and developmental conditions.

Rationale for Instrument Selection. All instruments were selected for their empirical validation in the Spanish population and relevance to Early Intervention practice. The FEIQoL provides an EI-specific measure of family well-being, the Con-Fam captures the multidimensional construct of family confidence, and the abbreviated ZBI allows for assessing caregiver burden efficiently while maintaining robust psychometric quality [34,35].

2.3. Procedure

This study was conducted as part of a larger research project examining caregiver burden in Early Intervention, with institutional IRB approval obtained prior to data collection. The broader project explores multiple dimensions of family experiences, including parental confidence, gender-related differences in burden perceptions, and family quality of life outcomes. The present analysis focuses specifically on the subset of participants for whom complete data on family quality of life and caregiver burden were available.

Data collection was facilitated through electronic surveys distributed by EI professionals and service providers to families enrolled in their programs. The survey integrated all measurement instruments along with sociodemographic questions into a single digital platform. Participation was entirely voluntary and confidential, with families accessing the questionnaires via a secure electronic link. Prior to survey completion, participants were required to review and provide consent through a mandatory informed consent statement embedded within the platform. Eligibility criteria included: (a) being a primary caregiver of a child aged 0–6 years receiving EI services; (b) having at least six months of service participation; and (c) providing informed consent. Families were excluded if the child had an acute medical condition or if the caregiver declined to participate. Given the distribution method through multiple service providers, the total number of families who received invitations could not be determined, precluding calculation of an exact response rate. For inclusion in the final analytical sample, cases were retained only if participants had completed at least 90% of scale items, ensuring data quality and reliability for subsequent analyses.

All participating EI centers across the four autonomous communities followed a shared professional framework. Specifically, these centers implement the DEC Recommended Practices and are integrated within the organizational network Plena Inclusión España, which provides common guidelines, professional development, and quality standards for service delivery. This shared framework contributes to a substantial degree of uniformity in the sampling frame across regions, despite potential administrative differences among autonomous communities.

The study was approved by the Research Ethics Committee of Catholic University of Valencia (Approval Code: UCV/2018-2019/111), adhering to the principles of the

Declaration of Helsinki. Electronic informed consent was obtained before participation, and confidentiality was guaranteed.

2.4. Data Analysis

Data were analyzed using fuzzy-set Qualitative Comparative Analysis (fsQCA), an approach suited to exploring how different combinations of conditions (i.e., psychosocial and contextual factors) jointly explain an outcome through the principle of equifinality. All analyses were performed using fsQCA software, version 4.1, following standard procedures for calibration, truth table construction, and solution derivation. Descriptive statistics (means, standard deviations, and correlations) were first computed to characterize the sample and contextualize the fuzzy-set calibration. Cases with more than 10% missing data were excluded; the remainder were analyzed using pairwise deletion, as missingness was random and minimal. Scale reliability was verified through both Cronbach's alpha and rho_A coefficients [36]. All conditions were calibrated into fuzzy sets (0 = full non-membership, 1 = full membership) using the 10th, 50th, and 90th percentiles as empirical anchors [37], following methodological recommendations for fsQCA [38]. Necessity analyses identified conditions systematically present or absent among cases with the outcome, using a consistency threshold of 0.90 to define strict necessity. Sufficiency analyses were performed using truth tables, applying a frequency cutoff of 1 and a minimum consistency threshold of 0.80. Three types of solutions (complex, parsimonious, and intermediate) were generated, with the intermediate solution selected for interpretation due to its balance between empirical robustness and theoretical coherence [27].

3. Results

To carry out the analysis using Fuzzy-set Qualitative Comparative Analysis (fsQCA), a descriptive analysis was initially performed and the corresponding calibration values were calculated (Table 1). The descriptive statistics show a sample of 117 participants with mean scores ranging from 0.95 for the number of sessions to 3.64 for the child's functional level. The variability observed across all variables provides an adequate basis for calibration into fuzzy sets, using the 10th, 50th, and 90th percentiles as anchor points to establish the thresholds for low, intermediate, and high membership to each condition.

Table 1. Descriptive statistics and calibration values.

		Nfuc	Sesc	Cafc	Canc	Burden
N		117	117	117	117	117
M		3.64	0.95	2.88	2.86	3.22
SD		0.88	0.28	0.61	0.67	0.84
Minimal		1.00	0.5	1.17	1.00	1.47
Maximum		5.00	2.00	4.00	4.00	5.00
Calibration Values						
Percentile	10	3.00	0.53	2.09	2.00	1.27
	50	4.00	1.00	3.00	2.95	2.08
	90	5.00	2.00	3.61	3.70	3.25

Note: Nfuc refers to the child's functioning level, Sesc to number of sessions, Cafc to confidence with helping the child, and Canc to confidence with helping the child. M = Mean; SD = Standard deviation.

3.1. Analysis of Necessary Conditions

The analysis of necessary conditions (Table 2) to explain both the presence and absence of burden shows that none of the evaluated conditions reaches the consistency threshold of 0.90 established by [39] as the criterion for considering a condition as necessary. The highest consistency values are observed for the child's low functioning level

(~Nfuc = 0.738) and the low levels of number of sessions (~Sesc = 0.765) in explaining low levels of burden, although neither reaches the critical threshold. These values indicate that none of the conditions alone is systematically common among cases with burden, which reinforces the need to analyze causal combinations through sufficiency analysis and confirms the configurational nature of the phenomenon under study.

Table 2. Analysis of necessary conditions for high and low burden levels.

	Burden			~Burden	
	Consistency	Coverage		Consistency	Coverage
Nfuc	0.492	0.649	~NFuc	0.738	0.596
Sesc	0.574	0.689	~Sesc	0. 765	0.646
Cafc	0.476	0.481	~Cafc	0. 495	0.490
Canc	0.581	0.581	~Canc	0. 589	0.588

Note: Nfuc refers to the child's functioning level, Sesc to number of sessions, Cafc to confidence with helping the child, and Canc to confidence with helping the child. ~ Refers to low levels.

3.2. Analysis of Sufficient Conditions

The sufficiency analysis identified combinations of causal conditions that lead to both high and low levels of caregiver burden. In constructing the truth table, a minimum consistency threshold of 0.80 was established, following a natural break in the distribution of consistency scores [39]. High levels of burden are explained by two sufficient configurations.

Regarding high levels of burden, two sufficient configurations were identified. In both, low family confidence (Cafc) emerges as a core and recurrent condition, highlighting its pivotal role in shaping caregivers' perceptions of burden. The first configuration (H1: ~Sesc and ~Cafc) combines few therapeutic sessions with low family confidence. This configuration (Raw coverage = 62.7%, Unique coverage = 12.6%, Consistency = 80.8%) shows that limited therapeutic contact, together with families' lack of perceived confidence, substantially contributes to increased levels of burden. Here, raw coverage represents the proportion of cases with high burden that are explained by this specific configuration, whereas unique coverage indicates the proportion explained exclusively by it, without overlapping with other configurations. Consistency, in turn, reflects the degree to which the configuration is a reliable subset of the outcome, that is, the extent to which the combination consistently leads to high burden. The second configuration (H2: ~Nfuc and ~Cafc) associates low child functional level with low family confidence (Raw coverage = 60.3%, Unique coverage = 10.2%, Consistency = 78.5%). This pathway suggests that when children exhibit reduced functional abilities and caregivers simultaneously feel unconfident in managing everyday challenges, the experience of burden intensifies. Taken together, both configurations achieve a solution coverage of 72.9% and a solution consistency of 78.0%, indicating that they jointly explain nearly three-quarters of the cases characterized by high burden, with a coherent and robust pattern of sufficiency.

In contrast, low levels of burden are explained by three consistent and theoretically meaningful configurations. Across these, family confidence with helping the family (Cafc) and family confidence with helping the child (Canc) appear as protective factors that mitigate caregivers' perceived burden, while functional level (Nfuc) and number of sessions (Sesc) act as contingent elements whose effects depend on their combination with the other conditions. The first configuration (L1: ~Nfuc and Cafc) (Raw coverage = 56.2%, Unique coverage = 13.7%, Consistency = 83.1%) shows that even when children have lower functioning levels, high family confidence compensates for this limitation, allowing caregivers to handle daily demands with less strain. The second configuration (L2: ~Nfuc and Sesc and Canc), showing a Raw coverage = 39.4%, Unique coverage = 3.9%, and Consistency = 83.2%, indicates that, under conditions of low child functioning, frequent therapeutic sessions combined with high confidence in helping the child act as a buffer against burden, reflecting the benefits of engagement and perceived self-efficacy. The third configuration (L3: ~Sesc and Cafc and Canc) (Raw coverage = 49.2%, Unique coverage = 8.4%, Consistency = 82.6%) suggests that fewer sessions do not necessarily lead to burden when both family and child confidence are high, implying that empowered and self-reliant family dynamics can offset the need for intensive professional support. Overall, these three configurations yield a solution coverage of 76.9% and a solution consistency of 79.9%, confirming that they jointly account for more than two-thirds of the cases with low levels of burden and display a high level of empirical reliability. A detailed summary of these configurations and their statistical indicators is presented in Table 3.

Table 3. Intermediate solution of the sufficiency analysis high and low levels of burden.

Group	Path	Nfuc	Sesc	Cafc	Canc	Coverage		Consistency
						Raw	Unique	
High levels of burden	H1		○	○		0.627	0.126	0.808
	H2	○		○		0.603	0.102	0.785
			Solution Coverage = 0.729; Solution Consistency = 0.780					
Low Levels of burden	L1	○		•		0.562	0.137	0.831
	L2	○	•		•	0.394	0.039	0.832
	L3		○	•	•	0.492	0.084	0.826
			Solution Coverage = 0.769; Solution Consistency = 0.799					

Note; • = presence of condition, ○ = absence of condition. Expected Vector for high levels of overbuden 1.1.1.1. (1 presence); expected Vector for low levels of buden 0.0.0.0 (0: absence) using the [40]. Nfuc refers to child's functioning level, Sesc = number of sessions, Cafc = family confidence with helping the family, and Canc = family confidence with helping the child.

Taken together, these findings reinforce the pivotal role of family confidence (Cafc) as a decisive condition in both directions of the outcome. Its absence consistently amplifies burden, while its presence, particularly when combined with child confidence (Canc), acts as a protective mechanism that reduces burden. Moreover, number of sessions (Sesc) and functional level (Nfuc) operate as situational moderators: reduced functioning or fewer sessions heighten burden only in the absence of family confidence, whereas strong family confidence mitigates these effects. This pattern underscores the importance of family empowerment and perceived competence as key levers for reducing caregiver strain.

These configurations are visually represented in Figures 1 and 2, which illustrate the causal patterns associated with high and low levels of caregiver burden, respectively. Figure 1 illustrates the causal configurations leading to high levels of caregiver burden. In both solutions, the absence of family confidence (Cafc) is central, reinforcing its key role in explaining burden. Configuration H1 combines few therapeutic sessions (Sesc) with low family confidence, while H2 links low child functional level (Nfuc) and low family confidence. Together, they show that insufficient confidence within the family system, whether accompanied by limited sessions or low child functioning, consistently leads to higher burden.

Figure 2 shows the causal configurations leading to low levels of caregiver burden. Across the three solutions, the presence of family confidence (Cafc) and child confidence (Canc) acts as a protective factor that reduces perceived burden. Configuration L1 combines low child functional level (Nfuc) with high family confidence, L2 joins low functional level, high number of sessions (Sesc), and high child confidence, and L3 integrates high family and child confidence with few sessions. Together, these configurations illustrate that strong family confidence buffers burden, even when functional limitations or limited service use are present.

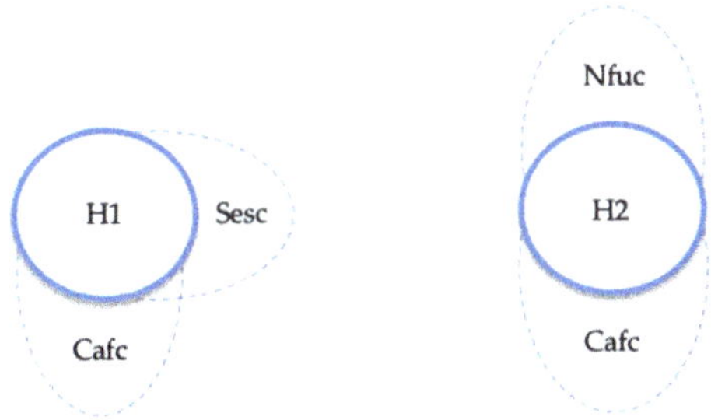

Figure 1. Causal configurations for high and low levels of burden. Note. Nfuc refers to functional level, Sesc = number of sessions, and Cafc = family confidence with helping the family. An ellipse outlined with a solid line signifies the presence of the condition, while an ellipse with a dotted line indicates its absence. If a condition is not pertinent to a given configuration, no ellipse is depicted.

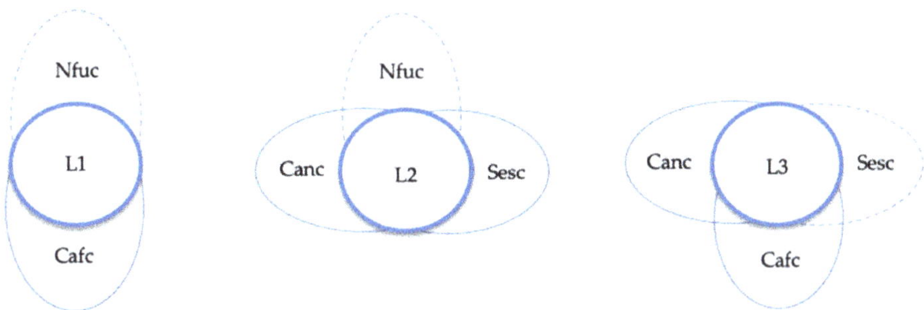

Figure 2. Causal configurations for low levels of burden. Note. Nfuc refers to functional level, Sesc to number of sessions, Cafc to family confidence, and Canc to child confidence. An ellipse outlined with a solid line signifies the presence of the condition, while an ellipse with a dotted line indicates its absence. If a condition is not pertinent to a given configuration, no ellipse is depicted.

4. Discussion

The results obtained through fuzzy-set qualitative comparative analysis (fsQCA) provide solid evidence of the complex and configurational nature of family burden in the Early Intervention (EI) context. This methodological approach goes beyond traditional linear associations, exploring how different combinations of conditions converge toward high or low levels of burden. The application of fsQCA confirms that caregiver burden can rarely be explained by a single variable, reinforcing the importance of considering causal configurations and equifinality in applied social research, particularly in family intervention.

The analysis of necessary conditions revealed that none of the evaluated variables—functional level, number of sessions, family confidence, and child confidence—reached the 0.90 consistency threshold required to be considered necessary. This aligns with previous research showing that family burden is a multidimensional phenomenon and that isolated effects are insufficient to explain the outcome [21]. The absence of necessary conditions highlights a distinction from correlation-based approaches, which typically identify independent linear predictors. By contrast, the fsQCA logic emphasizes equifinality: multiple causal paths can lead to the same outcome, a principle especially relevant in family contexts where interactions among child characteristics, resources, and family dynamics produce heterogeneous outcomes.

The sufficiency analysis identified two consistent configurations explaining high levels of burden, both with low family confidence as the central condition. The first combines a low number of sessions with low family confidence, suggesting that limited professional support and a perception of low competence create conditions conducive to burden. The second combines low confidence with a low functional level of the child, indicating that significant child needs exacerbate burden when caregivers feel less self-efficacy. This is consistent with studies showing that child functioning alone does not directly cause burden, but that its impact is mediated by parental confidence [21].

These findings are strongly supported by the literature. The centrality of low parental confidence/self-efficacy as a core factor in burden is consistent with the theoretical model of [19], which posits that capacity-building practices in EI services enhance parental self-efficacy, reducing stress and improving family quality of life. A recent study [41] also found burden to be negatively associated with caregivers' self-efficacy and quality-of-life dimensions. In addition, the first configuration corroborates findings in the Spanish context [13,29], where limited implementation of family-centered practices restricts participation and competence, intensifying perceived burden.

The analysis of configurations associated with low burden revealed three sufficient pathways, confirming greater diversity in protective strategies and reinforcing the principle of equifinality. The most prominent configuration combines low child functional level with high family confidence, underscoring the role of confidence as a protective factor even in contexts of functional dependence [4]. This supports empowerment-based approaches in EI [42]. The second configuration suggests that intervention frequency can reduce burden when needs are severe, while the third indicates that a low number of sessions does not necessarily increase burden if the family maintains high confidence—an outcome aligned with family-centered approaches promoting generalization and autonomy [13].

Configurations leading to low burden consistently include high levels of family or child confidence, reinforcing the idea that families who feel more competent implement intervention strategies more effectively [43]. This effective implementation generates a virtuous cycle: families adhere better to the plan, observe progress, and experience reduced burden [23]. A recent study in India [44] also showed that implementing family-centered practices improved caregiver strain and empowerment across contexts, with child severity being the only predictor of variation in benefit.

Some results diverge from previous studies that identified functional dependence as the main predictor of burden [45]. In our analysis, functional level appears only as part of specific configurations and never as a dominant condition. This discrepancy may reflect methodological differences: regression models assess net effects, whereas fsQCA shows that low functional level contributes to burden only when combined with additional unfavorable conditions. Our findings support the model of [9], where parental self-efficacy mediates the relationship between stressors and outcomes, and echo results showing that low confidence mediates the impact of stressors on Family Quality of Life [4]. Contextual factors may also contribute: families engaged with EI services may experience uniformly high caregiving demands, making psychological resources more explanatory than variations in daily care.

The results should be interpreted considering the heterogeneity of families receiving EI services. The identified configurations may vary depending on child characteristics, age at intervention onset, socioeconomic context, or cultural factors. Variables not included—such as informal support networks or differences in the implementation of family-centered practices—may also act as protective factors. Future research should incorporate measures of professional practices, community resources, and social support to refine the understanding of these configurations.

Our results also confirm a clear causal asymmetry between configurations leading to high versus low burden: the conditions explaining high levels are not simply the inverse of those predicting low levels. This finding, consistent with fsQCA principles, underscores the need for configurational approaches and suggests that preventing burden and reducing existing burden may require differentiated strategies tailored to each family's situation.

Several mechanisms may explain how the identified configurations lead to different levels of burden. Family confidence may act as a cognitive mediator shaping caregivers' appraisal of stressors, consistent with transactional stress theory. Confidence may facilitate more effective coping strategies, greater personal control, and better implementation of intervention plans. Although the literature is not unanimous regarding the primacy of psychological versus structural factors [46], our results suggest that the quality and empowerment focus of sessions may be more relevant than frequency [17].

Confidence in helping the child may also reflect perceptions of child progress, consistent with findings linking higher confidence to better perceptions of functioning and Family Quality of Life [13].

4.1. Implications for Future Practice and Research

We consider that our configurational analysis enriches and refines understanding of the phenomenon by positioning low family confidence not as the only factor, but as an indispensable catalyzing factor that, when interacting with other stressors, triggers the experience of burden. The configurations for low burden paint a hopeful and complex picture where there is no single recipe for family well-being, but rather a series of complementary strategies that EI services can implement: prioritizing empowerment as a cross-cutting element, adjusting session frequency according to needs, and working toward family autonomy with the goal that high confidence allows for a gradual reduction in service dependence without increasing burden.

These findings have direct implications for the design and delivery of EI services, highlighting the need for professionals to prioritize capacity-building practices that strengthen family confidence and competencies, going beyond merely providing direct therapy to the child [23,47]. There is no single solution, so services must evaluate each family's specific configuration to offer individualized supports to increase their sense of competence. These results provide strong arguments for advocating a family-centered and strengths-based EI model, even in contexts where it is not yet fully implemented [48], as is the case in Spain.

4.2. Limitations

Among the study's limitations are the sample size and the possible exclusion of other relevant variables such as formal and informal social support or financial stress. Future research should employ longitudinal designs to establish causality and observe the evolution of these configurations, include broader contextual variables to refine the models, and conduct in-depth qualitative studies to understand the subjective experience behind the identified configurations. This range of options reinforces the need for an individualized assessment of each family to identify which path toward burden reduction is most viable and appropriate, thus personalizing interventions in the most effective manner. Therefore, there is a need for EI services to assess and intervene in specific ways to strengthen parental self-efficacy, as this is the mechanism that can transform the way families perceive and manage caregiving demands, even when these are high.

5. Conclusions

In conclusion, this study uses an innovative configurational approach (fsQCA) to show that caregiver burden in Early Intervention is a multifaceted phenomenon shaped by the interaction of psychosocial and contextual factors rather than by the isolated effect of a single variable. The most consistent result is the central role of family confidence (Cafc): its absence characterizes pathways leading to high burden, while its presence underlies most protective configurations. This highlights empowerment and parental self-efficacy as core mechanisms that shape caregivers' experiences.

The findings also illustrate the principle of equifinality, demonstrating that there is no single path to preventing or mitigating burden. Different combinations of child functional level, intervention frequency, and confidence can lead to similar outcomes, underscoring the need for flexible, family-tailored interventions instead of standardized procedures.

Overall, this study provides empirical support for advancing EI practices toward family-centered, strengths-based models. Prioritizing the enhancement of caregivers' confidence and capabilities should be considered a central strategy for promoting child development and improving family quality of life.

Author Contributions: Conceptualization, P.G.-G. and R.J.G.-G.; methodology, P.G.-G.; software, P.G.-G.; validation, J.A.-T., G.M.-R. and R.J.G.-G.; formal analysis, P.G.-G.; investigation, P.G.-G.; resources, J.A.-T.; data curation, P.G.-G.; writing—original draft preparation, P.G.-G.; writing—review and editing, J.A.-T., G.M.-R. and R.J.G.-G.; visualization, P.G.-G.; supervision, R.J.G.-G.; project administration, G.M.-R.; funding acquisition, G.M.-R. All authors have read and agreed to the published version of the manuscript.

Funding: This research was funded by Spanish Ministry Projects: Knowledge Generation. State Program to Promote Research 2021–2023. ID: PID2022-142309OB-I00. Capacitas Research Group.

Institutional Review Board Statement: The study was conducted in accordance with the Declaration of Helsinki and approved by the Ethics Committee of the Catholic University of Valencia (protocol code CEI/UCV/111 2021; date 22 September 2022).

Informed Consent Statement: Informed consent was obtained from all subjects involved in the study.

Data Availability Statement: The original contributions presented in the study are included in the article, further inquiries can be directed to the corresponding authors.

Acknowledgments: The authors would like to thank as l'Alqueria-CAPACITAS early intervention professionals for their collaboration and participation in the study and data collection.

Conflicts of Interest: The authors declare no conflicts of interest.

Abbreviation

The following abbreviation is used in this manuscript:

EI Early Intervention

References

1. Xiong, C.; Biscardi, M.; Astell, A.; Nalder, E.; Cameron, J.I.; Mihailidis, A.; Colantonio, A. Sex and Gender Differences in Caregiving Burden Experienced by Family Caregivers of Persons with Dementia: A Systematic Review. *PLoS ONE* **2020**, *15*, e0231848. [CrossRef]
2. Zarit, S.H.; Todd, P.A.; Zarit, J.M. Subjective Burden of Husbands and Wives as Caregivers: A Longitudinal Study. *Gerontol* **1986**, *26*, 260–266. [CrossRef] [PubMed]
3. Badesha, M.; Thayanantha, A.; Shune, S.; Namasivayam-MacDonald, A. Caregiver Burden Interventions in Speech–Language Pathology: A Systematic Review. *Int. J. Lang. Commun. Disord.* **2023**, *58*, 1335–1356. [CrossRef] [PubMed]
4. García-Grau, P.; Martínez-Rico, G.; González-García, R.J.; Escorcia-Mora, C.T.; Cañadas-Pérez, M. Caregiver Burden and Family Quality of Life in Early Intervention: The Role of Mothers and Family Confidence. *Eur. J. Investig. Health Psychol. Educ.* **2024**, *14*, 1325–1337. [CrossRef]
5. Balbo, N.; Bolano, D. Child Disability as a Family Issue: A Study on Mothers' and Fathers' Health in Italy. *Eur. J. Public Health* **2024**, *34*, 79–84. [CrossRef]
6. Faden, S.Y.; Merdad, N.; Faden, Y.A. Parents of Children With Neurodevelopmental Disorders: A Mixed Methods Approach to Understanding Quality of Life, Stress, and Perceived Social Support. *Cureus* **2023**, *15*, e37356. [CrossRef] [PubMed]

7. Montorio Cerrato, I.; Fernández de Trocóniz, M.I.; López López, A.; Sánchez Colodrón, M. La Entrevista de Carga Del Cuidador. Utilidad y Validez Del Concepto de Carga. *An. Psicol.* **1998**, *14*, 229–248.
8. Evans, D.K.; Jakiela, P.; Knauer, H.A. The Impact of Early Childhood Interventions on Mothers. *Science* **2021**, *372*, 794–796. [CrossRef]
9. Dunst, C.J.; Raab, M.; Hamby, D.W. Interest-Based Everyday Child Language Learning. *Rev. Logop. Foniatr. Audiol.* **2016**, *36*, 153–161. [CrossRef]
10. Dunst, C.J. Family-Centered Practices: Birth Through High School. *J. Spec. Educ.* **2002**, *36*, 141–149. [CrossRef]
11. Dunst, C.J. Parents' Social Validity Appraisals of Early Childhood Intervention Practice Guides. *J. Educ. Dev. Psychol.* **2017**, *7*, 51–58. [CrossRef]
12. Bruder, M.B.; Dunst, C.; Maude, S.P.; Schnurr, M.; Van Polen, A.; Frolek Clark, G.; Winslow, A.; Gethmann, D. Practitioner Appraisals of Their Desired and Current Use of the 2014 Division for Early Childhood Recommended Practices. *J. Early Interv.* **2020**, *42*, 259–274. [CrossRef]
13. Montaño-Merchán, M.; Sanz-Ponce, R.; Padilla-Bautista, L.; Calero-Plaza, J. The Voice of Families: Perceptions of Family-Centred Practices and Natural Environments in Early Intervention in Spain. *Children* **2025**, *12*, 1068. [CrossRef] [PubMed]
14. Dunst, C.J.; Hamby, D.W.; Brookfield, J. Modeling the Effects of Early Childhood Intervention Variables on Parent and Family Well-Being. *J. Appl. Quant. Methods* **2007**, *2*, 268–288.
15. McWilliams, R. *Routines-Based Early Intervention: Supporting Young Children and Their Families*; Brookes Publishing Co: Baltimore, MD, USA, 2010.
16. Dunst, C.J.; Trivette, C.M.; Hamby, D.W. *Research Synthesis and Meta-Analysis of Studies of Family-Centered Practices*; Winterberry Press Monograph Series; ERIC; Winterberry Press: Morganton, NC, USA, 2008.
17. Dunst, C.J.; Trivette, C.M.; Hamby, D.W. Meta-analysis of Family-centered Helpgiving Practices Research. *Ment. Retard. Dev. Disabil. Res. Rev.* **2007**, *13*, 370–378. [CrossRef]
18. Dunst, C.J.; Trivette, C.M. Using Research Evidence to Inform and Evaluate Early Childhood Intervention Practices. *Top. Early Child. Spec. Educ.* **2009**, *29*, 40–52. [CrossRef]
19. Dunst, C.J.; Bruder, M.B.; Espe-Sherwindt, M. Family Capacity-Building in Early Childhood Intervention: Do Context and Setting Matter? *Sch. Community J.* **2014**, *24*, 37–48.
20. Swanson, J.; Raab, M.; Dunst, C.J. Strengthening Family Capacity to Provide Young Children Everyday Natural Learning Opportunities. *J. Early Child. Res.* **2011**, *9*, 66–80. [CrossRef]
21. Martínez-Rico, G.; García-Grau, P.; Cañadas-Pérez, M.; González-García, R.J. Does Family Confidence Bridge Child Functioning and Caregiver Burden in Early Intervention? *PLoS ONE* **2025**, *20*, e0321997. [CrossRef]
22. McWilliam, R.A.; García Grau, P. *Families in Early Intervention Quality of Life*; The University of Alabama: Tuscaloosa, AL, USA, 2017.
23. McWilliam, R.A. *Working with Families of Young Children with Special Needs*; Guilford Press: New York, NY, USA, 2010.
24. Bruder, M.B. Early Childhood Intervention: A Promise to Children and Families for Their Future. *Except. Child.* **2010**, *76*, 339–355. [CrossRef]
25. Espe-Sherwindt, M. Family-centred Practice: Collaboration, Competency and Evidence. *Support Learn.* **2008**, *23*, 136–143. [CrossRef]
26. Kurzrok, J.; McBride, E.; Grossman, R.B. Autism-Specific Parenting Self-Efficacy: An Examination of the Role of Parent-Reported Intervention Involvement, Satisfaction with Intervention-Related Training, and Caregiver Burden. *Autism* **2021**, *25*, 1395–1408. [CrossRef] [PubMed]
27. Ragin, C.C. *Redesigning Social Inquiry: Fuzzy Sets and Beyond*; University of Chicago Press: Chicago, IL, USA, 2009.
28. Schneider, C.Q.; Wagemann, C. *Set-Theoretic Methods for the Social Sciences: A Guide to Qualitative Comparative Analysis*; Cambridge University Press: Cambridge, UK, 2012.
29. García-Grau, P.; McWilliam, R.A.; Martínez-Rico, G.; Morales-Murillo, C.P. Rasch Analysis of the Families in Early Intervention Quality of Life (FEIQoL) Scale. *Appl. Res. Qual. Life* **2021**, *16*, 383–399. [CrossRef]
30. Zarit, S.H.; Reever, K.E.; Bach-Peterson, J. Relatives of the Impaired Elderly: Correlates of Feelings of Burden. *Gerontol* **1980**, *20*, 649–655. [CrossRef]
31. Pardo, X.M.; Cárdenas, S.J.; Cruz, A.V.; Venegas, J.M.; Magaña, I.M. Escala de Carga Del Cuidador de Zarit: Evidencia de Validez En México. *Psicooncología* **2014**, *11*, 71. [CrossRef]
32. Tartaglini, M.F.; Feldberg, C.; Hermida, P.D.; Heisecke, S.L.; Dillon, C.; Ofman, S.D.; Nuñez, M.L.; Somale, V. Escala de Sobrecarga Del Cuidador de Zarit: Análisis de Sus Propiedades Psicométricas En Cuidadores Familiares Residentes En Buenos Aires, Argentina. *Neurol. Argent.* **2020**, *12*, 27–35. [CrossRef]
33. García-Grau, P.; McWilliam, R.A.; Martínez-Rico, G.; Grau-Sevilla, M.D. Factor Structure and Internal Consistency of a Spanish Version of the Family Quality of Life (FaQoL). *Appl. Res. Qual. Life* **2018**, *13*, 385–398. [CrossRef]

34. Ballesteros, J.; Santos, B.; González-Fraile, E.; Muñoz-Hermoso, P.; Domínguez-Panchón, A.I.; Martín-Carrasco, M. Unidimensional 12-Item Zarit Caregiver Burden Interview for the Assessment of Dementia Caregivers' Burden Obtained by Item Response Theory. *Value Health* **2012**, *15*, 1141–1147. [CrossRef]
35. Higginson, I.J.; Gao, W.; Jackson, D.; Murray, J.; Harding, R. Short-Form Zarit Caregiver Burden Interviews Were Valid in Advanced Conditions. *J. Clin. Epidemiol.* **2010**, *63*, 535–542. [CrossRef] [PubMed]
36. *Multivariate Data Analysis: A Global Perspective*, 7th global ed.; Hair, J.F., Ed.; Pearson: Upper Saddle River, NJ, USA, 2010; ISBN 978-0-13-515309-3.
37. Woodside, A.G. Moving beyond Multiple Regression Analysis to Algorithms: Calling for Adoption of a Paradigm Shift from Symmetric to Asymmetric Thinking in Data Analysis and Crafting Theory. *J. Bus. Res.* **2013**, *66*, 463–472. [CrossRef]
38. Rasoolimanesh, S.M.; Ringle, C.M.; Sarstedt, M.; Olya, H. The Combined Use of Symmetric and Asymmetric Approaches: Partial Least Squares-Structural Equation Modeling and Fuzzy-Set Qualitative Comparative Analysis. *Int. J. Contemp. Hosp. Manag.* **2021**, *33*, 1571–1592. [CrossRef]
39. Rihoux, B.; Ragin, C.C. *Configurational Comparative Methods: Qualitative Comparative Analysis (QCA) and Related Techniques*; SAGE: Thousand Oaks, CA, USA, 2009; ISBN 978-1-4129-4235-5.
40. Fiss, P.C. Building Better Causal Theories: A Fuzzy Set Approach to Typologies in Organization Research. *Acad. Manag. J.* **2011**, *54*, 393–420. [CrossRef]
41. Lin, C.-Y.; Chang, S.-H.; Lin, C.-M.; Chang, Y.-Y. High-Burden and Self-Efficacy Are Associated with Quality of Life in Family Caregivers in Taiwan: A Cross-Sectional Study. *Sage Open Aging* **2025**, *11*, 30495334251365602. [CrossRef] [PubMed]
42. Dunst, C.J.; Trivette, C.M.; Raab, M. An Implementation Science Framework for Conceptualizing and Operationalizing Fidelity in Early Childhood Intervention Studies. *J. Early Interv.* **2013**, *35*, 85–101. [CrossRef]
43. MacKenzie, K.T.; Eack, S.M. Interventions to Improve Outcomes for Parents of Children with Autism Spectrum Disorder: A Meta-Analysis. *J. Autism Dev. Disord.* **2022**, *52*, 2859–2883. [CrossRef]
44. Muthukaruppan, S.S.; Cameron, C.; Campbell, Z.; Krishna, D.; Moineddin, R.; Bharathwaj, A.; Poomariappan, B.M.; Mariappan, S.; Boychuk, N.; Ponnusamy, R.; et al. Impact of a Family-Centred Early Intervention Programme in South India on Caregivers of Children with Developmental Delays. *Disabil. Rehabil.* **2022**, *44*, 2410–2419. [CrossRef] [PubMed]
45. Picardi, A.; Gigantesco, A.; Tarolla, E.; Stoppioni, V.; Cerbo, R.; Cremonte, M.; Alessandri, G.; Lega, I.; Nardocci, F. Parental Burden and Its Correlates in Families of Children with Autism Spectrum Disorder: A Multicentre Study with Two Comparison Groups. *Clin. Pract. Epidemiol. Ment. Health CP EMH* **2018**, *14*, 143. [CrossRef]
46. Whitehead, K.; Dorstyn, D.; Ward, L. Psychological Adjustment in Families Affected by Autism Spectrum Disorder. *J. Dev. Phys. Disabil.* **2015**, *27*, 703–717. [CrossRef]
47. McWilliam, R.A. The Routines-Based Model for Supporting Speech and Language. *Rev. Logop. Foniatría Audiol.* **2016**, *36*, 178–184. [CrossRef]
48. Ryan, A.K.; Miller, L.; Rose, T.A.; Johnston, L.M. Optimal Child-Led Goal Setting Practices for School-Aged Children with a Disability or Delay: An International Delphi Consensus Study. *Disabil. Rehabil.* **2025**, *47*, 3173–3181. [CrossRef]

healthcare

MDPI

Article

The Questions, Challenges, and Possibilities When Joining Critical Disabilities Studies and Healthcare Research

Madelyn Toman *, Meredith Atanasio and Pamela B. Teaster

Department of Human Development and Family Science, Virginia Polytechnic Institute and State University, Blacksburg, VA 24060, USA; matanasio@vt.edu (M.A.); pteaster@vt.edu (P.B.T.)
* Correspondence: maddie99@vt.edu

Abstract

Background/Objectives: Interdisciplinary research teams that include critical disability studies (CDS) scholars and Healthcare and Medical Researchers have the potential to investigate complex lived experiences and explore new opportunities to best serve disabled communities. However, individuals in these fields typically approach disability research in different ways. Throughout this manuscript, we refer to a hypothetical interdisciplinary research team as an example of how to integrate the questions, challenges, and possibilities into practice when joining CDS and Healthcare and Medical Research. **Discussion:** First, we raise three large and complex questions that researchers must address (and discuss) when conducting disability research: (a) what is (a) disability, (b) what does it mean to live with a disability, and (c) who is included in research samples/as research participants for disability research? Then, we discuss the colliding and harmful relationship history between CDS and Healthcare and Medical Research fields, and the continued oppositional training of professionals in both fields. Finally, we offer insights into how collaborative efforts and methods of interdisciplinary research teams can optimize success when tackling complex research questions to serve disabled communities. **Conclusions:** We suggest approaches for projects at the intersection of CDS and Healthcare and Medical Research: holistic, person-centered research, treating individuals in the disability community as experts, and collaborating with the community while conducting research. This manuscript serves as a starting point for researcher teams looking to conduct ethical, rigorous, and trustworthy research at the intersection of health, medicine, and disability.

Keywords: critical disability studies; healthcare and medical research; interdisciplinary research

1. Introduction

Interdisciplinary research is a popular approach to social science research [1,2]. When members of research teams have different disciplinary backgrounds and approaches, they can tackle complex, unexplored, or underexplored questions. Although interdisciplinary work can be exciting and is often desirable for academics, providers, funders, and policy makers, it is not necessarily easy or successful.

Challenges can arise when researchers attempt to bring together fields of research that do not naturally mix well. One example is the research fields of critical disability studies (CDS) and Healthcare and Medical Research—even though researchers in these fields serve the same population and ask similar questions, their approaches to research and knowledge come from different points of view (and are even at odds).

Throughout this article, we ask readers to reflect on the following research team scenario:

A team of four researchers have come together to investigate the symptoms, characteristics, and support needed for individuals with Down Syndrome who are diagnosed with early onset Alzheimer's disease (EOAD). Two of the team members are trained in CDS, one member is an MD/PhD specializing in research on neurodegenerative disorders, and the fourth team member is a physician.

Below we discuss the types of questions and challenges a research team such as this must address before designing a study as well as possibilities and opportunities that can be achieved when bringing together individuals with multiple points of view and expertise. The purpose of this manuscript is to offer suggestions for beginning a conversation between researchers, to provide examples of where clashes and tensions lay between CDS and Healthcare and Medical Research and offer concrete collaborative solutions for research teams.

2. Brief Overview of CDS and Healthcare and Medical Research

Combining the fields of CDS and Healthcare and Medical Research brings together contrasting "camps" or research fields, including laboratory, clinical, and epidemiological research and interventions. Healthcare and Medical Researchers often utilize physiological, behavioral, and participant self-report assessments, and engage in longitudinal methods to measure change in health status or disease trajectory over time [3]. The ultimate goal of medical research is to understand the general experience and trajectory of the patient and subsequently develop, test, and determine courses of care (e.g., pharmaceutical, physiological, psychological, etc.) to improve short- and long-term health outcomes [4]. In short, medical research has historically involved identifying clinical signs within a group of people and developing solutions to improve quality of life. However, newer approaches in medical research may make collaboration with CDS researchers more feasible, such as an emerging emphasis on patient health literacy that promotes patient agency and incorporates them into decision-making processes in both medical practice and clinical research [5].

The field of CDS is guided by Critical Disabilities Theory, as well as other critical perspectives such as feminist, crip, and queer theories [6–8]. CDS moves beyond relying on models that place disability within or outside of the individual, instead using a human rights approach that argues for equal access to all aspects of social life [9,10]. The "critical" in CDS translates to challenging structures, policies, and social norms that have worked in the past and that continue to oppress present and future generations of individuals with disabilities.

3. Questions

Based on the research team scenario described above, consider the primary conversations between the four scholars who are well-versed and trained in their respective fields. Although they may have similar motivations, research questions of interest, and overlapping general interests, the team members are likely to have vastly different approaches to research and service for disabled communities. In this section, we explore how these two "camps" of research respond to seemingly simple questions, yet in ways that are incongruent.

3.1. What Is (A) Disability?

As emphasized by influential disability rights activist Judy Heumann, disability is a normal part of life and a key aspect of the human experience [11]. Organizations in the

United States, such as the Centers for Disease Control, typically base their broad definitions of disability on that of the World Health Organization, which states:

> *Disability is part of being human. An estimated 1.3 billion people—about 16% of the global population—currently experience significant disability. This number is increasing in part due to population ageing and an increase in the prevalence of noncommunicable diseases. Disability results from the interaction between individuals with a health condition, such as cerebral palsy, Down syndrome and depression, with personal and environmental factors including negative attitudes, inaccessible transportation and public buildings, and limited social support.* [12]

Definitions of disability, like the one above, are typically broad and are highly subjective, reasons why individuals writing, teaching, and researching the topic of disability often rely on models of disability. Depending on the model used, the term disability can hold different meanings. Models of disability offer different ways to conceptualize disabilities, each model with its own strengths and weaknesses. While recognizing that CDS scholars intentionally look beyond only using models of disability to conceptualize and advocate for disability rights and research, the models offer a starting point for a conversation about the meaning of disability.

Models of Disability

The medical model of disability has the longest history and has two key components: pathology must be present, and pathologies are located within individuals [13] (Figure 1). This model reflects an understanding of disabilities as illnesses or diseases that individuals must overcome. With the goal to eradicate symptoms or traits of a disability, the medical model seeks to cure and 'normalize' individuals with disabilities [14]. This model has been useful in diagnosing and providing practical care for different types of disabilities, although there are clear weaknesses and shortcomings. For instance, pathologizing disability stigmatizes disabled communities and prioritizes the disability itself (or, more specifically, the diagnosis) over the individual. Furthermore, not all people with disabilities require care or desire cures.

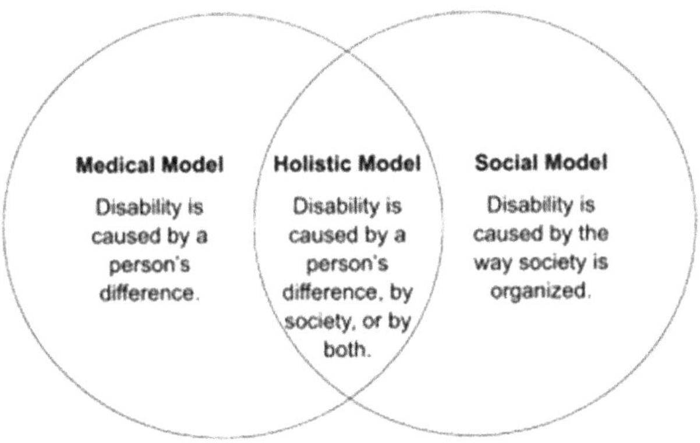

Figure 1. Model of Disability.

In 1970s, disabled communities began questioning and rejecting the medical model, thus, the social model of disability was developed as an alternative way to conceptualize disability [15]. The social model identifies a marked difference between impairment and disability. Individuals have/are diagnosed with impairments, and disability occurs when social practices and structural environments create barriers and disadvantage individuals with impairments [16,17]. Consequently, society plays a significant role in creating disability through stratification, determining hierarchies, and constructing societal norms [18]. While the social model of disabilities has been a useful tool for social-political movements and gaining civil rights for disabled populations, challenges or weaknesses to this conceptualization of disability exist [17,19]. For example, the social model of disabilities minimizes the embodiment of disability and overestimates the ability of societies to remove all barriers to individuals.

The medical model and the social model of disabilities have been the most prominent approaches that researchers, practitioners, activist groups, and politicians have used to conceptualize disability [20]. There are, however, alternative models of disability, such as the holistic model, economic model, charity model, and the social identity/cultural affiliation model [20,21]. Each offers different definitions of disability and informs policy, perceptions of needs, and disability identity. For the purposes of this manuscript, we describe the two most pertinent to the disability research field while acknowledging and highlighting the complexity that comes with conceptualizing what (a) disability is.

Conceptualizations of disability can use one particular model or a combination of models based on the researchers' interpretations and personal alignments. Although it is not necessary that all research team members (and researchers broadly) have the same conceptualization of disability, it is the responsibility of individuals conducting research at the intersection of CDS and Healthcare and Medical fields to be transparent and thorough in their descriptions of what disability means to them and in the context of their work.

It is also important to note that CDS scholars go beyond the models of disability when conceptualizing disability. In CDS research, disability is analyzed as a "cultural, historical, relative, social, and political phenomenon" [8]. Research centering disability in CDS highlights narratives of disabled communities and interprets lived experiences of disabled people to deconstruct and challenge binary assumptions of normality vs. abnormality. In doing so, CDS approaches disability through a social justice, person-centered framework.

3.2. What Does It Mean to Live with a Disability?

Once individuals identify with and/or are diagnosed with a disability, different types of support and services can be accessed. Not all disabilities are the same—there are many marked differences between an individual's disabilities (e.g., characteristics, symptomatology, presentation, outcomes). People with the same disabilities may have completely contrasting embodiments and experiences. Medical perceptions of disabilities do not necessarily align with ways that disabled communities view them [22].

An understanding of what it can mean to live with a disability is only possible when people with disabilities are sharing their understandings, stories, and perspectives with researchers, medical providers, policymakers, and others with the power to present disabled narratives. Thus, to truly understand what it means to live with a disability, critical qualitative methodologies, like narrative analysis, community participatory analysis, and phenomenology, should be used by research teams as opportunities to shift from clinical understanding of disability to experiential, contextual understandings of disability.

Individualization in lived experience with disabilities challenges medical discourse around "expectations" and "limitations" frequently explained when receiving diagnoses. Too often, medical professionals provide diagnoses and life expectations as warnings or limited expectations compared to others without those diagnoses. Examples of these types of conversations can be found in the narratives of adults with lifelong disabilities and families [23,24]. This is not to say that medical professionals should not offer knowledge and information about characteristics of diagnoses and a life with specific types of disabilities; however, all information provided to individuals (and families) about what living with a disability could mean upon diagnosis should be based on experiences of people who have similar diagnoses rather than perceptions made by able-bodied people.

3.3. Who Is Included in Research Samples/as Research Participants for Disability Research?

Who is included as research participants should depend on the research question(s) and outcome(s) being sought. These considerations have not always been the case. Disability research has been historically dominated by non-disabled voices, including those of medical providers, caretakers, and family members [25]. Research fields risk misrepresentation when they do not include the voices and experiences of the population they serve.

To combat the issue of misrepresentation in research, the popular disability social rights mantra, "Nothing About Us Without Us," should be extended to researchers intending to serve disabled communities. Disabled communities have expressed the need for inclusive research on disabilities where people with disabilities are more than just participants—they should also serve as consultants, experts, and partners during the research study [25]. Including disabled participants in disability health research allows medical providers and researchers the opportunity to work in partnership with disabled communities and enables the capability to meet their actual needs as opposed to their perceived needs by others [26]. Only by including participants with disabilities in disability research will it be possible to better understand the complexities, barriers, and lives of people with disabilities.

4. Challenges

After considering a few fundamental questions and working to consider both points of view, it is also necessary to understand the historical context and current challenges that face researchers aspiring to contribute meaningfully to intersectional work between CDS and healthcare. The history between the medical field and disabled communities has deep-rooted ableist scars and themes of dismissal and misrepresentation that go well beyond the brief description below [27,28]. Nonetheless, we offer specific instances of historical collision and difference in training between medical professionals and disabled communities in order to advance a conversation or explanation of why it is both difficult yet possible for these groups to meet in the middle, or compromise, when coming together in research arenas.

4.1. Relationship History

Historically, diagnoses and disabilities have been used against individuals with disabilities in the United States to justify discriminating, segregating, rejecting, and oppressing entire disabled populations [29]. Policies, statutes, and laws in the United States have conspired to strip people with disabilities of their civil and human rights. For example, the verdict from Buck vs. Bell [30] permitted involuntary sterilization of individuals deemed to be "feebleminded" and Ugly Laws in cities across the United States prohibited people with disabilities from appearing in public spaces [31].

Practices put forth by medical professionals (and political desires), such as eugenics and forced sterilization, have dehumanized disabled populations globally. Eugenic ideals and policies, practiced at a national and international level, have targeted disabled communities directly due to the general goal to reduce and eliminate "undesirable" traits for future generations [32,33]. Purposefully and unwittingly, medical and health professionals contributed to the discriminatory, ableist eugenics movement by "furnishing notions of health, diagnosing individuals with defects, and recommending and performing the sexual sterilizations" [33] (p. 3). Newer scientific advancements that serve medical fields, such as genetic testing [34], continue to promote similar ableist thinking. For instance, prenatal screening and genetic testing can be helpful when trying to know and understand more about the fetus; however, they become problematic and ableist in nature when used to identify and eliminate fetuses with disabilities.

The messy and frequently harmful relationship between medical fields and disabled communities is a significant contributor to the deep mistrust between individuals with disabilities and medical researchers [35]. Therefore, it is necessary to increase trustworthiness between researchers and the disabled community in order to conduct meaningful future research about disability [22]. CDS researchers have a particular advantage over medical researchers when recruiting and encouraging individuals with disabilities to participate in research because CDS focuses on empowering the community and challenges structural and historic ableism. Together, interdisciplinary research teams that include CDS scholars can promote trustworthiness in relationships between disabled communities and medical researchers [36,37] and, ultimately, in findings from research.

4.2. Opposing Trainings

A key difference between CDS scholars and Healthcare and Medical Research scholars lies in their training. Individuals conducting research in Healthcare and Medical Research fields are instructed to diagnose and treat diagnoses. CDS researchers are trained to challenge systemic ableism and empower individuals with disabilities. In short, medical researchers take a medical approach to disability while CDS scholars take a human rights approach to disability.

Consider how the two medical members of our interdisciplinary team might approach research on individuals with Down syndrome diagnosed with early onset Alzheimer's disease (EOAD). The medical professionals may be inclined to center their inquiry on an understanding of the pathological differences of this population, compared to those with EOAD who do not have comorbid Down syndrome, complications of differential diagnoses in the target population, and clinical trials, as has been the case in established medical research on the same populations [38]. Our two CDS researchers may voice concern that this approach is far too focused on diagnostics and take issue with the inherent 'othering' of the target population based on what they have predetermined to be 'typical.'

Another difference between these fields can be found in the communication of science and new knowledge, as variations exist in ways that each research field articulates research, largely dependent upon who is accessing information in scientific publications [39]. When discussing findings and implications, Healthcare and Medical Research articles are often filled with complex language and jargon. In contrast, CDS research articles typically use accessible language intentionally understandable by the populations they serve. Differences in accessibility and language can create challenges when disseminating research findings to high-impact journals and directly to disabled communities. While arguments can be made for both styles of academic reporting, products of research studies from these two fields are inherently different, and as a result, reach different audiences.

Due to continued differences in points of view and education, it is challenging for the fields of CDS and Healthcare and Medical Research to work together. Cooperation is not always possible. Individuals conducting intersectional research should not have to compromise their core beliefs and epistemologies when designing studies and describing outcomes. However, incorporating multiple points of view and acknowledging differences in approaches to research on disability can propel negotiation towards what possible research projects can be produced by intersectional teams.

5. Possibilities

Bringing together contrasting fields or research can be challenging but also rewarding. Combining the fields of CDS and Healthcare and Medical Research creates the opportunity to generate new knowledge and deeper understanding of the complexity of human disability experiences. Bringing together various disciplines for rich, meaningful research does not require reinventing the wheel—frameworks for integrating interdisciplinary research teams already exist, including the Integrated Model of the Interdisciplinary Research Process (IRP; [40]). This approach emphasizes that the different parties trying to collaborate should clearly lay out their respective approaches, including supporting literature and theoretical perspectives. Then, the researchers can work together to recognize the value in other insights, identify and resolve conflicts, integrate ideas, and ensure that participants have a clear understanding of the research plan and goals. Considering the research team scenario and the challenges they may face in collaboration, we propose several possibilities to promote such collaborative communication and concordance.

5.1. Holistic, Person-Centered Research

From a research perspective, the person-centered approach (PCA) identifies the individual as an expert of their own experiences and characteristics, where the individual is self-directing, self-maintaining, and seeking to further understand and enhance their perception of self [41]. Integral to the original conceptualization of PCA is that, even though a particular experience might be the topic of interest for any given research project, each individual is a complex being whose experiences inform the target experience [42,43]. Essentially, as an expert on themselves, an individual can provide unparalleled insights into a particular experience and provide feedback on what research topics/methods might be most relevant and inform researchers on the intersectional nature of their life experiences.

In the context of uniting the medical model and a CDS approach to disability research, using a PCA fosters an important collaborative methodology. CDS place significant emphasis on equal accessibility for everyone [9] and inherently acknowledges the intersectional experiences of each person. Consequently, the individual is just as essential as the larger group in informing and facilitating the goal of CDS research, which is to promote widespread, universal accessibility. Medical researchers can also draw upon the intersectional experiences of individuals with and without disabilities to inform research on their health and wellness. By centering the individual in the research, medical researchers are afforded the opportunity to understand unique medical needs, promote individual agency, and shape medical practices and advances, rather than project medical advances onto the larger group.

5.2. Inclusive Participation and Co-Production

Developing and employing unique research approaches and practices can help bridge the gap between the two CDS-trained researchers and the two physicians in the scenario and guide a more effective and holistic research approach. Action research emphasizes the agency of the individual as an active participant in research processes to facilitate improvements to their daily lives and experiences [44]. In particular, Kemmis et al. (2013) [44] identify that a defining characteristic of Critical Participatory Action Research (CPAR) research is the following:

> *Participants in social and educational life can do research for themselves. Others may also research social and educational life, but participants have special access to how social and educational life and work are conducted in local sites by virtue of being 'insiders' [p.5].*

Essentially, CPAR encourages the individual to define and lead research based on their own experiences, with academic researchers supporting them, following their cues, and recording processes and outcomes. Our research team might consider a qualitative study by Scott et al., (2014) [45], where researchers met with young adults with Down syndrome for both one-on-one and group interviews. One of the primary goals of their study was to understand participants' perspectives on different facilitators of and barriers to their general well-being. Through these interviews, researchers realized the need to align research of medical advancements meant to increase the lifespan of those with Down syndrome with an investment in understanding and facilitating quality of life based on direct feedback from participants [45]. Individuals within populations of interest are ready and willing to engage in research and to work with researchers to generate meaningful, relevant ideas regarding social autonomy and rights as well as clinical needs and experiences, serving as a point of reference to inform collaborative research between our CDS and medical researcher team.

The research team might also consider engaging more formal community stakeholders as a mechanism to inform the direction of the research and identify needs. A particularly pertinent example of this type of positive community stakeholder can be found in the presence of networks of community health workers (CHWs) and the populations they serve. CHWs are members of the community whose primary roles are to facilitate the accessibility of medical education and information to surrounding communities and serve as a mediator between the community and larger systems [46]. While CHWs are often trained in collaboration with various medical systems, CHW roles are often intentionally and inherently interdisciplinary in their training and purpose [47].

It is already documented that CHWs report engaging in community advocacy by communicating community needs and asking for assistance to meet those needs directly (e.g., in-person conversation, letters, etc.) to elected officials, healthcare systems, and social services [48], even though this may be outside of their scope of duty. As such, many CHWs are familiar with the experiences and needs of the community they serve and how to communicate those experiences and needs to other individuals and organizations. Inclusion of CHWs in disability research may also offer unique benefits to the success of research.

CHWs are often embedded and respected members of the community that they serve [49] and often engage with underserved communities, many previously harmed by or have reason to be wary of the medical system or research [46]. Because of their experience as bridges connecting communities and individuals to other resources in the context of public health, incorporating CHWs has the potential to facilitate a more positive relationship between individuals, the researchers, and the wider community, boosting participation and feedback and ultimately adding important perspectives for interdisciplinary research teams [50]. CHW's engagement in advocacy, commitment to disseminating information and resources to entire communities, and emphasis on social determinants of health [47] is well-aligned with the values of CDS researchers. CHWs, especially those serving in clinical roles, could be mobilized as collaborators in research to act as a liaison between disabled communities and researcher thus bridging gaps in CDS and medical model research.

5.3. Actionable Guidance for Collaboration in Practice

Communication will be key throughout collaborations and projects, but establishing expectations at the beginning is crucial to a successful and equitable experience for researchers and community members. Research teams might draw from collaborative frameworks such as the aforementioned IRP, or from current standards of collaborative research outlined by a bodies like the American Psychological Association [51]. Depending on the project, communication at the outset of the project should involve:

1. A mutual agreement on and understanding of the study goals and what the motivation of the research is.
2. What the desired outcome(s) of the research is.

3. Identifying differing points of view and ideas and working to resolve them through compromise.
4. Clearly stating the role each person will play (e.g., primary investigator, community liaison, data manager, etc.) and clearly outlining responsibilities.
5. Determining logistics of data collection: who will be recruited, how will they be recruited, what measures will be used, where will data be stored and managed, etc. Also, another thing to consider is who will primarily be in contact with participants: the researchers or the community experts?

These discussions should be kept in writing or recorded, and diseminated to all parties after each meeting. Record-keeping in this way can also serve to track how the project has evolved over time and hold all parties responsible for their contribitions. Teams should have regular check-ins over the course of the project, as research projects often evolve over time. Record-keeping in both in writing and auditory format is a good example of accessibility in the research process—using multiple formats and strategies to increase accessibility to all team members. Research teams should work to identify the needs of all members to ensure an experience that is accessible to all team members. This may include different ways of communication (written form, recording for revisiting later, real-time employment of an American Sign Language (ASL) translator, etc.) or different modes of attending research meetings or engaging in active data collection (transportation services for in-person meetings, options for joining via Zoom, etc.).

Individuals with disabilities, disabled communities, and community stakeholders should be considered experts and team members, not just consultants. This is particularly important in disability research collaboration, where participants and collaborators have historically been exploited and researchers have taken all credit. As such, the following should be established from the outset of a collaboration:

1. Regarding input from non-academic collaborators as equally valuable and actionable.
2. Formal credit for their contributions, including in project proposals, grant applications, and on publications and presentations.
3. Compensation as appropriate—for example, in the case of funded research, all collaborators should be compensated for their time and effort, not just the academic and/or medical researchers.
4. Ownership of the works—often times, the 'ownership' of research and data belongs to the funding body or the larger institution of the primary researchers. While this may be difficult to navigate, every effort should be made to ensure non-academic collaborators maintain access and rights to the data and research.

There are many other parts of the collaborative research process, and the afforementioned strategies are not exhaustive. However, communication is the bedrock of successful, accessible, and ethical collaborative research.

6. Conclusions

If the shared goal of any research team is to best serve the wants, needs, and interests of the population on which the research is focused, then an interdisciplinary research team can contribute enhanced depth to their fields by working together to create new knowledge. Using the hypothetical framework of a mixed research team as discussed above, different philosophical, methodological, and conceptual questions and ways of thinking can be addressed when bringing together contrasting research fields such as CDS and Healthcare and Medical Research. Future researchers who seek to join CDS and health fields should utilize creative research methods and intentionally include disabled partners and participants in every aspect of the research project. Engaging in participant- and community-centered research that supports the voices and experiences of disabled communities will increase rigor in research findings and trustworthiness in the partnership between researchers and disabled populations. Spending time in the gray/messy areas may be uncomfortable or difficult, but those are the precise areas where having multiple points of view and types of training will best serve the individuals and outcomes of research. Thinking critically and being transparent and descriptive throughout the research process enables opportunities to best serve disabled communities through research.

Author Contributions: Conceptualization, M.T.; Writing—original draft, M.T. and M.A.; Writing—review & editing, M.T., M.A. and P.B.T. All authors have read and agreed to the published version of the manuscript.

Funding: This research received no external funding.

Institutional Review Board Statement: Not applicable.

Informed Consent Statement: Not applicable.

Data Availability Statement: The original contributions presented in this study are included in the article. Further inquiries can be directed at the corresponding author.

Conflicts of Interest: The authors declare no conflicts of interest.

Abbreviations

The following abbreviations are used in this manuscript:

CDS	Critical Disability Studies
EOAD	Early Onset Alzheimer's Disease
PCA	Person-Centered Approach
CPAR	Critical Participatory Action Research
CHW	Community Health Workers

References

1. Guerreiro, J.A. Interdisciplinary Research in Social Sciences: A two way process. In Proceedings of the International Congress on Interdisciplinarity in Social and Human Sciences, Faro, Portugal, 5–6 May 2016; pp. 209–213.
2. Klein, J.T. Interdisciplinary approaches in social science research. In *The SAGE Handbook of Social Science Methodology*; SAGE Publications: Los Angeles, CA, USA, 2007; pp. 32–50.
3. Kiani, A.K.; Naureen, Z.; Pheby, D.; Henehan, G.; Brown, R.; Sieving, P.; Sykora, P.; Marks, R.; Falsini, B.; Capodicasa, N.; et al. Methodology for clinical research. *J. Prev. Med. Hyg.* **2022**, *63*, E267–E278. [CrossRef]
4. Sacristan, J.A. Clinical research and medical care: Towards effective and complete integration. *BMC Med. Res. Methodol.* **2015**, *15*, 4. [CrossRef] [PubMed]
5. Bader, M.; Zheng, L.; Rao, D.; Shiyanbola, O.; Myers, L.; Davis, T.; O'Leary, C.; McKee, M.; Wolf, M.; Assaf, A.R. Towards a more patient-centered clinical trial process: A systematic review of interventions incorporating health literacy best practices. *Contemp. Clin. Trials* **2022**, *116*, 106733. [CrossRef] [PubMed]
6. Devlin, R.F.; Pothier, D. (Eds.) *Critical Disability Theory: Essays in Philosophy, Politics, Policy, and Law*; UBC Press: Vancouver, BC, Canada, 2006.
7. Goodley, D. *Disability Studies: An Interdisciplinary Introduction*; SAGE Publications: Los Angeles, CA, USA, 2016.
8. Hall, M.C. Critical Disability Theory. 2019. Available online: https://plato.stanford.edu/ENTRIES/disability-critical/ (accessed on 1 September 2025).
9. Gillies, J. Critical disability theory. In *Encyclopedia of Quality of Life and Well-Being Research*; Springer International Publishing: Cham, Switzerland, 2024; pp. 1495–1497.
10. Goodley, D.; Lawthom, R.; Liddiard, K.; Runswick-Cole, K. Provocations for critical disability studies. *Disabil. Soc.* **2019**, *34*, 972–997. [CrossRef]
11. Jackson, M.; Volion, A. *The Impact of Judy Heumann's Legacy Within the Disability Community*; Rewriting the Narrative; Women Enabled International: Washington, WA, USA, 2023; Available online: https://medium.com/rewriting-the-narrative/the-impact-of-judy-heumanns-legacy-within-the-disability-community-8be0e6a67fa4 (accessed on 1 September 2025).

12. Centers for Disease Control (CDC). *Disability and Health*; Centers for Disease Control (CDC): Atlanta, Georgia, 2025. Available online: https://www.cdc.gov/disability-and-health/index.html (accessed on 1 September 2025).
13. Smart, J. Models of disability: The juxtaposition of biology and social construction. In *Handbook of Rehabilitation Counseling*; Springer Publishing Company: Princeton, NJ, USA, 2004; pp. 25–49.
14. Zaks, Z. Changing the medical model of disability to the normalization model of disability: Clarifying the past to create a new future direction. *Disabil. Soc.* **2024**, *39*, 3233–3260. [CrossRef]
15. Oliver, M. The social model of disability: Thirty years on. *Disabil. Soc.* **2013**, *28*, 1024–1026. [CrossRef]
16. Mercer, G.; Shakespeare, T. *Exploring Disability: A Sociological Introduction*; Polity: Cambridge, UK, 1999.
17. Shakespeare, T. Chapter 13: The social model of disability. In *The Disability Studies Reader*, 5th ed.; Davis, L.J., Ed.; Routledge, Taylor & Francis Group: Oxford, UK, 2016; pp. 195–203.
18. Shifrer, D.; Frederick, A. Disability at the intersections. *Sociol. Compass* **2019**, *13*, e12733. [CrossRef]
19. Owens, J. Exploring the critiques of the social model of disability: The transformative possibility of Arendt's notion of power. *Sociol. Health Illn.* **2015**, *37*, 385–403. [CrossRef]
20. Retief, M.; Letšosa, R. Models of disability: A brief overview. *HTS Teol. Stud./Theol. Stud.* **2018**, *74*, a4738. [CrossRef]
21. Twardowshi, A. Controversies around the social model of disability. *Kult.-Społeczeństwo-Eduk.* **2019**, *2*, 7–21. Available online: https://www.ceeol.com/search/article-detail?id=880842 (accessed on 1 September 2025).
22. Aguirre, A.; Lee, S.S.J.; Callier, S.; Spicer, P.; Sabatello, M. Towards trustworthiness of precision medicine research for people with disabilities. *Nat. Genet.* **2025**, *57*, 1321–1324. [CrossRef] [PubMed]
23. Tannila, A.; JÄrvelin, M.R.; Kokkonen, J. Parental guidance and counselling by doctors and nursing staff: Parents' views of initial information and advice for families with disabled children. *J. Clin. Nurs.* **1998**, *7*, 505–511. [CrossRef] [PubMed]
24. Toman, M.; Wesche, R.; Shivers, C.M. Narratives of personal health and sexual education experiences of emerging adults with disabilities. *Sex. Disabil.* **2024**, *42*, 851–880. [CrossRef]
25. Kitchin, R. The researched opinions on research: Disabled people and disability research. *Disabil. Soc.* **2000**, *15*, 25–47. [CrossRef]
26. Hogan, A.; Jain, N.R.; Peiris-John, R.; Ameratunga, S. Disabled people say 'Nothing about us without us'. *Clin. Teach.* **2020**, *17*, 70–75. [CrossRef]
27. Lindsay, S.; Fuentes, K.; Ragunathan, S.; Lamaj, L.; Dyson, J. Ableism within health care professions: A systematic review of the experiences and impact of discrimination against health care providers with disabilities. *Disabil. Rehabil.* **2023**, *45*, 2715–2731. [CrossRef]
28. Longmore, P.K. Medical decision making and people with disabilities: A clash of cultures. *J. Law Med. Ethics* **1995**, *23*, 82–87. [CrossRef]
29. Bayton, D.C. Chapter 2: Disability and the justification of inequality in American history. In *The Disability Studies Reader*, 5th ed.; Davis, L.J., Ed.; Routledge, Taylor & Francis Group: Oxford, UK, 2016; pp. 33–57.
30. U.S. Supreme Court. *Buck vs. Bell 274. US, 200*; U.S. Supreme Court: Washington, WA, USA, 1927.
31. Schweik, S.M. *The Ugly Laws: Disability in Public*; New York University Press: New York, NY, USA, 2009.
32. Wilson, R.A. Eugenics, disability, and bioethics. In *The Disability Bioethics Reader*; Routledge: Oxfordshire, UK, 2022; pp. 21–29.
33. Wilson, R.A. Eugenic thinking in medicine, healthcare, and bioethics. In *Handbook of the Philosophy of Medicine*; Springer: Dordrecht, The Netherlands, 2025; pp. 1–14.
34. Berube, M. Disability, democracy, and the new genetics. In *The Disability Studies Reader*; Routledge: Oxfordshire, UK, 2013; pp. 105–118.
35. Smirnoff, M.; Wilets, I.; Ragin, D.F.; Adams, R.; Holohan, J.; Rhodes, R.; Winkel, G.; Ricci, E.M.; Clesca, C.; Richardson, L.D. A paradigm for understanding trust and mistrust in medical research: The community VOICES study. *AJOB Empir. Bioeth.* **2018**, *9*, 39–47. [CrossRef]
36. Kraft, S.A.; Cho, M.K.; Gillespie, K.; Halley, M.; Varsava, N.; Ormond, K.E.; Luft, H.S.; Wilfond, B.S.; Lee, S.S.J. Beyond consent: Building trusting relationships with diverse populations in precision medicine research. *Am. J. Bioeth.* **2018**, *18*, 3–20. [CrossRef]
37. Wilkins, C.H. Effective engagement requires trust and being trustworthy. *Med. Care* **2018**, *56*, S6–S8. [CrossRef]
38. Hartley, D.; Blumenthal, T.; Carrillo, M.; DiPaolo, G.; Esralew, L.; Gardiner, K.; Granholm, A.-C.; Iqbal, K.; Krams, M.; Lemere, C.; et al. Down syndrome and Alzheimer's disease: Common pathways, common goals. *Alzheimer's Dement.* **2015**, *11*, 700–709. [CrossRef]
39. Devolder, B. *The Faces of Disability and Disability Health Research*; Disabilities Health Research Network (DHRN): Kelowna, BC, Canada, 2010; Available online: https://www.dhrn.ca/files/DHRN%20PrimerBook-Final.pdf (accessed on 1 September 2025).
40. Repko, A.F.; Szostak, R. *Interdisciplinary Research: Process and Theory*; SAGE Publications: Los Angeles, CA, USA, 2020.
41. Lux, M.; Motschnig-Pitrik, R.; Cornelius-White, J. The essence of the person-centered approach. In *Interdisciplinary Handbook of the Person-Centered Approach: Research and Theory*; Springer: New York, NY, USA, 2013; pp. 9–21.
42. Rogers, C.R. *Client-Centered Therapy*; original work published in 1951; Constable: London, UK, 1995.

43. van der Gaag, M.A. A person-centered approach in developmental science: Why this is the future and how to get there. *Infant Child Dev.* **2023**, *32*, e2478. [CrossRef]
44. Kemmis, S.; McTaggart, R.; Nixon, R. *The Action Research Planner: Doing Critical Participatory Action Research*; Springer Science & Business Media: Berlin/Heidelberg, Germany, 2013.
45. Scott, M.; Foley, K.R.; Bourke, J.; Leonard, H.; Girdler, S. "I have a good life": The meaning of well-being from the perspective of young adults with Down syndrome. *Disabil. Rehabil.* **2014**, *36*, 1290–1298. [CrossRef]
46. Love, M.B.; Gardner, K.; Legion, V. Community health workers: Who they are and what they do. *Health Educ. Behav.* **1997**, *24*, 510–522. [CrossRef]
47. Malcarney, M.B.; Pittman, P.; Quigley, L.; Horton, K.; Seiler, N. The changing roles of community health workers. *Health Serv. Res.* **2017**, *52*, 360–382. [CrossRef]
48. Ingram, M.; Sabo, S.; Rothers, J.; Wennerstrom, A.; De Zapien, J.G. Community health workers and community advocacy: Addressing health disparities. *J. Community Health* **2008**, *33*, 417–424. [CrossRef]
49. American Public Health Association. *Community Health Workers*; APHA: Washington, WA, USA, 2025; Available online: https://www.apha.org/apha-communities/member-sections/community-health-workers (accessed on 1 September 2025).
50. Lloyd, J.; Davis, R.; Moses, K. *Recognizing and Sustaining the Value of Community Health Workers and Promotores*; Center for Health Care Strategies: Hamilton Township, NJ, USA, 2020; Volume 13.
51. American Psychological Association. Transparency and Communication Are Key to Building Successful Research Collaborations. 2023. Available online: https://www.apa.org/monitor/2023/09/building-successful-research-collaborations (accessed on 1 September 2025).

healthcare

MDPI

Article

The Impact of Support Intensity Needs on Person-Centred Case Management

Paolo Bianchi [1,*], Marco Lombardi [2], Luigi Croce [3], Antonio Caserta [4] and Roberta Speziale [4]

1 Nottingham University Business School China, University of Nottingham Ningbo China, Ningbo 315100, China
2 EQUALTY Research Collective, HOGENT, University of Applied Sciences and Arts, 9000 Ghent, Belgium; marco.lombardi@hogent.be
3 Dipartimento di Pedagogia, Università Cattolica del Sacro Cuore, 25121 Brescia, Italy; luigi.croce@unicatt.it
4 ANFFAS, 00179 Rome, Italy; acaserta@anffas.net (A.C.); roberta.s@anffas.net (R.S.)
* Correspondence: paolo.bianchi@nottingham.edu.cn

Abstract

Background: International and national policies increasingly call for person-centred approaches in disability services, yet little is known about how support intensity needs influence the allocation of resources for individuals with intellectual and developmental disabilities (IDDs). In Italy, where integrated socio-health systems operate within a human rights framework, this quantitative study investigates how individual and contextual factors shape resource use in individualized support planning. **Methods:** We analyzed data from 1152 adults with IDDs enrolled in 23 service centres across 13 Italian regions. Case managers developed Individualized Support Plans (ISPs) informed by the Supports Intensity Scale and socio-ecological variables. Resource use was measured as weekly counts of adaptive skills training, community participation supports, habilitation services, prosthetics, and assistive technologies. We applied multivariate count models (Sarmanov–Lee) to capture the interdependence across support types. **Results:** Findings show that gender and level of intellectual functioning did not significantly affect resource allocation. However, individuals with the highest support intensity needs often received fewer supports, particularly in adaptive skills and community participation. Residential settings were associated with higher levels of support provision compared to family or independent living. Assistive technologies and prosthetics were linked with more comprehensive support packages. **Conclusions:** While person-centred planning frameworks are being implemented, systemic inequities remain, with those at the highest levels of need at risk of receiving fewer enabling supports. Multivariate modelling provides a robust tool for understanding resource use and highlights the importance of equity-focused planning. These findings support policy and practice reforms that operationalize human rights principles and align with the UNCRPD, ensuring more inclusive and responsive systems of support.

Keywords: intellectual and developmental disability; person-centred care; resource use; support needs

1. Introduction

The sector of social care and related healthcare services for people with intellectual and developmental disabilities (IDDs) has experienced a paradigmatic transition in the last few decades. The gradual shift from the medical model and the growing acceptance of the socio-ecological model of disability and human rights have accompanied the emergence of a person-centred approach, where assistance and support plans aim to overcome individual-specific disabling barriers [1,2], to fulfil the empowerment of the person with a disability, warrant independent life, and the enjoyment of human rights [3,4].

The main aim of this study was to investigate the impact of socio-ecological factors on resource use in person-centred case management for adults with IDDs. The associated aim was to evaluate a flexible multivariate approach to model the pattern of resource use in complex care, contributing to the debate on the comparative usefulness between univariate and multivariate approaches in such a context [5]. In contrast to previous research based on single case studies, we used anonymized individual data from a large national study [6]. Our sample included both individuals residing in service communities and individuals living within their family households; the former group has been usually excluded from traditional statistical surveys and empirical studies [7].

In Italy, care services for people with IDDs are provided within an integrated socio-health system. The Italian disability services sector is characterized by the presence of both public and private organizations; inspired by the idea of welfare pluralism and human rights as self-determination and independent life, people with IDDs may be assisted in residential facilities or receive home and community-based care [8]. Under law 104/1992, an individual's disability and related needs are assessed by a multi-disciplinary board of specialists. The evaluation is derived from a health model of disability and focused on assessing the degree of inability to work. Local units of the Italian National Health System (INHS) are the referral points and supervise the process, where the board compiles a diagnostic report informed by the ICD-10 guidelines from the World Health Organization.

In addition, individuals with IDDs in Italy receive a national cash allowance, designed to facilitate the direct purchase of care instead of directly provided care services. In practice, this cash allowance is used to integrate family income and is akin to a compensation for family members providing care [9]. While this cash-for-care scheme carries the risk of marketization and commodification of care services, people with IDDs and their families have been able to exercise freedom of choice, creating an incentive for providers to implement efficient and sustainable service solutions aligned with human rights requirements [10]. The INHS has been entrusted with the provision of habilitation services, either by directly establishing so-called social-rehabilitation centres or through accreditation and monitoring of private organizations. Supports are typically provided in the following:

- Day centres (for lower and higher support needs);
- Residential centres (for lower and higher support needs);
- Supports at home.

Fea noted that although each region in Italy has its own set of requirements over such centres, all have to conform to national law [11]. Services are required to meet the quality criteria of the funding institution and must be designed to support the person with disability wherever it seems necessary and reasonable [12]. Moreover, the INHS must guarantee the provision of a list of assistive technology and prosthetics supports that are included in the so-called "essential levels of care". Italian support provisions for people with intellectual and developmental disabilities are framed by European policy through alignment with the UN Convention on the Rights of Persons with Disabilities (UNCRPD) and the EU Charter of Fundamental Rights, and are further guided by the EU's Strategy for the Rights of Persons with Disabilities 2021–2030 and the Next Generation EU (NGEU) funds. The traditional Italian system has been called for renovation and paradigm change with Italy's national reforms, such as the Law on Disability and the implementation of deinstitutionalisation projects using NGEU grants, which aim to strengthen community-based services and promote social inclusion in line with these European frameworks.

The system is inspired by person-centred care with the aim to provide person-centred planning. Person-centred planning refers to a structured, collaborative approach to support provision that prioritizes the individual's aspirations and strengths, with the overarching goal of enhancing community inclusion, meaningful relationships, self-determination, and personal competence [13–15]. Paradigmatic is the introduction of the policy reform by Legislative Decree n.62 in 2024. The recent reforms, particularly in disability services, focus heavily on personalizing support and empowering individuals to determine their own needs, a shift from previous models that largely centred around service providers' offerings. This transformation places individuals at the heart of their own care and support planning, which aligns with global movements advocating for self-determination and independence for people with disabilities. The reform highlights the importance of tailoring services to individual preferences and needs, with an emphasis on the use of personal budgets. These budgets enable people with disabilities to directly control the financial resources allocated to their care, enabling more flexible and customized services.

The shift towards individualized services and the autonomy to make decisions about one's support needs is crucial in fostering a sense of empowerment and improving life satisfaction. Research consistently shows that when people with disabilities can choose and manage their supports, it enhances their quality of life and participation in society [16,17]. This reform can be seen as a critical step towards making Italy's disability policies more inclusive and responsive to the actual needs and aspirations of people with disabilities, moving away from the one-size-fits-all solutions. By shifting the focus from provider-driven budgets to user-controlled resources, the reform fosters a system where individuals can define their own life goals and determine the type and level of support they need [18].

This approach aligns with broader international trends in disability policy, including those seen in the UK, Sweden, and other European countries, where individualization and self-determination have been shown to significantly improve outcomes for people with disabilities [19–22]. Accordingly, this study aims to examine how socio-ecological factors influence resource allocation in person-centred case management for adults with intellectual and developmental disabilities (IDDs), and to assess the utility of a flexible multivariate modelling approach for capturing patterns of resource use in complex support provision.

2. Materials and Methods

This study employs a cross-sectional observational design, utilizing data from an experimental project funded by the Italian Ministry of Labor and Social Policy aimed at promoting social inclusion and quality of life (QOL) of adults with IDDs. The project had been instrumental to create ISPs for more than 1000 people with disabilities. Disability case managers composed the individual profile of service users and formulated a person-centred plan of supports aligned with individual needs. All case managers received an initial training in the best evidence-based practices aimed at improving quality of life [23] of people with IDDs, and were selected among experienced staff at the service centres.

Participants were recruited among clients of 23 ANFFAS NGO services in 13 Italian regions and selected by case managers to provide a representative sample of adults associated with their service. Data were collected between November 2014 and January 2015 in electronic format using the protocol developed by ANFFAS (Rome, Italy) "Matrici Ecologiche" (http://www.matriciecologiche.net)" (accessed 24 October, 2025, designed to support the creation of a person-centred plan within a QOL-oriented framework. The software aligns in a logical framework data collected from the assessment, with personal outcomes and supports to achieve the outcomes. It accounts the type and number of supports used to create an Individualized Support Plan in a person-centred way. In addition, an on-line community of practice was created, encompassing other service centres.

The analytic sample comprised 1152 adults with intellectual and developmental disabilities (IDDs) recruited from 23 ANFFAS NGO service centres across 13 Italian regions. Participants ranged in age from 16 to 88 years (M = 41.5, SD = 14.1), with 62% male (n = 705) and 38% female (n = 441). Levels of intellectual functioning were distributed as follows: mild (9%), moderate (24%), severe (26%), and no impairment reported (41%). Regarding living arrangements, 75% of participants resided with their families or independently, 12% lived in small residential facilities (<10 residents), and 13% in larger residential facilities (>10 residents). Approximately 31% were engaged in work, volunteering, or day centre activities.

Inclusion criteria required participants to be aged 16 years or older, formally registered with one of the participating service centres, and to have an Individualized Support Plan (ISP) developed by a trained case manager. Exclusion criteria were limited to incomplete records, particularly missing values on key socio-demographic variables or Supports Intensity Scale scores, which resulted in the final analytic sample of 1152 individuals [19]. ANFFAS head office collected the information and provided data anonymized to researchers. Case managers recorded personal characteristics, environmental variables, and formulated support plans framed within a person-centred approach and the QOL paradigm [23,24].

We measured resource use within ISPs by the weekly number of provided supports. We categorized supports and services according to the classification proposed in Claes, Van Hove, Vandevelde, van Loon, and Schalock [14] and in Lombardi et al. [25]:

- Community participation supports (COM.PART) intend to facilitate social integration;
- Adaptive skills supports (AD.SKILLS) develop positive behavioural skills and motivate clients toward capability and knowledge acquisition;
- Habilitation professional services (HABIL) address specific functional needs;
- PROSTHETICS enable and facilitate sensory–motor functioning;
- Technology (TECH) includes assistive and information technology to enhance cognitive functioning.

The key explanatory variables included the client's intensity of support needs, extraordinary behavioural and medical support needs, and level of intellectual functioning.The Supports Intensity Scale (SIS; [26]) used in this study was the Italian adaptation validated by Leoni and Croce in 2008 and further tested for measurement invariance and reliability in Italian populations by Shaw et al. in 2022 [27,28]. The instrument has demonstrated strong internal consistency (Cronbach's α ranging between 0.89 and 0.96 across domains) and robust construct validity for adults with intellectual and developmental disabilities. Although the SIS is standardized for adult respondents, our sample included a wide age range (16–88 years). While the tool is considered appropriate for adults across the life span, potential differences in how younger and older adults interpret or experience support needs were acknowledged when interpreting results. The SIS assesses the supports needed to participate in typical activities within ordinary environments, including home and community living, lifelong learning, employment, health and social activities, health and safety, as well as protection and advocacy. Case managers also recorded scores for extraordinary BEHAVIOURAL and MEDICAL needs. Level of intellectual functioning was collected from client's INHS files.

Remaining control variables included client's characteristics, family and client desires for improvement, living arrangement, and working status. All regression models controlled for the number of QOL domains represented among the desires and goals for improvement were expressed as priorities in ISPs by clients and their families. Recorded information also included living arrangements:

- independent;

- with family;
- residential service with <10 clients;
- residential service with >10 clients;

and working status:

- no activity;
- paid job;
- volunteering;
- day care centre activities.

The analysis was conducted using multivariate count regression models to account for the joint determination of different types of supports included in Individualized Support Plans (ISPs). We first fitted univariate models (Poisson, negative binomial, and Poisson-lognormal) to each support category—adaptive skills training, community participation, and habilitation services—selecting the best-fitting models based on Bayesian Information Criterion (BIC). These marginals were then combined within the Sarmanov–Lee multivariate framework, which allows flexible modelling of correlations and heterogeneity across support types. This approach enabled us to identify associations among supports while controlling for socio-ecological variables such as support intensity, living arrangements, working status, and assistive technologies. The methodology ensured that the analysis captured the interdependence of supports, providing a more accurate understanding of resource allocation in complex support provision contexts.

Table 1 shows definition and summary statistics of variables used in the empirical analysis. Composition by gender is displayed, but excluded from the reported results because it did not show a significant impact in the analysis. Mean number of AD.SKILLS in ISPs was 4.1 (SD = 2.61), while clients received 1.02 (SD = 1.09) HABIL services on average. In addition, the average counts of COM.PART supports, PROSTHETICS, and assistive TECH were 1.65 (SD = 1.65), 0.25 (SD = 0.57), and 1.62 (SD = 1.37), respectively. Interestingly, counts of adaptive skills training and community participation are overdispersed, while counts of habilitation interventions, prosthetics, and assistive technology are roughly equidispersed.

Information on the level of impairment of intellectual functioning was used to construct three dummy variables: MILD (n = 98, 8.51%), MODERATE (n = 273, 23.70%), and SEVERE (n = 303, 26.30%), with "no impairment" (n = 478, 41.49%) as the reference category. Support needs of the participants were on average in the 63rd percentile (SD = 16.4) as measured with the SIS. With regard to exceptional support needs, the participants displayed on average 3.66 (SD = 4.04) BEHAVIOUR and 1.63 (SD = 2.52) MEDICAL as measured by the respective sub-scales. The participants expressed on average DESIRES in 6.53 (SD = 2.41) out of 8 domains of QOL. Additionally, 31% of participants were involved in some forms of WORKING activities.

Those residing in SMALL residential facilities were 12%, and a similar percentage resided in LARGE contexts (13%), while the majority (75%) lived with their families or independently.

Table 1. Summary of Individual Characteristics.

Variable	Mean	SD	Maximum
Supports count			
Adaptive skills	4.10 (4.43) [a]	2.61	14
Community participation	1.65 (19.44) [a]	1.65	13
Habilitation	1.02 (36.28) [a]	1.09	7
Prosthetic supports	0.25 (80.90) [a]	0.57	4
Technology-based supports	1.62 (23.09) [a]	1.37	7

Table 1. *Cont.*

Variable	Mean	SD	Maximum
Female	0.38	0.49	
Age	41.5	14.1	
Intellectual disability			
Mild	0.09	0.28	
Moderate	0.24	0.43	
Severe	0.26	0.44	
SIS percentile	63.4	16.4	
Specialized support need scale			
Behavioural	3.66	4.04	
Medical	1.63	2.52	
QOL desires and expectations	6.53	2.41	
Working	0.31	0.46	
Residential context			
Small (<10)	0.12	0.33	
Large (>10)	0.13	0.34	

Note. n = 1152; SIS = Supports Intensity Scale percentile; QOL = quality of life [a] Frequency of zero counts.

3. Econometric Framework and Model Selection

Given the features of the case management process, we considered the use of supports to be jointly determined. We employed a flexible multivariate count model allowing for positive, negative, or no association among the counts. Specially, we adopted the approach by Sarmanov and Lee to obtain multivariate distributions by given marginal [29,30]. Miravete showed that the Sarmanov model avoids overestimating the degree of association between uncorrelated count variables in small samples [31]. A valuable feature of the Sarmanov–Lee count models is that correlation and unobserved heterogeneity depend on different parameters, allowing for overdispersion and equidispersion (or underdispersion) in the marginals [30]. We took the following steps to find a good multivariate model of the form of the second equation: First, we fitted univariate models for each of the support counts and selected the best marginal models based on information criteria. Then, we estimated Sarmanov–Lee multivariate models combining maintained marginals and tested for association among the counts. Finally, we evaluated overall model specification through conditional moments tests.

Considering that the Poisson regression model (PRM) can be nested within the three mixed Poisson alternatives, namely negative binomial-1 (NB1), negative bino-mial-2 (NB2), and Poisson-lognormal (PLN), while the other models are not nested, we computed the Bayesian Information Criteria (BIC) to identify the best marginal model. Quasi-maximum likelihood (QML) and numerical optimization routines were employed for all the estimation procedures.

For two-part models, we assumed independence between the hurdle and the positive component, so the log-likelihood can be factored into two terms and separately maximized. When the likelihood of the mixed Poisson model required the evaluation of an integral, this was performed with Gauss–Hermite quadrature.

Our specific-to-general modelling approach calls for a rigorous evaluation of the maintained model. The goodness of fit of the multivariate models was assessed through conditional moment comparisons as developed in Andrews [32].

4. Empirical Results

4.1. Marginal Model Selection

Modelling multivariate count data with Sarmanov–Lee distributions enables the selection of models separately for each marginal. For counts of AD.SKILLS and COM.PART, it was possible to estimate one-part and two-part regression models for over-dispersed data, whereas attempts to fit mixing models for HABIL resulted in the convergence of numerical routines to the baseline PRM and hurdle probit zero-truncated Poisson. We used the Bayesian Information Criterion (BIC) to select the best marginal models. These are the negative binomial-1 for AD.SKILLS, the hurdle probit zero-truncated Poisson-lognormal (PLN) for COM.PART, while the standard Poisson regression model is enough for modelling HABIL, given the explanatory variables. We conducted the flexible multivariate count distributions analysis adopting the three above selected count data regression models.

4.2. Tests of Independence and Goodness of Fit of Multivariate Models

Computing Kendall's τ statistics to evaluate the degree of dependence between the key count variables yielded all positive and statistically significant results, i.e., τ(AD. SKILLS, COM. PART) = 0.1154, z = 6.30, τ(AD. SKILLS, HABIL) = 0.1430, z = 7.74, τ(COM. PART, HABIL) = 0.0676, z = 3.72. We computed standard errors for z statistics with *somersd* Stata 16 package. The association was strongest between AD.SKILLS and HABIL, while COM.PART and HABIL showed the weakest degree of association. These results suggested that AD.SKILLS, COM.PART, and HABIL supports are considered functional complements in the socio-ecological logic of person-centred case management. Nonetheless, the detected bivariate associations in our sample are merely unconditional in nature and, for instance, cannot control for observed heterogeneity.

Table 2 displays estimates of association coefficients and goodness-of-fit measures for the multivariate Sarmanov–Lee models. Where bivariate association is allowed for only one pair of count variables, bivariate models 1–3, all three estimated coefficients are positive, with the association between COM.PART and HABIL significant at 1% level, and the other two models capturing associations at 5% significance level. The above results establish positive pairwise associations between the three counts.

Table 2. Estimates of association coefficients and goodness-of-fit measures for the multivariate Sarmanov–Lee models.

Association Coefficient	Bivariate Model 1	Bivariate Model 2	Bivariate Model 3	Trivariate Model 1	Trivariate Model 2
ω_{12}	1.0418 *			1.2357 **	1.2887 *
	(0.4619)			(0.4738)	(0.5329)
ω_{13}		0.7999 *		0.9630 **	0.8817 **
		(0.3737)		(0.3647)	(0.3392)
ω_{23}			0.7493 **	0.7861 **	0.7254 **
			(0.2564)	(0.2556)	(0.2568)
ω_{123}					−3.2026 *
					(1.4364)
χ^2_{CM}	69.823 ***	49.021 ***	43.852 ***	28.78	28.263
df	17	16	12	28	28

Note: y_1: AD.SKILLS, y_2: COM.PART, y_3: HABIL; χ^2_{CM} = goodness-of-fit test; df = degrees of freedom of the goodness-of-fit test; QML robust standard errors in parentheses. * $p < 0.05$. ** $p < 0.01$. *** $p < 0.001$.

Table 2 also reports the chi-square goodness-of-fit statistics calculated for the bivariate and trivariate Sarmanov–Lee count regression models. While all three bivariate regression models do not pass the goodness-of-fit test, the hypotheses that the two trivariate models are correctly specified cannot be rejected at standard significance levels. Taking into consideration these results and the statistical significance of the third order association coefficient, ω_{123}, we adopted the trivariate model with full Sarmanov–Lee dependence structure for the computation of the marginal effects.

4.3. Marginal Effects

In this section, we present results based on the trivariate regression model with full Sarmanov–Lee dependence structure; this is the model denoted Trivariate Model 2 in Table 2. First, we discuss the age utilization gradient and marginal effects at the mean for prosthetics, assistive technologies, working status, and type of living arrangements. Then, results are presented for the supports intensity need utilization gradient and marginal effects of levels of intellectual functioning, exceptional behavioural and medical support needs, and expressed desires of the clients and their families.

Figure 1 illustrates the expected number of supports included in the ISPs as a function of the age of the client. AD.SKILLS training is provided consistently to younger clients, but we found a negative utilization gradient for middle-age and older clients. COM.PART has also a marked non-monotonic relation with age; the expected supports in this area reach a maximum for individuals aged 45 years. Interestingly, resource use on HABIL supports is not related to age in our model, once we control for a measure of support needs; to find otherwise could expose an "illusion of necessity" [33].

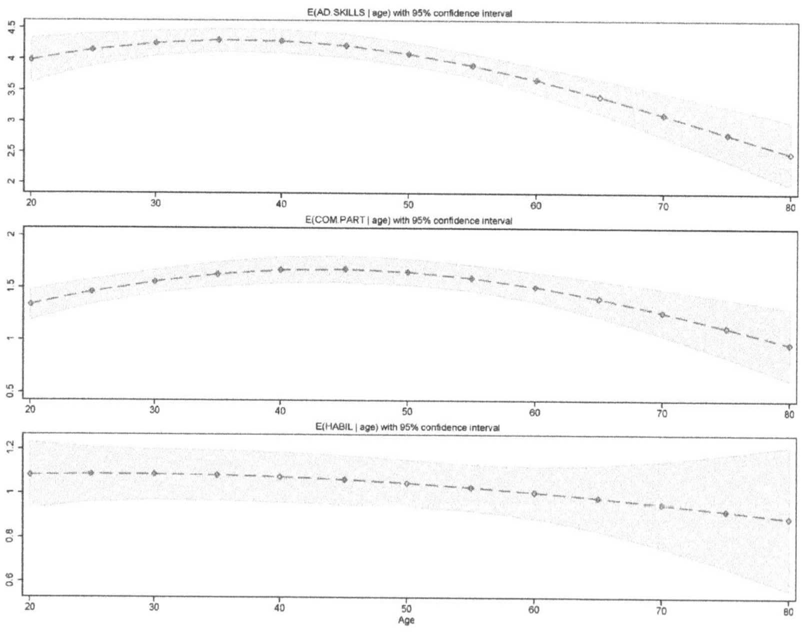

Figure 1. Expected number of supports included in Individual Support Plans (ISPs) as a function of client age. Grey color represents the 95% confidence interval.

Table 3 shows that the presence of prosthetics has a positive impact on the inclusion of supports in ISPs. Compared to no prosthetics, having one PROSTHETIC support is associated with 0.71, 0.42, and 0.2 more supports in AD.SKILLS, COM.PART, and HABIL, respectively. Similarly, having one assistive technology device is associated with 0.41 and 0.1 more supports in AD.SKILLS and HABIL, while there is no significant impact on COM.PART. Working status only has direct influence on the number of AD.SKILLS training. Being involved in productive activities either inside or outside of the service centres is associated with 1.03 additional supports in adaptive skills.

Table 3. Marginal effects on the expected number of supports included in the ISPs.

Variable	Supports in ISPs		
	Adaptive Skills	Community Participation	Habilitation
PROSTHETICS [a]	0.709 *** (0.120)	0.422 *** (0.093)	0.200 *** (0.055)
TECH [a]	0.409 *** (0.045)	0.004 (0.032)	0.101 *** (0.020)
BEHAVIOUR	−0.059 ** (0.019)	−0.026 * (0.011)	0.033 *** (0.007)
MEDICAL	−0.036 (0.029)	−0.055 † (0.031)	−0.004 (0.020)
Level of Intellectual Disability			
None	Ref.	Ref.	Ref.
MILD	−0.338 (0.251)	0.190 (0.137)	−0.084 (0.122)
MODERATE	0.288 (0.182)	0.395 *** (0.115)	−0.056 (0.082)
SEVERE	0.333 † (0.179)	0.331 ** (0.103)	−0.054 (0.076)
DESIRES [b]	0.200 *** (0.034)	0.121 *** (0.020)	0.040 ** (0.013)
Working status			
Not working	Ref.	Ref.	Ref.
WORKING	1.033 *** (0.188)	0.110 (0.086)	0.011 (0.078)
Living arrangements			
Living at home	Ref.	Ref.	Ref.
SMALL	1.292 *** (0.243)	0.354 * (0.143)	0.572 *** (0.102)
LARGE	1.510 *** (0.240)	0.489 ** (0.167)	0.211 * (0.090)

Notes: For continuous variables, the table reports the effect of a (unitary) change in the variable on the expected number of supports included in the ISPs. For each dummy variable, the table reports the effect of the dummy variable going from 0 to 1 on the expected number of supports included in the ISPs. Standard errors in parentheses, computed with 200 draws from the covariance matrix of QML estimator. † $p < 0.10$, * $p < 0.05$, ** $p < 0.01$, *** $p < 0.001$. [a] Discrete change effect, one unit increase compared to zero count of supports [b] Considered as a continuous variable.

Finally, results show that clients living in residential contexts have more supports included in their ISPs over all three categories, compared to clients living with families or independently. Living in small residential contexts (SMALL) is associated with 1.29 more AD.SKILLS, 0.35 more COM.PART, and 0.57 more HABIL. Similarly, living in larger residential contexts (LARGE) implies 1.51 more AD.SKILLS, 0.49 more COM.PART, but only 0.21 more HABIL.

The three panels in Figure 2 show the expected number of supports included in the ISPs as a function of the SIS percentile. The relationship between the number of AD.SKILLS and intensity of support needs is non-monotonic. Clients near the 65th percentile of the SIS measurement receive the highest number of adaptive skills training. Strikingly, individuals with the most intense needs do not receive more supports in this area. COM.PART shows a monotone relationship with SIS; clients with low levels of support needs see around 0.8 community participation supports in their ISPs, while clients in the higher spectrum of support intensity needs on average see 2.1 COM.PART included in their ISP. The number of HABIL supports are at their highest for clients in the 55th to 60th SIS percentile. Again, somewhat surprisingly, individuals in the top percentiles of the SIS measurement receive significantly fewer supports in this area.

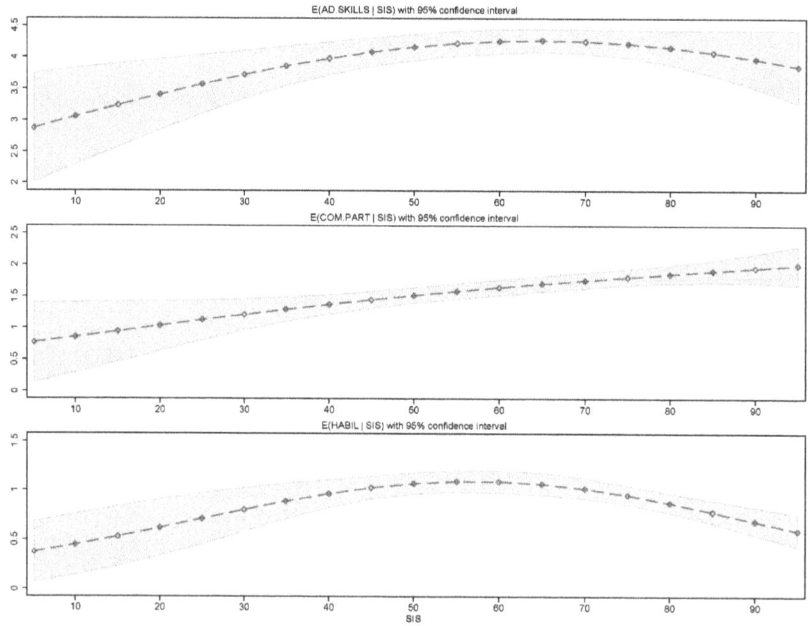

Figure 2. Expected number of support measures included in Individual Support Plans (ISPs) as a function of client's SIS score. Grey color represents the 95% confidence interval.

Inspecting the marginal effects of intellectual functioning, reported in Table 3, clients with MODERATE impaired intellectual functioning receive 0.39 more COM.PART. Individuals with SEVERE intellectual impairment have 0.33 more AD.SKILLS and COM.PART included in their ISPs. For participants with MILD intellectual impairment, the joint model suggests no significant differences with the comparison group (no intellectual disability reported). Clients with extraordinary needs related to their BEHAVIOUR receive on average fewer AD.SKILLS and COM.PART supports, but their ISPs include more HABIL services. While extraordinary MEDICAL needs are not related to the composition of ISPs, this result arises once unobserved heterogeneity is allowed into the model. The number of DESIRES for improvements in the QOL domains when expressed by the clients and their families are positively associated with the average number of AD.SKILLS and HABIL supports, while they are negatively related to the counts of COM.PART supports.

5. Discussion

This study aimed to evaluate public policy outcomes in terms of services and supports provided and determine the social return on investment of social enterprises investigating how socio-ecological factors shape resource allocation in person-centred case management for adults with intellectual and developmental disabilities [4,34,35]. The data were collected in 2015 and are discussed in the context of the ongoing reform of Italy's national support system. Thus, this study offers relevant evidence on how the traditional system of support allocation operated in sight of the current paradigm shift towards a human rights and QOL outcomes driven system. Given the study's cross-sectional observational design, the findings provide a snapshot of the traditional system of support allocation at a specific point in time, offering valuable insights but also reflecting the inherent limitations of such a design, particularly in establishing causal relationships or tracking longitudinal trends.

The findings reveal several important patterns. First, there is a non-monotonic relationship between resources allocated in Individualized Support Plans (ISPs) and measured support intensity needs, indicating that individuals with intermediate levels of need tend to receive more supports than those with higher or lower levels of need. Second, person-centred support planning does not discriminate by gender or intellectual functioning once needs and contextual factors are controlled. Third, individuals in residential settings receive, on average, more supports—particularly oriented toward adaptive skills and habilitation within the service context—than toward community participation. Finally, the multivariate model accurately predicts how resources are distributed across community participation, adaptive skills training, and habilitation services.

These results align with international research linking QOL to support prov ision [14,19,36,37]. However, the purposive sampling approach introduces important considerations. While the sample was designed to reflect the diversity of service users, it was not randomly or statistically stratified. This approach may limit the generalizability of the findings, as the sample could overrepresent individuals whose needs align with the priorities or capacities of the participating centres. Importantly, the findings suggest that current systems may inadequately serve the most vulnerable individuals—those with the highest support needs—while focusing disproportionately on clients with average levels of need. This imbalance raises concerns about equity and effectiveness, particularly given that individuals with extraordinary behavioural needs appear to receive fewer supports for adaptive skills and community participation, even though their ISPs include more habilitation-oriented interventions. As Brady et al. observed, such gaps risk leaving the most vulnerable individuals, often with limited communication skills, underserved [38]. Conversely, clients with lower support needs may also be underserved in community-oriented supports, leaving them at risk of segregation [39]. Together, these findings indicate that although person-centred frameworks are being implemented, they still reflect traditional habilitation-oriented models rather than fully inclusive, socio-ecological approaches.

Interestingly, the finding that clients living with their families account for fewer supports may be explained by the tendency to include only formal supports in ISPs. This organizational bias could contribute to a system that remains service-centred rather than truly person-centred [40]. Consistent with a socio-ecological view, effective planning should sequence interventions from personal priorities to environmental and system accommodations, reflecting evidence that QOL applications are context-dependent and rights-anchored rather than service-centric [20,25].

Client-level implications.

Persons with disabilities, families, and case managers should incorporate a structured equity review into ISP development. In particular, plans for people in the upper decile of support intensity or with extraordinary behavioural needs should demonstrate balanced allocations across adaptive skills, community participation, and habilitation supports. For instance, if a plan emphasizes habilitation due to behavioural concerns, it should still include at least one community-participation activity to prevent social isolation. Given the negative age gradient in adaptive skills supports, reductions in training for middle-aged and older adults should be explicitly justified. It is essential to emphasize that individuals with disabilities (e.g., intellectual or motor) should actively cultivate their abilities, as skill development can progress over time regardless of impairment [41]. Early assistive technology reviews are recommended, as prosthetics and technology supports in our data were associated with richer, more enabling support packages.

Provider-level implications.

Provider organizations should formalize a community–connector function responsible for brokering inclusive roles, transportation solutions, and natural supports. In residential settings, rebalancing from service-internal habilitation toward externally oriented participation goals is warranted. Standard workflows should include assistive technology screening, environmental and community asset mapping, and transport/access supports before defining time-limited skill-building interventions, followed by a planned fading of personnel-driven supports where feasible. This perspective emphasizes naturally available supports and contextual facilitators that foster human functioning and participation in community life as any other citizen, not as a "disabled person." The ultimate goal should be to build environments that are universally accessible [42,43].

System-level implications.

At the system level, organizations and policymakers should adopt case-mix-adjusted, outcomes-linked financing mechanisms supported by transparent equity audits. The literature has shown that data analysis and integration can help identify predictors, mediators, and moderators of QOL outcomes [19,24,44]. The present findings demonstrate that using data-driven approaches—such as our multivariate model to establish expected ranges for adaptive skills, community participation, and habilitation supports—can assist in identifying inequities in service provision. This reinforces an evidence- and value-based perspective: there is a need to operationalize human rights, foster full citizenship and inclusion, and employ evidence-based supports to achieve those outcomes [45]. Accordingly, contracting standards should include minimum inclusion criteria (e.g., at least one community-participation support per plan) and public reporting of a Support Equity Index by support needs tier and living arrangement. The Friuli Venezia Giulia region in Italy provides a relevant example of reform, where individualized project budgets are tied to personal goals rather than fixed service types (Regional Law 22/2019; Regional Law 16/2022). Such systems shift responsibility toward co-designed, outcome-oriented supports, allowing accredited organizations to manage flexible budgets that reflect real needs rather than standardized allocations. This approach highlights the potential of person-centred, data-informed models to replace service-driven systems and foster innovation in community-based supports.

6. Limitations

Nevertheless, the study is not without limitations. First, the cross-sectional design precludes causal inferences or the examination of longitudinal trends. Second, the participating organizations were not randomly selected, but were part of one single network of support providers (ANFFAS), and inclusion was voluntary. This may have introduced bias, as organizations more committed to self-assessment and outcome measurement were overrepresented, potentially limiting generalizability. Additionally, participant selection by case managers may affect both internal and external validity. Third, many organizations were unfamiliar with QOL and socio-ecological frameworks of support, leading to a predominance of staff-based supports in ISPs (particularly in adaptive skills training). This may reflect providers' current orientations more than actual needs, and constrains the conclusions that can be drawn about the breadth of support provision. Fourth, a further limitation concerns the time frame of data collection (2014–2015), which preceded recent national disability reforms, including Legislative Decree n.62/2024 and the implementation of the Next Generation EU (NGEU) framework. Although the age of the data may limit direct comparability with current service models, they provide an important historical baseline for understanding how person-centred principles were operationalized before the policy transition toward individualized budgets and community inclusion. Future research using post-reform datasets will be crucial to evaluate whether these systemic changes have effectively addressed the equity gaps observed in this study. Future research should include longitudinal and experimental designs comparing standard and innovative support models to identify practices that most effectively promote personal outcomes [24].

7. Conclusions

In conclusion, understanding the interaction between contextual factors, support provision, and client outcomes is essential for effective and equitable systems [46]. At the micro level, person-centred case management should ensure individualized supports aligned with personal goals and participation in community life [25]. At the meso level, organizations and service providers have the opportunity to use evidence-based algorithms and flexible funding to match supports to actual needs while minimizing inequalities. At the macro level, policymakers should prioritize sustainable, data-driven systems that integrate personal and community resources. Taken together, the findings of this study, while subject to limitations, offer guidance for reducing discrepancies between assessed needs and provided supports, and for fostering collaborative, equitable, and innovative support ecosystems.

Author Contributions: Conceptualization, M.L. and L.C.; Methodology, P.B.; Formal analysis, M.L.; Investigation, R.S.; Writing—original draft, P.B.; Writing—review and editing, M.L.; Visualization, P.B.; Funding acquisition, A.C. All authors have read and agreed to the published version of the manuscript.

Funding: This research was funded by the Italian Ministry of Labour and Social Policies, grant number 383, 07.12.00, addressing lines 2013, project F.

Institutional Review Board Statement: Not applicable.

Informed Consent Statement: Not applicable.

Data Availability Statement: The data presented in this study are available on request from the corresponding author due to personal and health information that does not allow public availability for privacy reasons.

Conflicts of Interest: The authors declare no conflicts of interest.

References

1. Oliver, M. The social model of disability: Thirty years on. *Disabil. Soc.* **2013**, *28*, 1024–1026. [CrossRef]
2. Shakespeare, T. The social model of disability. In *The Disability Studies Reader*; Davis, L.J., Ed.; Routledge: Abingdon, UK, 2006; Volume 2, Chapter 16; pp. 197–204.
3. Verdugo, M.; Navas, P.; Gómez, L.; Schalock, R.L. The concept of quality of life and its role in enhancing hu-man rights in the field of intellectual disability. *J. Intellect. Disabil. Res.* **2012**, *56*, 1036–1045. [CrossRef] [PubMed]
4. Lombardi, M.; Vandenbussche, H.; Claes, C.; Schalock, R.L.; De Maeyer, J.; Vandevelde, S. The Concept of Quality of Life as Framework for Implementing the UNCRPD. *J. Policy Pract. Intellect. Disabil.* **2019**, *16*, 180–190. [CrossRef]
5. Blumenthal, D.; Abrams, M.K. Tailoring complex care management for high-need, high-cost patients. *JAMA* **2016**, *316*, 1657–1658. [CrossRef] [PubMed]
6. Ratti, V.; Hassiotis, A.; Crabtree, J.; Deb, S.; Gallagher, P.; Unwin, G. The effectiveness of person-centred planning for people with intellectual disabilities: A systematic review. *Res. Dev. Disabil.* **2016**, *57*, 63–84. [CrossRef]
7. European Commission. *Progress Report on the Implementation of the European Disability Strategy (2010–2020)*; European Commission: Brussels, Belgium, 2017. Available online: https://www.europarl.europa.eu/thinktank/en/document/EPRS_ATA(2017)614586 (accessed on 5 August 2020).
8. Longo, F.; Notarnicola, E.; Tasselli, S. A framework to assess welfare mix and service provision models in health care and social welfare: Case studies of two prominent Italian regions. *BMC Health Serv. Res.* **2015**, *15*, 152. [CrossRef]
9. Pavolini, E.; Ranci, C.; Lamura, G. Long-term care in Italy. In *Long-Term Care for the Elderly in Europe*; Routledge: London, UK, 2016; pp. 89–106.
10. United Nations. Convention on the Rights of Persons with Disabilities. 2006. Available online: https://www.ohchr.org/en/hrbodies/crpd/pages/conventionrightspersonswithdisabilities.aspx (accessed on 10 September 2021).

11. Fea, F. Services for Persons with Intellectual and Developmental Disabilities in Italy. In *Health Care for People with Intellectual and Developmental Disabilities Across the Lifespan*; Springer: Berlin/Heidelberg, Germany, 2016; pp. 555–561.
12. Bacherini, A.; Pierluigi, I.; Balboni, G. Healthcare for people with intellectual and developmental disabilities in Italy. *J. Policy Pract. Intellect. Disabil.* **2024**, *21*, e12490. [CrossRef]
13. O'Brien, C.; O'Brien, J. The origins of person-centered planning. In *Person Centered Planning: Research, Practice and Future Directions*; Holburn, S., Vietze, P.M., Eds.; Brookes: Baltimore, MD, USA, 2002; pp. 3–27.
14. Claes, C.; Van Hove, G.; Vandevelde, S.; van Loon, J.; Schalock, R. The influence of supports strategies, environmental factors, and client characteristics on quality of life- related personal outcomes. *Res. Dev. Disabil.* **2012**, *33*, 96–103. [CrossRef]
15. Wilson, G.; Hutchison, J.S. In pursuit of a person-centered approach to care delivery: A qualitative descriptive study of the patient experience of a long-term conditions clinic in general practice. *Qual. Health Res.* **2025**, *35*, 680–696. [CrossRef]
16. Cirulli, F.; Venerosi, A. A focus on the rights to self-determination and quality of life in people with mental disabilities. Editorial. *Ann. Ist. Super. Sanità* **2020**, *56*, 133–134. [CrossRef]
17. Prandini, R.; Orlandini, M. The morphogenesis of disability policies and the personalisation of social services. A case study from Italy. *Int. Rev. Sociol.* **2018**, *28*, 86–109. [CrossRef]
18. Thompson, J.R.; Bradley, V.J.; Buntinx, W.H.; Schalock, R.L.; Shogren, K.A.; Snell, M.E.; Wehmeyer, M.L.; Borthwick-Duffy, S.; Coulter, D.L.; Craig, E.P.M.; et al. Conceptualizing supports and the support needs of people with intellectual disability. *Intellect. Dev. Disabil.* **2009**, *47*, 135–146. [CrossRef] [PubMed]
19. Lombardi, M.; Croce, L.; Claes, C.; Vandevelde, S.; Schalock, R.L. Factors predicting quality of life for people with intellectual disability: Results from the ANFFAS study in Italy. *J. Intellect. Dev. Disabil.* **2016**, *41*, 338–347. [CrossRef]
20. Luckasson, R.; Schalock, R.L.; Bradley, V.J. Diffusion of the Shared Citizenship Paradigm: Strategies and next steps. *Am. J. Intellect. Dev. Disabil.* **2024**, *129*, 362–376. [CrossRef]
21. Power, A.; Lord, J.; DeFranco, A. *Active Citizenship and Disability: Implementing the Personalisation of Support*; Cambridge University Press: Cambridge, UK, 2013.
22. Schalock, R.L.; Luckasson, R.; Tassé, M.J.; Shogren, K.A. The IDD paradigm of shared citizenship: Its opera-tionalization, application, evaluation, and shaping for the future. *Intellect. Dev. Disabil.* **2022**, *60*, 426–443. [CrossRef]
23. Gómez, L.E.; Schalock, R.L.; Verdugo, M.A. The role of moderators and mediators in implementing and evaluating intellectual and developmental disabilities-related policies and practices. *J. Dev. Phys. Disabil.* **2020**, *32*, 375–393. [CrossRef]
24. Buntinx, W.H.; Schalock, R.L. Models of disability, quality of life, and individualized supports: Implications for professional practice in intellectual disability. *J. Policy Pract. Intellect. Disabil.* **2010**, *7*, 283–294. [CrossRef]
25. Lombardi, M.; Claes, C.; Bradley, V.J.; Schalock, R.L. The influence of context on the conceptualization, measurement, and application of the concept of quality of life. *J. Policy Pract. Intellect. Disabil.* **2024**, *21*, e12508. [CrossRef]
26. Thompson, J.R.; Hughes, C.; Schalock, R.L.; Silverman, W.; Tassé, M.J.; Bryant, B.; Craig, E.M.; Campbell, E.M. Integrating supports in assessment and planning. *Ment. Retard.* **2002**, *40*, 390–405. [CrossRef]
27. Leoni, M.; Croce, L. Italian translation of the supports intensity scale. In *International Implementation of the Supports Intensity Scale*; Schalock, R.L., Thompson, J.R., Tassé, M.J., Eds.; American Association on Intellectual and Developmental Disabilities: Washington, DC, USA, 2008.
28. Shaw, L.A.; Thompson, J.R.; Lombardi, M.; Croce, L.; Speziale, R.; Gomiero, T.; Shogren, K.A. The Italian translation of the Supports Intensity Scale-Children (SIS-C Italian): Measurement invariance and differences. *J. Int. Spec. Needs Educ.* **2022**, *25*, 37–47. [CrossRef]
29. Sarmanov, O.V.E. Generalized normal correlation and two-dimensional Fréchet classes. In *Doklady Akademii Nauk*; Academy of Sciences: Moscow, Russia, 1966; Volume 168, pp. 32–35.
30. Lee, M.-L.T. Properties and applications of the Sarmanov family of bivariate distributions. *Commun. Stat. Theory Methods* **1996**, *25*, 1207–1222. [CrossRef]
31. Miravete, E.J. Testing for complementarities among countable strategies. *Empir. Econ.* **2014**, *46*, 1521–1544. [CrossRef]
32. Andrews, D.W. Chi-square diagnostic tests for econometric models: Introduction and applications. *J. Econom.* **1988**, *37*, 135–156. [CrossRef]
33. Mason, T.; Sutton, M.; Whittaker, W.; Birch, S. Exploring the limitations of age-based models for health care planning. *Soc. Sci. Med.* **2015**, *132*, 11–19. [CrossRef] [PubMed]
34. Cordes, J.J. Using cost-benefit analysis and social return on investment to evaluate the impact of social enterprise: Promises, implementation, and limitations. *Eval. Program Plan.* **2017**, *64*, 98–104. [CrossRef] [PubMed]
35. Yates, B.T.; Marra, M. Introduction: Social return on investment (SROI). *Eval. Program Plan.* **2017**, *64*, 95–97. [CrossRef]
36. Gómez, L.E.; Peña, E.; Arias, B.; Verdugo, M.A. Impact of individual and organizational variables on quality of life. *Soc. Indic. Res.* **2016**, *125*, 649–664. [CrossRef]
37. Simões, C.; Santos, S. The impact of personal and environmental characteristics on quality of life of people with intellectual disability. *Appl. Res. Qual. Life* **2017**, *12*, 389–408. [CrossRef]

38. Brady, N.C.; Bruce, S.; Goldman, A.; Erickson, K.; Mineo, B.; Ogletree, B.T.; Siegel, E. Communication services and supports for individuals with severe disabilities: Guidance for assessment and intervention. *Am. J. Intellect. Dev. Disabil.* **2016**, *121*, 121–138. [CrossRef]
39. Adair, B.; Ullenhag, A.; Keen, D.; Granlund, M.; Imms, C. The effect of interventions aimed at improving participation outcomes for children with disabilities: A systematic review. *Dev. Med. Child Neurol.* **2015**, *57*, 1093–1104. [CrossRef]
40. Nuri, R.P.; Piccone, C.; Gaurav, N.; Thomson, D.; Pauls, R.; Perry, L.; Aldersey, H.M. The limits and contributions of formal support: Service providers' perspectives on balancing formal and natural support for people with disabilities and their families in Canada. *J. Dev. Phys. Disabil.* **2025**, *37*, 129–156. [CrossRef] [PubMed]
41. Cavaggioni, L.; Trecroci, A.; Formenti, D.; Hogarth, L.; Tosin, M.; Alberti, G. Seasonal Changes in Breathing Pattern, Trunk Stabilization, and Muscular Power in Paralympic Swimmers. *Adapt. Phys. Act. Q.* **2021**, *38*, 215–231. [CrossRef]
42. Shogren, K.A.; Luckasson, R.; Schalock, R.L. The Responsibility to Build Contexts That Enhance Human Functioning and Promote Valued Outcomes for People with Intellectual Disability: Strengthening System Responsive-ness. *Intellect. Dev. Disabil.* **2018**, *56*, 287–300. [CrossRef]
43. Shogren, K.A.; Luckasson, R.; Schalock, R.L. Using a Multidimensional Model to Analyze Context and Enhance Personal Outcomes. *Intellect. Dev. Disabil.* **2020**, *58*, 95–110. [CrossRef]
44. Blanco-López, J.L.; Fernández-Lázaro, D.; Sánchez-Valdeón, L.; Seco-Calvo, J. Quality of life predictors for individuals with intellectual disability: Cross-sectional proxy-report data from a multicentre study. *J. Intellect. Dev. Disabil.* 1–16, *in press*. [CrossRef]
45. Claes, C.; Schalock, R.L.; Van Hove, G. The Shared Citizenship Paradigm and Its Measurement. *J. Policy Pract. Intellect. Disabil.* **2025**, *22*, e70017. [CrossRef]
46. Verdugo, M.Á.; Schalock, R.L.; Gómez, L.E. The quality of life supports model as a major component in ap-plying the quality of life paradigm. *J. Policy Pract. Intellect. Disabil.* **2024**, *21*, e12468. [CrossRef]

healthcare

MDPI

Article

Aging Unequally: Functional Age Disparities Between Developmental and Non-Developmental Disabilities

Ji Ung Jeong

Department of Disability Studies, Daegu University, Gyeongsan-si 38453, Republic of Korea; jiungjeong987@gmail.com

Abstract

Background: Adults with developmental disabilities often experience accelerated aging, but the magnitude of this phenomenon is not well quantified. This study aimed to measure the disparity in functional ability and chronic illness prevalence between adults with developmental and other disabilities. **Methods**: A "functional age" was calculated for adults with developmental disabilities. This metric, designed as a statistical index of disparity, was derived from normative regression models of ADL and IADL based on a reference group of adults with other disabilities. **Results**: A profound gap was found between chronological and functional age. On average, a 44-year-old individual with a developmental disability exhibited a level of functional limitation equivalent to a person over 100 years older in the reference population for both ADL and IADL ($p < 0.001$). **Conclusions**: Accelerated aging in this population manifests as a severe, early onset functional disadvantage rather than an elevated burden of general chronic disease. Policies should shift toward function-based, not age-based, models of care to address these lifelong support needs.

Keywords: developmental disabilities; accelerated aging; functional age; health disparities; functional limitation

1. Introduction

A central paradox of modern healthcare is that increased longevity does not always equate to an extended period of health [1,2]. This is particularly true for individuals with developmental disabilities—a broad category encompassing intellectual disabilities, autism spectrum disorder, and cerebral palsy—who are now living longer than ever before [3,4]. This demographic shift has created an aging population with a unique and complex health profile, characterized by the long-observed clinical phenomenon of "accelerated aging" [5]. This phenomenon describes the earlier onset of age-related health conditions, premature functional decline, and mortality compared to the general population [6,7]. Research shows that many individuals with developmental disabilities experience physical changes and mobility limitations in their 40s and 50s, mirroring patterns typically seen in neurotypical adults decades older [8]. This apparent disconnect between chronological and biological age suggests that standard age-based models of care are inadequate, highlighting a critical need to understand the specific nature and timing of the aging process in this group [9].

The concept of accelerated aging is supported by extensive, multidimensional evidence that spans biological, clinical, and functional domains. Biologically, the phenomenon is often attributed to factors inherent in certain conditions—such as increased oxidative stress and chronic low-grade inflammation in Down syndrome—combined with a higher prevalence of lifestyle risks like physical inactivity and obesity across the broader developmental disability population [10–12]. These underlying mechanisms are believed to hasten the onset of cellular senescence and contribute to a state of increased physiological vulnerability [13].

Clinically, this leads to an earlier emergence of conditions typically associated with old age. For individuals with Down syndrome, the genetic overexpression of amyloid precursor protein means the neuropathological hallmarks of Alzheimer's disease are nearly universal by age 40, with corresponding declines in adaptive functioning occurring decades earlier than in the general population [14]. Beyond this specific example, adults with intellectual and developmental disabilities (IDD) as a whole show a higher burden of multimorbidity, including an earlier onset of osteoporosis, sensory impairments, and cardiovascular disease [15,16].

This decline is typically assessed through limitations in Activities of Daily Living (ADLs), which refer to basic self-care activities like eating and bathing, and Instrumental Activities of Daily Living (IADLs), which encompass more complex tasks necessary for independent community living, such as managing finances or shopping [17,18]. Hilgenkamp et al. [19] reported that adults with intellectual disabilities exhibit significantly impaired performance on ADL and IADL by their 50s. Similarly, adults with cerebral palsy often encounter age-related declines in strength, increased pain, and new mobility limitations—so-called "secondary health conditions"—at a much younger age than their peers, often leading to a loss of independent ambulation in early to middle adulthood [20,21]. This evidence collectively paints a consistent picture of a population facing the functional and health challenges of old age while still in their middle years.

These physiological declines are deeply intertwined with social determinants of health that create a "cascade of disparities" [5]. As individuals with developmental disabilities age, they are more likely to experience poverty, social isolation, and inadequate healthcare, which together heighten physiological vulnerability [22]. This is often exacerbated by "diagnostic overshadowing," a pervasive cognitive bias wherein clinicians mistakenly attribute physical symptoms of a co-occurring condition to the primary developmental disability, leading to missed or delayed diagnoses [23,24]. Although mortality rates remain higher in this population, those surviving into midlife often face levels of functional impairment far greater than would normally be expected for their chronological age [11,25]. This phenomenon has profound implications, impacting everything from individual quality of life and caregiver burden to the design of long-term support services and public health policy [26,27].

Yet a comprehensive, population-level understanding of this disparity remains limited by methodological challenges that restrict accurate assessment of accelerated aging. Much of the research to date is based on narrowly defined clinical cohorts or restricted to specific diagnostic groups, such as Down syndrome or intellectual disability. While such studies have provided foundational insights—such as the early emergence of Alzheimer's pathology in individuals with Down syndrome [28], or midlife declines in ADL/IADL functioning in those with intellectual disabilities [19]—their findings are often not generalizable to the broader and more diverse developmental disability population. This is particularly problematic given the variability in functional status, comorbidity profiles, and support needs across different subgroups [5,29]. In addition, comparisons to the general population—though valuable for identifying broad disparities—often fail to disentangle the effects of early onset, lifelong disability from those of later-acquired impairments. Such approaches risk obscuring critical differences in developmental trajectories, health risks, and service needs [16,24].

To disentangle these factors, a more insightful comparison—pitting adults with developmental disabilities against their peers with other, later-onset disabilities—is necessary. This comparison is crucial for isolating the unique impact of a condition present from early life, a principle central to the life course health development model, which posits that the timing and duration of health exposures fundamentally shape long-term outcomes [30]. By using adults with other disabilities as a reference, it becomes possible to control for the general experience of disability and focus specifically on the "accelerated" component attributable to developmental conditions. Yet, such direct comparisons, especially using quantitative functional metrics, are notably uncommon in large-scale research. Consequently, a clear, quantitative assessment of this specific "health gap" using nationally representative data is needed to move beyond the limitations of clinical observation and inform evidence-based practice at a population level [3].

The present study addresses this gap by utilizing nationally representative data and a functional aging framework that enables direct, empirically grounded comparisons. By calculating "functional age" based on normative models of aging from a reference group, this approach moves beyond descriptive comparisons to offer a quantifiable measure of health disparity. In doing so, this study provides the kind of rigorous, population-level evidence needed to inform inclusive health policy, targeted service provision. Therefore, the primary research aims are to determine: whether adults with developmental disabilities exhibit functional limitations in ADL and IADL that are disproportionate to their chronological age; and whether this pattern of accelerated aging applies equally to the prevalence of chronic illness. This study proposes a shift toward function-based aging metrics as a more equitable foundation for care planning, health screening, and resource allocation. In doing so, it aims to contribute to a more just and evidence-informed understanding of aging in the developmental disability population.

2. Method

2.1. Data and Sample

This study utilizes data from the 18th wave of the Korean Welfare Panel Study (KOWEPS), a nationally representative longitudinal survey conducted in 2023 [31]. KOWEPS is jointly managed by the Korea Institute for Health and Social Affairs and Seoul National University since 2006. The survey is designed to track the economic, social, and health conditions of households and individuals across South Korea, with a particular emphasis on low-income and vulnerable populations. The analysis leverages the main survey data in conjunction with the supplemental survey on persons with disabilities, which contains detailed information on disability characteristics, health, and functional status. The target population of KOWEPS includes all private households in South Korea as of 2022, excluding special facilities and island regions. The sample was drawn using a two-stage stratified sampling method based on the 2005 Korean Population and Housing Census. From this pool, 7000 households (3500 general and 3500 low-income) were chosen to ensure balanced representation across income levels and enhance the statistical efficiency of the panel.

To quantify the phenomenon of accelerated aging, this study employed a two-part sampling strategy to compare the functional health status of adults with developmental disabilities to their peers. As this study utilized a pre-existing, nationally representative dataset, an a priori sample size calculation was not performed. The eligibility criteria for the sample included all adults with a registered disability in the KOWEPS dataset. The reference group, used to build the normative aging models for ADL and IADL, consisted of all 1364 individuals in the dataset with non-developmental disabilities. The focal group for the primary analysis comprised all individuals with a registered developmental disability

($N = 93$). To ensure analytical consistency, one case with missing data on key variables was excluded, making the final analytical sample for the paired-samples t-tests 92 individuals from this focal group.

This study was a secondary analysis of cross-sectional data using publicly available, de-identified data from the KOWEPS. Therefore, it was exempt from institutional review board approval. The original KOWEPS survey was conducted in accordance with the Declaration of Helsinki, and the protocol was approved by the Institutional Review Board of the Korea Institute for Health and Social Affairs.

2.2. Measures

The first dependent variable, ADL, measured functional limitation using a 12-item scale assessing an individual's ability to perform basic self-care tasks such as dressing, bathing, and eating. Each item was rated on a 3-point scale from 1 ("Completely Independent") to 3 ("Needs Complete Assistance"). The responses were summed to create a total ADL score ranging from 12 to 36, where a higher score indicates a greater level of functional dependence. The second dependent variable, IADL, assessed the capacity for more complex independent living tasks like managing finances or preparing meals via a 10-item scale. Responses of "Not Applicable" were treated as missing data, while remaining items were rated on the same 3-point scale as the ADL. A total IADL score was computed by summing the valid responses, with a higher score signifying greater difficulty with instrumental tasks. The third dependent variable, Presence of Chronic Illness, measured general health status using an item assessing the duration of treatment for a chronic condition. This variable was treated as an ordinal outcome with four levels: "No Illness," "Treatment for less than 3 months," "Treatment for 3–6 months," and "Treatment for 6 months or more."

The primary independent variable was Disability Type, a dichotomous variable where individuals with intellectual or autism spectrum disorders were coded as 1 ("Developmental Disability"), and individuals with all other disability types served as the reference group (coded as 0).

To isolate the relationship between disability type, age, and health outcomes, several key sociodemographic and economic variables were included as controls. Age was included as a continuous variable. Sociodemographic controls included Sex (1 = Male, 0 = Female), Education Level (an ordinal scale), and Marital Status (1 = Partnered, 0 = Other). Economic status was controlled for using the natural logarithm of the household's annual disposable income. Finally, a dummy variable for Disability Severity (1 = Severe, 0 = Mild) was included to account for baseline differences in health status.

2.3. Analytical Strategy

A multi-stage analytical strategy was employed, tailored to the measurement level of each dependent variable.

2.3.1. Analysis of Functional Limitations (ADL and IADL)

For the continuous outcome variables (ADL and IADL), a two-stage "functional age" model was used. This approach was constructed to create a quantifiable index of health disparity, following the precedent of similar "biological age" metrics in other health fields, such as "lung age" in pulmonology [32] and "brain age" in neuroimaging [33]. The first stage involved establishing a covariate-adjusted normative aging trajectory by estimating a multiple linear regression model on the reference population of individuals with non-developmental disabilities. The general form of this normative model was:

$$\text{Predicted Score}_i = \beta_0 + \beta_1 (\text{Age}_i) + \beta_2 (\text{Sex}_i) + \ldots + \beta_n (\text{Covariate}_{ni}) + \varepsilon_i$$

In the second stage, a "functional age" was calculated for each individual in the developmental disability group. This was achieved by inverting the regression equation and using it to solve for the age at which a person in the reference group would be expected to have the same functional score, after accounting for all other covariates. The general formula for this calculation was:

$$\text{Functional Age}_i = ([\text{Actual Score}_i - \Sigma(\beta_n \times \text{Covariate\_Value}_{ni})] - \beta_0)/\beta_1$$

Finally, a paired-samples *t*-test was conducted to determine if there was a statistically significant difference between the chronological age and the calculated functional age for the developmental disability group.

2.3.2. Analysis of Chronic Illness Prevalence

As the "Presence of Chronic Illness" variable is ordinal, a different analytical approach was required. First, an ordinal logistic regression model was estimated to assess the relationship between the predictor variables and the likelihood of being in a higher category of chronic illness duration. The general form of the underlying linear model is:

$$\text{Logit}(P(Y \leq j)) = \text{Threshold}_j - (\beta_1\ (\text{DisabilityType}_i) + \beta_2\ (\text{Age}_i) + \ldots + \beta_n\ (\text{Covariate}_{ni}))$$

Second, to illustrate the practical magnitude of the effect of disability type, the coefficients from this model were used to calculate and compare the predicted probabilities of having a chronic illness for a "typical" individual profile (e.g., based on the sample mean/mode for covariates), once for each disability group. This comparison serves to quantify any observed health gap in an intuitive, probabilistic framework.

All analyses were conducted using SPSS version 28, with statistical significance set at $p < 0.05$.

2.3.3. Patient and Public Involvement

It was not possible to involve patients or members of the public in the design, conduct, or reporting of this research. This study is a secondary analysis of a pre-existing, de-identified public-use dataset. As such, the research questions and analytical strategy were formulated based on the available data, and there was no direct contact with the study participants. The findings of this study will be disseminated through academic publication to reach clinicians, policymakers, and advocacy groups working with this population.

3. Results

3.1. Descriptive Characteristics of the Sample

The descriptive statistics of the study sample are presented in Table 1. The final sample comprised 1457 individuals with disabilities, of whom 93 (6.4%) were identified as having a developmental disability and 1364 (93.6%) had other types of disabilities.

An independent samples *t*-test revealed significant demographic and socioeconomic differences between the two groups. The developmental disability group was substantially younger on average (M = 44.17, SD = 14.63) compared to the group with other disabilities (M = 72.76, SD = 12.52), a difference that was statistically significant, $t(101.41) = 18.40$, $p < 0.001$. Conversely, the average annual household disposable income was significantly higher for the developmental disability group (M = 44.68 million KRW) than for the other disabilities group (M = 31.42 million KRW), $t(103.94) = -4.06$, $p < 0.001$. Regarding the dependent variables, there was no statistically significant difference in the level of ADL limitation between the developmental disability group (M = 13.75) and the other disabilities group (M = 13.03), $t(102.74) = -1.82$, $p = 0.072$. However, a significant difference was observed for IADL limitations. The developmental disability group reported a significantly higher mean IADL limitation score (M = 16.99, SD = 5.98) than the other disabilities group (M = 12.62, SD = 4.71), indicating greater difficulty with instrumental daily tasks, $t(99.46) = -6.86$, $p < 0.001$.

Table 1. Descriptive Characteristics of the Study Sample by Disability Type.

Characteristic	Developmental Disability (*n* = 93)	Other Disabilities (*n* = 1364)	Test Statistic	*p*-Value
Continuous Variables (*Mean ± SD*)			***t*-test**	
Age (years)	44.17 ± 14.63	72.76 ± 12.52	18.40	**<0.001**
Household Income (10,000 KRW/year)	4467.86 ± 3057.49	3141.92 ± 2940.20	−4.06	**<0.001**
ADL Limitation Score	13.75 ± 3.69	13.03 ± 3.42	−1.82	0.072
IADL Limitation Score	16.99 ± 5.98	12.62 ± 4.71	−6.86	**<0.001**
Categorical Variables *n* (%)			**χ^2-test**	
Sex			10.80	**0.001**
Female	33 (35.5)	724 (53.1)		
Male	60 (64.5)	640 (46.9)		
Education Level			43.51	**<0.001**
No Schooling	5 (5.4)	197 (14.4)		
Elementary School	23 (24.7)	509 (37.3)		
Middle School	10 (10.8)	244 (17.9)		
High School	47 (50.5)	291 (21.3)		
University or Higher	8 (8.6)	123 (9.0)		
Marital Status			57.26	**<0.001**
Unpartnered (Single, Divorced, etc.)	81 (87.1)	635 (46.6)		
Partnered (Married, etc.)	12 (12.9)	729 (53.4)		
Disability Severity			186.71	**<0.001**
Mild	0 (0.0)	951 (69.7)		
Severe	93 (100.0)	413 (30.3)		
Chronic Illness Status			69.59	**<0.001**
No Illness	33 (35.5)	117 (8.6)		
<3 months of treatment	2 (2.2)	18 (1.3)		
3–6 months of treatment	0 (0.0)	10 (0.7)		
6+ months of treatment	58 (62.4)	1219 (89.4)		
Total Sample	**93 (100.0)**	**1364 (100.0)**		

Further analysis using chi-square tests showed significant differences in the distribution of categorical variables between the two groups (see Table 1). The proportion of males was significantly higher in the developmental disability group (64.5%) compared to the other disabilities group (46.9%), $\chi^2(1, N = 1457) = 10.80$, $p = 0.001$. Significant differences were also found in educational attainment, $\chi^2(4, N = 1457) = 43.51$, $p < 0.001$. A notable concentration of individuals with developmental disabilities was observed at the high school level (50.5%), whereas the other disabilities group was most concentrated at the elementary school level (37.3%). Marital status also differed significantly between the groups, $\chi^2(1, N = 1457) = 57.26$, $p < 0.001$. Most individuals with developmental disabilities were single/unpartnered (87.1%), while the other disabilities group was more evenly split between being partnered (53.4%) and unpartnered (46.6%). A stark and highly significant difference was found in disability severity, $\chi^2(1, N = 1457) = 186.71$, $p < 0.001$. All individuals (100.0%) in the developmental disability group were classified as having a severe disability, compared to only 30.3% in the other disabilities group. Finally, the prevalence of chronic illness differed significantly, $\chi^2(3, N = 1457) = 69.59$, $p < 0.001$. A larger proportion of the other disabilities group reported long-term treatment (6+ months) for a chronic condition (89.4%) compared to the developmental disability group (62.4%). Conversely, a higher percentage of the developmental disability group reported having no chronic illness (35.5%) compared to the other group (8.6%).

3.2. Functional Age Analysis for ADL

To quantify the functional health disparity suggested by the descriptive data, the "functional age" methodology was employed. This analysis first established a normative aging trajectory for ADL limitations and then used this benchmark to evaluate the developmental disability group.

3.2.1. Normative Model of ADL Limitation

A multiple linear regression was estimated using the reference group of 1364 individuals with non-developmental disabilities. The model predicted the ADL limitation score from chronological age and a set of sociodemographic and economic covariates. The results are presented in Table 2.

Table 2. Regression Model for Normative ADL Limitation Trajectory (Reference Group Only).

Predictor	B	Std. Error	β	*t*	*p*-Value
(Constant)	4.689	1.637		2.864	0.004
Age (years)	0.048	0.010	0.171	4.913	<0.001
Sex (Male)	0.005	0.205	0.001	0.024	0.980
Education Level	0.035	0.101	0.012	0.344	0.731
Marital Status (Partnered)	0.053	0.218	0.008	0.242	0.809
Household Income (ln)	0.530	0.165	0.109	3.208	0.001
Disability Severity (Severe)	2.018	0.206	0.272	9.799	<0.001

Note: Dependent Variable = ADL Limitation Score. $N = 1251$. $R^2 = 0.086$.

The overall model was statistically significant, $F(6, 1244) = 19.45$, $p < 0.001$, and explained 8.6% of the variance in ADL scores ($R^2 = 0.086$). In this model, both chronological age ($B = 0.048$, $p < 0.001$) and disability severity ($B = 2.018$, $p < 0.001$) were significant positive predictors of ADL limitation, indicating that greater age and having a severe disability were associated with worse functional outcomes. Household income also emerged as a significant predictor ($B = 0.530$, $p = 0.001$).

3.2.2. Comparison of Chronological and Functional Age

Using the coefficients from the normative model, a functional age was calculated for each of the 92 individuals in the developmental disability group. A paired-samples *t*-test was then conducted to compare their mean chronological age with their mean calculated functional age.

The results, shown in Table 3, revealed a profound and statistically significant disparity. The mean chronological age of the developmental disability group was 44.25 years (SD = 14.69). In stark contrast, their mean functional age based on ADL limitations was 188.77 years (SD = 76.94). This difference of −144.52 years was highly significant, $t(91) = -17.11, p < 0.001$.

Table 3. Paired-Samples *t*-Test of Chronological Age vs. ADL-Based Functional Age (Developmental Disability Group).

Variable	Mean	Std. Deviation	*N*	*t*-Statistic	*df*	*p*-Value (2-Tailed)
Chronological Age	44.25	14.69	92			
Functional Age (ADL)	188.77	76.94	92	−17.11	91	<0.001
Mean Difference	−144.52	80.10	92			

This finding indicates that an average 44-year-old with a developmental disability exhibits a level of functional limitation in basic daily activities that is comparable to a person aged 188 years in the reference population. While the calculated age is outside the human lifespan, it serves as a powerful metric illustrating the extreme severity of the functional health gap between the two groups.

3.3. Functional Age Analysis for IADL

To determine if the pattern of accelerated aging extends to more complex daily tasks, the same functional age analysis was repeated for IADL.

3.3.1. Normative Model of IADL Limitation

A multiple linear regression was estimated on the reference group to establish a normative trajectory for IADL limitations. The results of this model are detailed in Table 4.

Table 4. Regression Model for Normative IADL Limitation Trajectory (Reference Group Only).

Predictor	B	Std. Error	β	*t*	*p*-Value
(Constant)	0.345	2.167		0.159	0.874
Age (years)	0.107	0.013	0.278	8.313	<0.001
Sex (Male)	0.142	0.271	0.015	0.525	0.600
Education Level	−0.004	0.134	−0.001	−0.032	0.974
Marital Status (Partnered)	−0.263	0.289	−0.028	−0.908	0.364
Household Income (ln)	0.443	0.219	0.066	2.025	0.043
Disability Severity (Severe)	3.665	0.273	0.359	13.443	<0.001

Note: Dependent Variable = IADL Limitation Score. $N = 1251$. $R^2 = 0.158$.

The overall model was highly significant, $F(6, 1244) = 38.97, p < 0.001$, explaining 15.8% of the variance in IADL scores ($R^2 = 0.158$). Similarly to the ADL model, both chronological age (B = 0.107, $p < 0.001$) and disability severity (B = 3.665, $p < 0.001$) were strong, positive predictors of IADL limitation. Household income was also a significant predictor (B = 0.443, $p = 0.043$). The coefficients from this model were used to derive the normative formula for calculating IADL-based functional age.

3.3.2. Comparison of Chronological and Functional Age

The IADL-based functional age was subsequently calculated for each of the 92 individuals in the developmental disability group. A paired-samples *t*-test was then performed to compare their chronological age with their newly calculated functional age.

As shown in Table 5, the results confirmed a significant and substantial gap, consistent with the ADL findings. The mean chronological age of the group was 44.25 years (SD = 14.69), while their mean functional age based on IADL limitations was 155.55 years (SD = 55.88). The mean difference of −111.30 years was highly statistically significant, $t(91) = -17.86$, $p < 0.001$.

Table 5. Paired-Samples *t*-Test of Chronological Age vs. IADL-Based Functional Age (Developmental Disability Group).

Variable	Mean	Std. Deviation	*N*	*t*-Statistic	*df*	*p*-Value (2-Tailed)
Chronological Age	44.25	14.69	92			
Functional Age (IADL)	155.55	55.88	92	−17.86	91	<0.001
Mean Difference	−111.30	59.78	92			

This result demonstrates that the functional disadvantage extends robustly to instrumental tasks. On average, a 44-year-old with a developmental disability shows a level of functioning in complex daily activities comparable to that of a 155-year-old with another type of disability. This provides a second, powerful line of evidence supporting the concept of accelerated aging.

3.4. *Analysis of Chronic Illness Prevalence*

Finally, the analysis shifted from functional health to general health status, as measured by the presence and duration of a chronic illness. Given the ordinal nature of this outcome, the analytical approach differed from the functional age model. An ordinal logistic regression was first employed to assess the relationship between the predictor variables and the likelihood of reporting a longer duration of chronic illness.

3.4.1. Ordinal Logistic Regression Model

The results of the ordinal logistic regression are presented in Table 6. The overall model was statistically significant, indicating that the set of predictors reliably distinguished between levels of chronic illness ($\chi^2(8) = 25.40$, $p = 0.001$). Chronological age ($p = 0.004$), education level ($p = 0.008$), and household income ($p = 0.021$) were all significant predictors.

Table 6. Ordinal Logistic Regression Model Predicting Duration of Chronic Illness.

Predictor	Estimate (B)	Std. Error	Wald	*df*	*p*-Value
Threshold [Illness = 0]	−4.396	2.231	3.882	1	0.049
Threshold [Illness = 1]	−4.271	2.230	3.667	1	0.055
Threshold [Illness = 2]	−4.253	2.230	3.638	1	0.056
Location					
Age (centered)	0.063	0.022	8.297	1	0.004
Education Level	0.443	0.167	7.026	1	0.008
Household Income (ln)	−0.588	0.254	5.359	1	0.021
Disability Type (Non-Dev)	−0.210	0.420	0.249	1	0.617
Sex (Female)	0.280	0.280	1.002	1	0.317
Marital Status (Unpartnered)	−0.347	0.369	0.882	1	0.348
Disability Severity (Mild)	−0.325	0.339	0.920	1	0.337

Note: $N = 283$. Model −2 Log Likelihood = 395.156. Nagelkerke $R^2 = 0.111$.

Crucially, the main effect for Disability Type was not statistically significant ($p = 0.617$). This finding suggests that, after controlling for age, severity, and other socioeconomic factors, there is no significant difference in the underlying likelihood of having a long-term chronic illness between the developmental disability group and the reference group.

3.4.2. Comparison of Predicted Probabilities

To illustrate the practical implications of this non-significant finding, predicted probabilities were calculated based on the model for a representative individual: a 50-year-old male with a severe disability, a high school education, and an average household income.

As shown in Table 7, the results confirm the lack of a substantial health gap for this outcome. For an individual with a developmental disability, the predicted probability of having a chronic illness lasting six months or more was 63.5%. For an otherwise identical individual with a non-developmental disability, the corresponding probability was 58.5%. This small, 5-percentage-point difference aligns with the statistical non-significance of the disability type variable in the regression model.

Table 7. Predicted Probability of Chronic Illness Status by Disability Type.

Chronic Illness Status	Developmental Disability	Other Disabilities
No Illness	33.3%	38.1%
<3 months of treatment	2.8%	3.0%
3–6 months of treatment	0.4%	0.4%
6+ months of treatment	63.5%	58.5%

Note: Probabilities calculated for a 50-year-old male with severe disability, average income, and high school education.

Thus, while the analyses for ADL and IADL provide strong evidence for accelerated functional aging, this pattern does not extend to the general prevalence of long-term chronic illness.

4. Discussion

4.1. Interpretation of Key Findings

The most striking result of this study is the massive gap in functional age between adults with developmental disabilities and the normative trajectory derived from individuals with other types of disabilities. While the average chronological age of the developmental disability group was just 44.25 years, their functional age based on ADL limitations was 188.77 years, and 155.55 years based on IADL limitations. Both differences were highly significant (ADL: $t(91) = -17.11, p < 0.001$; IADL: $t(91) = -17.86, p < 0.001$). This indicates that a middle-aged adult with a developmental disability exhibits a level of functional limitation comparable to someone over 100 years older in the reference population—a finding that powerfully operationalizes the concept of accelerated functional aging [19]. It is critical to interpret this "functional age" not as a literal biological prediction but as a statistical index of disparity. The extreme values serve to quantify the immense scale of the functional health gap when mapped against a normative trajectory, illustrating a severe, early onset functional disadvantage.

Notably, this disparity is not simply a product of disease accumulation in old age. The descriptive data revealed that, although individuals with developmental disabilities were significantly younger on average than their peers ($p < 0.001$), they nonetheless reported significantly worse IADL scores ($p < 0.001$) and similar, albeit not statistically different, ADL limitations ($p = 0.072$). When age, income, and other confounders were controlled for in the functional age model, these underlying disparities became even more pronounced, suggesting a persistent and severe functional disadvantage that begins early in the life course.

These findings align with extensive clinical research indicating that people with developmental disabilities often experience early and persistent functional impairment that differs from typical aging patterns [16,19,20]. Down syndrome provides a key example, where the manifestation of functional regression and neurodegenerative symptoms can commence as early as the third decade of life [12,34,35]. These impairments are often lifelong and may be compounded by a "cycle of disadvantage," including limited access to habilitative services, social exclusion, and inadequate aging-in-place supports, which further exacerbates health inequities [24,36,37]. Building upon the argument that midlife is a critical period for study [38], this research demonstrates that for adults with developmental disabilities, it is a period in which significant health inequities are already firmly established.

In contrast to the profound functional limitations, the prevalence of chronic illness did not differ significantly between groups after controlling for age and other covariates (p = 0.617). The predicted probability analysis confirmed this, showing only a small and statistically non-significant difference in the likelihood of reporting long-term illness between the groups. At first glance, this might suggest that individuals with developmental disabilities do not bear an elevated general health burden. However, this interpretation warrants significant caution, as it may reflect systemic healthcare inequities rather than true health parity.

A substantial body of literature has highlighted that diagnostic overshadowing—where clinicians attribute physical symptoms to an individual's primary disability rather than investigating for co-occurring conditions—can lead to the underdiagnosis of treatable illnesses in this population [5,23]. This is a well-documented barrier that can suppress reported prevalence rates of common conditions like hypertension, diabetes, and gastrointestinal disorders [39]. Additionally, communication challenges, limited health literacy, and systemic barriers to preventive care further distort the accurate reporting and diagnosis of chronic conditions [26,40].

Moreover, the demographic differences between the groups must be considered. The developmental disability group was, on average, nearly 30 years younger than the comparison group. Therefore, the very fact that they had statistically comparable levels of long-term illness, despite this large age gap, could itself be interpreted as evidence of an earlier onset of chronic conditions that remains statistically undetected due to the limitations of cross-sectional data or the competing risk of premature mortality. These findings reinforce the idea that accelerated aging appears clearly in functional limitations but not consistently across all areas of health. The functional disadvantage appears early and is severe, likely reflecting both inherent developmental factors and cumulative disadvantage, while the lack of disparity in chronic illness prevalence may be an artifact of underdiagnosis and other systemic barriers.

4.2. Implications for Policy

The findings of this study, particularly the profound gap between chronological and functional age highlight the need for the prudent reform and targeted strengthening of existing support structures to enhance their efficiency. The results underscore three key policy applications:

First, the findings challenge the efficacy of using chronological age as a primary gateway for accessing long-term services and supports. A shift to a function-based eligibility model is not a call for expanded entitlement, but a fiscally responsible measure to ensure that public resources are directed with precision to individuals with demonstrated need.

By aligning support with functional status rather than an arbitrary age, policymakers can better steward taxpayer funds, prevent waste, and ensure that interventions have the greatest possible impact.

Second, the early entrenchment of severe functional limitations calls for proactive, integrated support models that begin well before the conventional threshold of old age. This approach also aligns with principles of individual empowerment, allowing for more tailored, consumer-directed support packages that can adapt to changing needs over the life course [41]. Such systems are essential for upholding the rights of persons with disabilities, as outlined in the UN Convention on the Rights of Persons with Disabilities (CRPD), particularly Article 28 (right to an adequate standard of living and social protection).

Finally, the potential for underdiagnosis of chronic illness points to a critical need to improve diagnostic practices within the existing healthcare system. Diagnostic overshadowing leads to poor health outcomes and often results in more costly emergency interventions down the line. A prudent, low-cost strategy to address this is to promote the widespread adoption of evidence-based clinical guidelines and enhance provider education for the primary care of adults with developmental disabilities [39]. Investing in the capacity of the current healthcare infrastructure to provide competent care—thereby fulfilling Article 25 of the CRPD (right to health)—is a more sustainable solution than creating separate, parallel systems. By improving diagnostic accuracy, the existing system can operate more effectively, improve long-term health, and reduce the future fiscal burden associated with managing unaddressed chronic conditions.

4.3. Limitations and Future Research

While this study provides important insights, several limitations must be acknowledged. First, the analysis is based on cross-sectional data from a single wave of the KOWEPS. Although the functional age methodology provides a robust snapshot, longitudinal data tracking the same individuals over time would be necessary to definitively measure the rate of decline and confirm the trajectories suggested here. Second, the measure of chronic illness was based on self-report of treatment duration, which may not capture undiagnosed conditions. The findings regarding chronic illness should therefore be interpreted with caution, as they may reflect disparities in healthcare access as much as true prevalence. Third, the developmental disability category is heterogeneous, encompassing a wide range of conditions and support needs. The current analysis, while informative, could not disaggregate between different types of developmental disabilities (e.g., intellectual disability vs. autism spectrum disorder) due to sample size constraints. Fourth, a formal sensitivity analysis was not performed to test the robustness of the model estimates. Collectively, these limitations, including the small focal group size and potential for survivorship bias, mean the findings should be viewed as indicative of a profound disparity rather than as definitive, generalizable estimates.

Future research should prioritize longitudinal analysis to track health and functional trajectories over time. Additionally, studies incorporating direct health measures (e.g., biomarkers) alongside self-reported data could help disentangle the effects of inherent functional limitations from the impact of undiagnosed chronic disease, providing a clearer picture of the mechanisms driving the health disparities observed in this study. Lastly, the finding that chronic illness prevalence is not higher among people with developmental disabilities deserves further investigation—especially into diagnostic access, survivorship bias, and cause-of-death data.

5. Conclusions

This study set out to examine whether adults with developmental disabilities exhibit signs of accelerated aging compared to individuals with other types of disabilities. The analysis revealed a pronounced and statistically significant disparity in functional ability, but not in general morbidity. Adults with developmental disabilities demonstrated functional profiles consistent with individuals several decades older, despite their relatively young chronological age. In contrast, the study did not find significant differences in the prevalence or duration of chronic illness between the developmental disability group and the reference group. This divergence suggests that the aging process in individuals with developmental disabilities may follow a unique path—marked more by a severe disadvantage in daily functioning than by an elevated burden of traditional chronic diseases.

Taken together, these findings emphasize the need to reconceptualize aging in the context of developmental disability. The results support a model of early onset functional decline, showing that limitations arise earlier and progress more severely, warranting earlier intervention, proactive support planning, and age-independent access to services. Standard age-based models of care and policy may be insufficient or even exclusionary when applied uniformly. This study reframes the concept of accelerated aging from a simple measure of a faster rate of decline to a more complex picture of early and severe functional disadvantage.

Funding: This research received no external funding.

Institutional Review Board Statement: The original data collection was conducted in accordance with the Declaration of Helsinki and approved by the Korea Institute for Health and Social Affairs (KIHASA) P202400045 (approved date 6 February 2024).

Informed Consent Statement: Informed consent was obtained from all subjects involved in the original study by the primary data collection team.

Data Availability Statement: The data analyzed in this study are available from the Korean Welfare Panel Study (KOWEPS) data repository. Access can be requested at: https://www.koweps.re.kr:442/login.do (accessed on 6 September 2024).

Acknowledgments: The author would like to express sincere gratitude to the Korea Institute for Health and Social Affairs and Seoul National University for providing the valuable data used in this research.

Conflicts of Interest: The author declares no conflicts of interest.

References

1. Garmany, A.; Yamada, S.; Terzic, A. Longevity leap: Mind the healthspan gap. *NPJ Regen. Med.* **2021**, *6*, 57. [CrossRef]
2. Hansen, M.; Kennedy, B.K. Does longer lifespan mean longer healthspan? *Trends Cell Biol.* **2016**, *26*, 565–568. [CrossRef]
3. Havercamp, S.M.; Scott, H.M. National health surveillance of adults with disabilities, parents with disabilities, and their children. *Disabil. Health J.* **2015**, *8*, 165–172. [CrossRef]
4. Torr, J.; Strydom, A.; Patti, P.; Jokinen, N. Aging in Down syndrome: Morbidity and mortality. *J. Policy Pract. Intellect. Disabil.* **2010**, *7*, 70–81. [CrossRef]
5. Krahn, G.L.; Hammond, L.; Turner, A. A cascade of disparities: Health and health care access for people with intellectual disabilities. *Ment. Retard. Dev. Disabil. Res. Rev.* **2006**, *12*, 70–82. [CrossRef]
6. van Heumen, L.; Munly, K.; Heyn, P. Aging with intellectual and developmental disabilities: A critical examination of supports for healthy aging. *Innov. Aging* **2021**, *5* (Suppl. 1), 224. [CrossRef]
7. McCarron, M.; Swinburne, J.; Burke, E.; McGlinchey, E.; Mulryan, N.; Andrews, V. *Growing Older with an Intellectual Disability in Ireland 2013: First Results from the Intellectual Disability Supplement to the Irish Longitudinal Study on Ageing*; Trinity College Dublin: Dublin, Ireland, 2013.

8. Stephens, M.M.; Herge, E.A.; Rene, R. Aging in adults with intellectual disabilities and severe and persistent mental illness. In *Reichel's Care of the Elderly: Clinical Aspects of Aging*; Busby-Whitehead, J., Durso, S.C., Arenson, C., Elon, R., Palmer, M.H., Reichel, W., Eds.; Cambridge University Press: Cambridge, UK, 2022; pp. 604–619.
9. Santos, F.H.; Zurek, J.; Janicki, M.P. Efficacy of healthy aging interventions for adults with intellectual and developmental disabilities: A systematic review. *Gerontologist* **2022**, *62*, e235–e252. [CrossRef] [PubMed]
10. Rimmer, J.H.; Yamaki, K. Obesity and intellectual disability. *Ment. Retard. Dev. Disabil. Res. Rev.* **2006**, *12*, 22–27. [CrossRef] [PubMed]
11. Tyrer, F.; Smith, L.K.; McGrother, C.W. Mortality in adults with moderate to profound intellectual disability: A population-based study. *J. Intellect. Disabil. Res.* **2007**, *50*, 520–527. [CrossRef]
12. Lott, I.T.; Head, E. Dementia in Down syndrome: Unique insights for Alzheimer disease research. *Nat. Rev. Neurol.* **2019**, *15*, 135–147. [CrossRef] [PubMed]
13. Widerström-Noga, E.; Finlayson, M.L. Aging with a disability: Physical impairment, pain, and fatigue. *Phys. Med. Rehabil. Clin. N. Am.* **2010**, *21*, 309–321. [CrossRef] [PubMed]
14. Fortea, J.; Zaman, S.H.; Hartley, S.; Rafii, M.S.; Head, E.; Carmona-Iragui, M. Alzheimer's disease associated with Down syndrome: A genetic form of dementia. *Lancet Neurol.* **2021**, *20*, 930–942. [CrossRef] [PubMed]
15. O'Leary, L.; Cooper, S.A.; Hughes-McCormack, L. Early death and causes of death of people with intellectual disabilities: A systematic review. *J. Appl. Res. Intellect. Disabil.* **2018**, *31*, 325–342. [CrossRef] [PubMed]
16. Hermans, H.; Evenhuis, H.M. Multimorbidity in older adults with intellectual disabilities. *Res. Dev. Disabil.* **2014**, *35*, 776–783. [CrossRef]
17. Katz, S.; Ford, A.B.; Moskowitz, R.W.; Jackson, B.A.; Jaffe, M.W. Studies of illness in the aged. The index of ADL: A standardized measure of biological and psychosocial function. *JAMA* **1963**, *185*, 914–919. [CrossRef]
18. Lawton, M.P.; Brody, E.M. Assessment of older people: Self-maintaining and instrumental activities of daily living. *Gerontologist* **1969**, *9*, 179–186. [CrossRef]
19. Hilgenkamp, T.I.M.; van Wijck, R.; Evenhuis, H.M. (Instrumental) activities of daily living in older adults with intellectual disabilities. *Res. Dev. Disabil.* **2011**, *32*, 1977–1987. [CrossRef]
20. Peterson, M.D.; Ryan, J.M.; Hurvitz, E.A.; Mahmoudi, E. Chronic conditions in adults with cerebral palsy. *JAMA* **2015**, *314*, 2303–2305. [CrossRef]
21. Majnemer, A.; Shevell, M.; Hall, N.; Poulin, C.; Law, M. Developmental and functional abilities in children with cerebral palsy as related to pattern and level of motor function. *J. Child. Neurol.* **2010**, *25*, 1236–1241. [CrossRef]
22. Strax, T.E.; Luciano, L.; Dunn, A.M.; Quevedo, J.P. Aging and developmental disability. *Phys. Med. Rehabil. Clin. N. Am.* **2010**, *21*, 419–427. [CrossRef]
23. Jopp, D.A.; Keys, C.B. Diagnostic overshadowing reviewed and reconsidered. *Am. J. Ment. Retard.* **2001**, *106*, 416–433. [CrossRef] [PubMed]
24. Krahn, G.L.; Fox, M.H. Health disparities of people with intellectual disabilities: What do we know and what can we do? *J. Appl. Res. Intellect. Disabil.* **2014**, *27*, 431–446.
25. McCarron, M.; Haigh, M.; McCallion, P. *Health, Wellbeing and Social Inclusion: Ageing with an Intellectual Disability in Ireland*; Trinity College Dublin: Dublin, Ireland, 2017.
26. Griffith, G.M.; Hastings, R.P. 'He's hard work, but he's worth it.' The experience of caregivers of individuals with intellectual disabilities and challenging behaviour: A meta-synthesis of qualitative research. *J. Appl. Res. Intellect. Disabil.* **2014**, *27*, 401–419. [CrossRef]
27. Murthy, S.; Parker Harris, S.; Hsieh, K. Formal support and service needs of family caregivers of adults with intellectual and/or developmental disabilities in India. *J. Appl. Res. Intellect. Disabil.* **2024**, *37*, e13235. [CrossRef]
28. Strydom, A.; Shooshtari, S.; Lee, L.; Raykar, V.; Torr, J.; Tsiouris, J.; Jokinen, N.; Courtenay, K.; Bass, N.; Sinnema, M.; et al. Dementia in older adults with intellectual disabilities—Epidemiology Presentation, and Diagnosis. *J. Policy Pract. Intellect. Disabil.* **2010**, *7*, 96–110. [CrossRef]
29. Haak, P.; Majnemer, A.; Rosenbaum, P.; Abrahamowicz, M. Development of functional abilities in children with cerebral palsy. *Dev. Med. Child. Neurol.* **2009**, *51*, 890–897.
30. Halfon, N.; Hochstein, M. Life course health development: An integrated framework for developing health, policy, and research. *Milbank Q.* **2002**, *80*, 433–479. [CrossRef]
31. Korea Institute for Health and Social Affairs; Seoul National University. *User's Guide for the 18th Wave of the Korean Welfare Panel Study*; Korea Institute for Health and Social Affairs: Sejong, Republic of Korea; Seoul National University: Seoul, Republic of Korea, 2023.
32. Morris, J.F.; Temple, W. Spirometric "lung age" estimation for motivating smoking cessation. *Prev. Med.* **1985**, *14*, 655–662. [CrossRef]

33. Cole, J.H.; Franke, K. Predicting age using neuroimaging: Innovative brain ageing biomarkers. *Trends Neurosci.* **2017**, *40*, 681–690. [CrossRef] [PubMed]
34. Bittles, A.H.; Glasson, E.J. Clinical, social, and ethical implications of changing life expectancy in Down syndrome. *Dev. Med. Child Neurol.* **2004**, *46*, 282–286. [CrossRef] [PubMed]
35. Silverman, W.P.; Zigman, W.B.; Krinsky-McHale, S.J.; Ryan, R.; Schupf, N. Intellectual disability, mild cognitive impairment, and risk for dementia. *J. Policy Pract. Intellect. Disabil.* **2013**, *10*, 245–251. [CrossRef] [PubMed]
36. Bigby, C.; Frawley, P. A new paradigm for the social inclusion of people with developmental disability across the life course. In *Social Inclusion and People with Developmental Disability*; Routledge: Abingdon, UK, 2020; pp. 1–24.
37. Emerson, E.; Hatton, C. The socio-economic circumstances of children at risk of disability in Britain. *Disabil. Soc.* **2007**, *22*, 563–580. [CrossRef]
38. Wang, S.; Phillips, D.; Lee, J. Disability prevalence in midlife (aged 55–65 years): Cross-country comparisons of gender differences and time trends. *Womens Midlife Health* **2021**, *7*, 1. [CrossRef]
39. Sullivan, W.F.; Berg, J.M.; Bradley, E.; Cheetham, T.; Denton, R.; Heng, J.; Hennen, B.; Joyce, D.; Kelly, M.; Korossy, M.; et al. Primary care of adults with developmental disabilities: Canadian consensus guidelines. *Can. Fam. Physician* **2011**, *57*, 541–553. [PubMed]
40. Ali, A.; Scior, K.; Ratti, V.; Strydom, A.; King, M.; Hassiotis, A. Discrimination and other barriers to accessing health care: Perspectives of patients with mild and moderate intellectual disability and their carers. *PLoS ONE* **2013**, *8*, e70855. [CrossRef] [PubMed]
41. Braddock, D.L.; Hemp, R.E.; Tanis, E.S.; Wu, J.; Haffer, L. *The State of the States in Intellectual and Developmental Disabilities*, 11th ed.; American Association on Intellectual and Developmental Disabilities: Silver Spring, MD, USA, 2017.

healthcare

MDPI

Article

Enhancing Inclusive Social, Financial, and Health Services for Persons with Disabilities in Saudi Arabia: Insights from Caregivers

Ghada Alturif [1], Wafaa Saleh [2,*], Hessa Alsanad [1] and Augustus Ababio-Donkor [3]

1 Department of Social Work, College of Humanities and Social Sciences, Princess Nourah bint Abdulrahman University, P.O. Box 84428, Riyadh 11671, Saudi Arabia; gaaltarif@pnu.edu.sa (G.A.); hassanad@pnu.edu.sa (H.A.)

2 School of Computing, Engineering and the Built Environment, Edinburgh Napier University, 10 Colinton Road, Edinburgh EH10 5DT, UK

3 Regional Transport Research and Education Centre, Kumasi (TRECK), Department of Civil Engineering, Kwame Nkrumah University of Science & Technology, Kumasi PMB UPO, Ghana; aadonkor@knust.edu.gh

* Correspondence: w.saleh@napier.ac.uk

Abstract

Background: Social and financial services are essential for the inclusion and well-being of people with disabilities (PWDs), who often rely on family caregivers to access these systems. In Saudi Arabia, where disability inclusion is a strategic goal under Vision 2030, understanding caregiver experiences is crucial to identifying service gaps and improving accessibility. **Objectives:** This study aimed to explore caregivers' perspectives on awareness, perceived barriers, and accessibility of social and financial services for PWDs in Saudi Arabia. The analysis is grounded in Andersen's Behavioural Model of Health Service Use and the WHO's International Classification of Functioning, Disability and Health (ICF) framework. **Methods:** A cross-sectional survey was conducted with 3353 caregivers of PWDs attending specialised day schools. The survey collected data on demographic characteristics, service awareness, utilisation, and perceived obstacles. Exploratory Factor Analysis (EFA) identified latent constructs, and Structural Equation Modelling (SEM) was used to test relationships between awareness, barriers, and accessibility. **Results:** Findings reveal that over 70% of caregivers lacked awareness of available services, and only about 3% had accessed them. Key challenges included technological barriers, complex procedures, and non-functional or unclear service provider platforms. Both User Barriers and Service Barriers were negatively associated with Awareness and Accessibility. Awareness, in turn, significantly predicted perceived Accessibility. Caregiver demographics, such as age, education, gender, and geographic location, also influenced awareness and service use. **Conclusions:** There is a pressing need for targeted awareness campaigns, accessible digital service platforms, and simplified service processes tailored to diverse caregiver profiles. Inclusive communication, decentralised outreach, and policy reforms are necessary to enhance service access and promote the societal inclusion of PWDs in alignment with Saudi Arabia's Vision 2030.

Keywords: people with disabilities (PWDs); caregivers; Saudi Arabia; service accessibility; structural equation modelling; vision 2030; social inclusion; disability services

1. Introduction, Background and the Literature Review

The United Nations Convention on the Rights of Persons with Disabilities (UNCRPD) defines individuals with disabilities as those experiencing long-term physical, mental, intellectual, or sensory impairments that, in interaction with various barriers, hinder their full and equal participation in society [1]. Approximately 15% of the global population—around 1 billion people—live with some form of disability [2]. People with disabilities (PWDs) often require support in navigating daily life and accessing essential services, with family members frequently assuming the role of primary caregivers [3,4].

Despite the growing recognition of the role caregivers play in supporting PWDs, their perspectives, particularly in relation to service accessibility, remain underexplored in the literature. Understanding these experiences is critical for developing inclusive policies and support systems that address the needs of both PWDs and their caregivers. This study addresses this gap by exploring caregivers' perceptions of financial and social service accessibility in Saudi Arabia.

To conceptually organise the key dimensions of service access and barriers, this study draws on two theoretical frameworks: the Andersen Behavioural Model of Health Services Use [5] and the World Health Organization's International Classification of Functioning, Disability and Health (ICF) [6].

The Andersen model suggests that the use of health and related services is influenced by three core components: predisposing characteristics, enabling resources, and perceived or evaluated need [5]. Informed by this model, the constructs Services Awareness (Awareness) and Service Accessibility (ServAcc) are conceptualised as representing enabling factors that facilitate or hinder service utilisation. Awareness captures caregiver awareness of support services such as financial aid or vocational training programs, while ServAcc reflects the structural and administrative ease or difficulty with which these services are accessed, including perceptions of availability and quality.

The ICF framework complements this by emphasising the interaction between individual health conditions and contextual factors, including environmental and personal influences, that shape functioning and participation [6]. Guided by this perspective, the constructs Service Barriers (ServBarrier) and User Barriers (UserBarrier) reflect external environmental constraints (e.g., bureaucratic processes, physical inaccessibility) and personal-level limitations (e.g., low income, lack of information), respectively.

Although these four constructs were initially derived through exploratory factor analysis, their categorisation is theoretically supported. Awareness and ServAcc, while both linked to enabling factors, are conceptually distinct: awareness is a prerequisite for access, and perceived service quality can influence uptake. Similarly, ServBarrier and UserBarrier align with the ICF's distinction between external and personal determinants of access. This theoretical grounding enhances the construct validity of the measurement model, as recommended in the scale development literature [7,8].

Previous studies also support this conceptual structure. For example, Turnbull and Turnbull [9], Dunst et al. [10], and Scherer et al. [11] emphasise the importance of empowering families of PWDs through awareness and family-centred service models. Hashemi et al. [12] and Mitra et al. [13] demonstrate structural and attitudinal barriers in health and transport service systems, particularly in low- and middle-income countries. Other research has identified barriers to financial inclusion, such as limited financial literacy, inaccessible environments, and discriminatory policies [14,15]. Other studies emphasised the cultural perceptions of disability and caregiving, which are critical to understanding the broader context of service access and utilisation. For example, persistent misconceptions that disabilities, particularly cognitive or intellectual disabilities, are caused by familial shame may discourage families from seeking formal diagnoses or support services. Caregivers, especially mothers, could also face social judgment as caregiving is often seen as a private family responsibility rather than a shared societal obligation. Such stigma can lead to delays in diagnosis, underutilisation of services, and reluctance to engage with public support systems. These situations highlight the importance of culturally sensitive policy and outreach strategies that not only expand service provision but also challenge deep-rooted social attitudes toward disability and caregiving [4].

In Saudi Arabia, similar issues have been identified. Alqahtani and Al-Jifree [16] examine barriers to social inclusion related to education and employment, while Alshaigi and Naji [17] highlight limited financial access for PWDs. Alshammari et al. [18] further explore employment discrimination and the lack of accommodations in the workplace and further explored employment discrimination and the lack of accommodations in the workplace. Other research [19,20] emphasise healthcare access challenges and stigma-related service limitations.

Despite ongoing reforms and increasing attention to disability inclusion in Saudi Arabia under Vision 2030, caregivers of people with disabilities (PWDs) continue to face considerable challenges in navigating social and financial support systems. While several programs and services exist, access to and effective utilisation of these services remain uneven and poorly understood from the perspective of caregivers, who often act as critical intermediaries in securing support for PWDs. This study seeks to address a central research question: What are the perspectives and experiences of caregivers of PWDs in Saudi Arabia regarding the accessibility and effectiveness of financial and social services? To investigate this question, we adopt Andersen's Behavioural Model of Health Service Use as a guiding conceptual framework. This model emphasises the role of predisposing, enabling, and need-related factors in shaping service utilisation behaviours. In doing so, we aim to explore how individual caregiver characteristics (e.g., age, gender, education), environmental barriers, and systemic factors influence both awareness of and access to disability-related services. Using a large-scale survey of 3353 caregivers of PWDs attending specialised day schools across the Kingdom, we apply a mixed-methods quantitative approach. We first use Exploratory Factor Analysis (EFA) to identify latent constructs related to service awareness, accessibility, and user- or system-level barriers. These constructs are then tested using Structural Equation Modelling (SEM) to analyse the relationships among key factors, providing a robust empirical basis to understand accessibility challenges and their policy implications.

Study Context: Saudi Arabia and Vision 2030

The study was conducted within the Kingdom of Saudi Arabia (KSA), a Middle Eastern country known for its vast oil reserves and significant geopolitical influence in the region, with Riyadh as its capital. The population is predominantly Arab and Sunni Muslim, with a significant expatriate community. Saudi society is deeply rooted in Islamic traditions, though recent reforms under the country's Vision 2030 aim to diversify the economy and promote sectors like tourism and technology, alongside enhancing women's rights and participation [21].

Vision 2030 also aims to provide equal opportunities for everyone, including PWDs, who make up 7.1% of the Saudi population [22]. The vision seeks to empower PWDs by ensuring their rights to health and personal care, rehabilitation services, and education through inclusive education, specialised services, and accessible infrastructure to ensure their independence and effective participation in Saudi society. This reflects the Kingdom's commitment to improving the quality of life for all its citizens to receive financial, social, and job opportunities [21].

According to statistics, in Saudi Arabia, there are 355,289 individuals with hearing disabilities, 30,155 with hyperactivity and distractions, 136,833 with motor disabilities, 23,282 with autism spectrum disorder, 19,428 with Down syndrome, and 610 with visual impairments, totalling 2,036,966 individuals with disabilities in the country [22]. This highlights the importance of implementing programs that protect and support their health, social care, education, and employment opportunities. In line with this, the 2030 Vision for Support to Persons with Disabilities has initiated several projects to promote their rights and enhance services for them.

Saudi Arabia's Vision 2030 is a transformative initiative aimed at diversifying the economy and enhancing the quality of life for all citizens, including PWDs. The vision emphasises inclusivity, accessibility, and empowerment to ensure that PWDs can participate fully in society across multiple dimensions. Additionally, Vision 2030 aims to enhance the quality and reach of social services by increasing financial assistance, expanding disability pensions and housing aid, improving rehabilitation services and specialised medical care, and addressing the stigma around disabilities through public education about PWD rights. Policy and governance reforms have also been considered to further strengthen disability rights through legislation and enforcement.

By integrating disability inclusion into its national agenda, Vision 2030 aims to create a more equitable and empowered society for PWDs. The success of these initiatives will depend on policy implementation, private sector collaboration, and sustained public awareness efforts.

This study distinguishes itself by focusing on the perspectives of carers and caregivers of PWDs in Saudi Arabia, a viewpoint that has been underrepresented in existing research. By employing a mixed-methods approach, the study integrates qualitative insights from caregivers with quantitative data analysis, offering a comprehensive understanding of the challenges faced in accessing social and financial services. The methodology provides a holistic view of the systemic barriers impacting both PWDs and their support networks.

Furthermore, the study aligns with Saudi Arabia's Vision 2030, which emphasises social inclusion and support for PWDs. The research evaluates the effectiveness of initiatives such as the national strategy featuring 23 initiatives for PWDs, the national program for the diagnosis and classification of disabilities, and the creation of a unified national registry and statistics database. By assessing these initiatives from the caregivers' perspectives, the study offers valuable insights into their implementation and impact, contributing to the ongoing efforts to enhance service accessibility and inclusivity for PWDs in the Kingdom.

2. Material and Methods

2.1. Introduction

This study draws upon two foundational models to guide its conceptual and analytical structure: the Andersen Behavioral Model of Health Services Use [5] and the World Health Organization's International Classification of Functioning, Disability and Health (ICF) [6]. These frameworks informed the identification and interpretation of the four constructs derived through exploratory factor analysis: Awareness of Services (Awareness), Service Barriers (ServBarrier), User Barriers (UserBarrier), and Service Accessibility (ServAcc).

Consistent with Andersen's model, Awareness and ServAcc represent enabling resources and perceived dimensions of access, which facilitate or hinder service utilisation. ServBarrier and UserBarrier correspond to external and personal contextual factors, respectively, which can constrain access, reflecting structural and individual-level challenges. The ICF framework further supports this categorization by highlighting how both environmental and personal elements interact to shape disability-related experiences and influence service engagement. Together, these theoretical foundations enhance the construct validity of our measurement model and ensure alignment with internationally recognized approaches to disability and service access research.

2.2. Data Collection

Data collection involved structured surveys designed to gather qualitative and quantitative data on various aspects related to caregivers and persons with disabilities (PWDs). To ensure that only one caregiver per child participated, we implemented unique identifiers and screening questions at the beginning of the survey. Additionally, recruitment was managed through service organisations that helped verify eligibility and avoid duplicate participation. We have now explicitly stated these measures in the methods section for clarity. Caregivers play a pivotal role in navigating the support systems available for PWDs, making their insights invaluable for assessing service gaps and barriers. The questionnaire is implemented in Arabic, the native language of respondents in the Kingdom of Saudi Arabia (KSA), and is organised into distinct sections to collect comprehensive information aligned with the research objectives:

1. Socio-Economic Variables: This section collects demographic and socio-economic data about the person with a disability (PWD), including age, gender, type of disability, and other relevant characteristics.
2. Caretaker Information: This section gathers details about the primary caretaker, such as age, gender, relationship to the PWD, income level, educational background, location and type of residence, and household structure.
3. Awareness of Available Services: This section assesses the respondent's awareness of services accessible to PWDs, encompassing educational, financial, civil, and legal services.
4. Accessibility of Services: This section evaluates the ease with which PWDs and their caretakers can access available services, considering factors such as physical accessibility, transportation, and communication.
5. Acceptability of Services: This section examines the suitability and cultural appropriateness of the services provided, including the attitudes of service providers and the perceived quality of services.
6. Barriers to Service Utilisation: This section identifies obstacles that hinder the effective use of available services by PWDs and their caretakers, such as financial constraints, lack of information, or discriminatory practices.

This structured approach ensures a comprehensive understanding of the factors influencing service utilisation among PWDs and their caretakers. In addition to the quantitative data collected from caregivers, this research also gathered qualitative insights from 70 service providers working in disability-related institutions. These qualitative data, while highly valuable, are not the focus of the current manuscript, which is centred on analysing caregiver perspectives through a quantitative context. The findings from the service providers are being analysed separately and will be presented in a forthcoming publication. This separation allows for a focused interpretation of each dataset. Future studies will aim to integrate both perspectives, caregivers and service providers, to offer a more holistic understanding of the barriers, needs, and service dynamics within the disability support system in Saudi Arabia.

2.3. Study Population and Sampling

The study targeted caregivers of PWDs attending specialised day schools across Saudi Arabia. These schools provide individualised education and therapeutic services, making them an ideal setting for capturing rich caregiver insights into service access and barriers. A stratified cluster sampling method was employed:

Phase 1 (Stratification): The country was divided into five regions, north, south, east, west, and central.

Phase 2 (Clustering): Educational and rehabilitation institutions within each region were treated as clusters.

Phase 3 (Random Sampling): Random selection of centres/schools, followed by random selection of caregiver respondents.

This multi-stage sampling approach yielded a final sample of 3353 respondents from 375 centres nationwide. The sampling ensured broad geographic coverage and high representativeness.

An electronic questionnaire was used to ensure anonymity and ease of participation. Informed consent was obtained digitally, and all ethical considerations, including confidentiality, voluntary participation, and data protection, were strictly observed in accordance with institutional research ethics.

2.4. Data Analysis

Data were analysed using SPSS version 26, AMOS version 23, and Microsoft Excel 365. The analytic strategy included descriptive and inferential statistics, Factor Analysis, and Structural Equation Modelling (SEM). Descriptive statistics were used to profile socio-demographics. An Exploratory Factor Analysis (EFA), Confirmatory Factor Analysis (CFA), and SEM were performed using SPSS and AMOS to validate the factor structure and test the hypothesised relationships among constructs. The model fit was assessed using Average Variance Extracted (AVE), Composite Reliability (CR), and Discriminant Validity through square root AVE comparison, in addition to Model Fit Indices such as CFI, TLI, RMSEA, and SRMR [23–25]. This robust analytical approach, supported by established psychological and methodological frameworks [26–28], ensured rigorous construct validation. Furthermore, the AMOS analysis was enhanced using the Master Validity plugin Tool to systematically test validity thresholds [29], providing insights into the multidimensional factors influencing service accessibility for PWDs in Saudi Arabia. In addition, the study is informed by broader literature on caregiver well-being, stigma, and inclusive practices [30–34], which provided conceptual grounding for interpreting key findings related to caregiver burden, systemic discrimination, and regional service disparities.

3. Analysis and Results

3.1. Descriptive

The study analysed data from 3353 responses of caregivers of PWDs of various Day Care Centres. The majority of respondents were males (62.2%), while females accounted for 37.8%. The distribution of the respondents' age is shown in Table 1. The majority of respondents are aged between 36 and 50 years (54.2%). Education levels among respondents (care takers) were relatively high, with the majority holding a university degree (43.5%). Secondary education (31.4%) and primary education (7.9%) were also represented. This suggested that many respondents had a certain level of education. The majority of respondents resided in cities (78.5%), with those in the villages constituting the minority (21.5%). The monthly household income of respondents varied, with the majority (38%) earning between SAR 5000 and 10,000.

Table 1. Characteristics of caregivers.

Item	Description	Frequency	Percentage
Gender	Female	1268	37.8
	Male	2085	62.2
Age	Under 20	97	2.9
	21–35 yrs	992	29.6
	36–50 yrs	1816	54.2
	51 yrs and Older	448	13.4
Education	Primary	266	7.9
	Secondary	1052	31.4
	Average	347	10.3
	University	1460	43.5
	Uneducated	117	3.5
	Other	111	3.3
Income	<5000 SAR	1120	33.4
	6000–10,000 SAR	1274	38.0
	11,000–15,000 SAR	679	20.3
	>16,000 SAR	280	8.4

As shown in Figure 1a, the types of disabilities among persons with disabilities (PWDs) were varied, with Autism being the most common (34.5%), followed by mental disabilities (17.9%) and physical activity-related disabilities (14.6%). Figure 1b illustrates the relationship between caregivers and PWDs, which was predominantly familial: mothers accounted for 68.6% and fathers for 19.8%. Other caregivers included siblings (5.7%) and other relatives (4.5%). It is important to note here that while a majority of the reported primary caregivers were mothers of persons with disabilities (PWDs), a substantial portion of the survey responses were submitted by male household members. This reflects a common practice in the Saudi context, where male guardians often act as the official respondents in formal or online interactions, even when the day-to-day caregiving responsibilities are primarily undertaken by female family members. As such, the gender of the respondent does not always align with the actual caregiver's identity. Figure 1c presents the age distribution of PWDs, with the highest proportion aged 6–10 years (41.4%), indicating a young population among those surveyed.

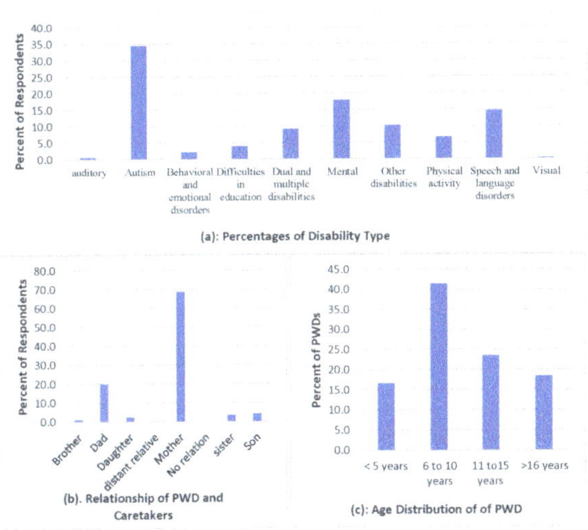

Figure 1. Demographics.

Figure 2 presents the level of awareness of the respondents of the available social services. The Figure shows a severe awareness gap, across various social and health services, which threatens progress toward Saudi Vision 2030 goals. To gain an in-depth understanding necessary to close this gap, the study investigates this observation further through cross-tabulations, factor analysis and structural equation modelling.

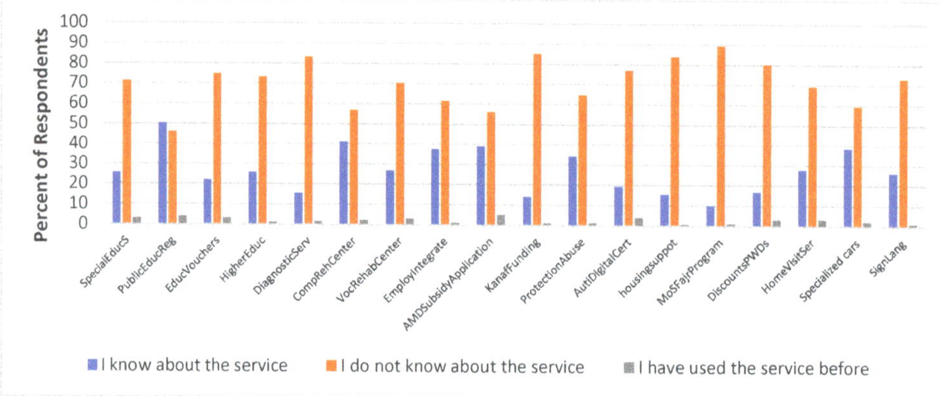

Figure 2. Awareness level of existing social services.

The study also revealed a general lack of awareness about educational services, such as the provision of educational vouchers in cooperation with private education for PWDs. A total of 74.7% of respondents (caretakers) indicated a lack of awareness of the availability of this service, with only 3.3% indicating they have used the service before. Older respondents exhibited significantly lower levels of awareness of these services, highlighting the need for targeted campaigns among this age group. Additionally, the study found that 73.1% of respondents were unaware of higher education and scholarship opportunities for PWDs at private colleges and universities. This observation was not considered a major issue since all the PWDs in this study are still below the higher education age. Meanwhile, there is a need for increased promotion and awareness of these opportunities among the families of PWDs for future eventualities.

The high level of knowledge gap regarding existing educational support programmes for PWDs presents a significant challenge to the achievement of Vision 2030 of Saudi Arabia, which states that "We will also enable those of our people with disabilities to receive the education and job opportunities that will ensure their independence and integration as effective members of society. They will be provided with all the facilities and tools required to put them on the path to commercial success" [35].

The survey also revealed a significant lack of awareness regarding key social and health services among caregivers, as illustrated in Figure 2. Specifically, 83% were unaware of measurement and diagnostic services, 56.9% were unaware of comprehensive rehabilitation centre services, 70.2% lacked awareness of vocational rehabilitation centre services, and 61.5% were unaware of programmes aimed at integrating PWDs into the labour market. This substantial knowledge gap not only limits access to essential support but also contributes to the continued marginalisation of persons with disabilities. Particularly concerning is the limited awareness of employment inclusion programmes, which may partly explain the disproportionately high unemployment rates among PWDs in Saudi Arabia [3]. 29.8% A comprehensive awareness campaign is therefore crucial to educate the public about the available social services and promote inclusion and accessibility in all aspects of life, ultimately bridging the gap towards a more equitable society. Moreover, the study found that 56% of respondents were unfamiliar with subsidy applications for assistive medical devices, with females and university graduates showing significantly higher usage. This suggests that there is a need for targeted awareness campaigns among males and those with lower levels of education, who may face additional barriers to accessing these services. The survey also revealed a lack of awareness about Kanaf funding for PWDs (85% unaware), protection from abuse services for PWDs (64.6% unaware), digital certification services for Autism (76.8% unaware), housing support services for PWDs (83.8% unaware), and the Ministry of Sports' Fajr Program for sports rehabilitation (89.1% unaware). These findings highlight the need for increased awareness and education about these services among the general population and for targeted campaigns to reach those who may be most in need of these services.

The survey found that 80.1% of respondents were unaware of special offers and discounts for PWDs, with rural residents showing significantly lower awareness. Overall, the survey findings highlight the need for a comprehensive awareness campaign to educate the public about the various social and financial services available to PWDs, and to promote inclusion and accessibility in all aspects of life. All service centres could be equipped to educate or create awareness about all the available services, while also providing hotlines for seeking assistance. A more inclusive and equitable society for all could be worked towards by addressing these knowledge gaps and promoting awareness and understanding.

Modern technology, for instance, intended to facilitate access to these services was found to pose a significant barrier for 29.8% of respondents (Figure 3), with a notable 31.5% remaining indifferent. This suggested a lack of understanding or familiarity with modern technology among a substantial family of PWDs. In their study [36], the researchers made a similar observation, which indicated that technology designed to provide assistance for PWDs and their caretakers rather presented significant barriers owing to the complexities and poor design quality. Previous research has noted that the simplest of assistive technologies were more likely to be successfully integrated into the daily routines of PWDs and their caretakers [37–39]. The literature recommends several measures to enhance the adoption and effective use of assistive technologies by PWDs and their caretakers in accessing support services. These measures include short courses or workshops, online learning platforms, demonstrations of technology for families, hands-on practice with technology usage prior to implementation, support networks for post-implementation troubleshooting, and designated "super-users" at various levels for continued support and mentorship [40,41].

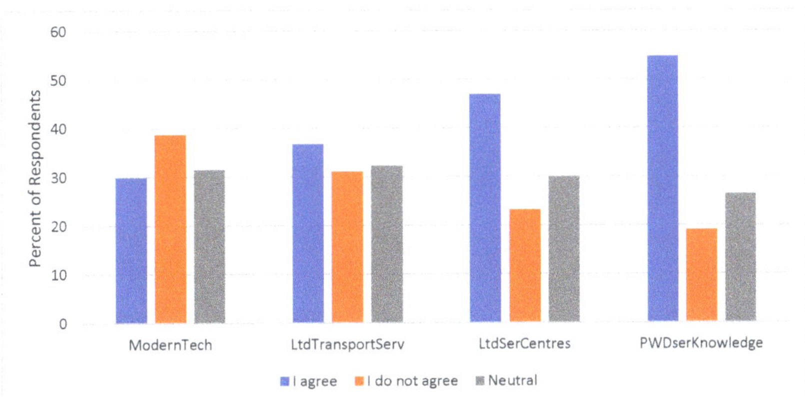

Figure 3. Perception of user barriers.

The education level of caretakers emerged as a critical factor in modern technology usage, with those with lower education more likely to struggle with modern technology. Similarly, Older respondents (51 and above) also faced significant challenges with modern technology usage. The struggle with modern technology usage due to age and low education is widely reported in the literature [42,43], emphasising the importance of age-friendly solutions or developing alternative solutions to digital technology deficiency.

Lack of transportation to service providers was another significant barrier, affecting 36.7% of respondents. University-educated individuals were less likely to face this challenge. It is believed that members of this group could be in employment and consequently have access to transportation. The availability of service providers in the area was a significant concern, with 46.9% of respondents citing fewer branches or distant locations as a barrier. Rural residents (villages) were more likely to face this challenge, emphasising the need for decentralised service provision and outreach programs to bridge the gap.

The results indicate that while the majority (45.8% of respondents) had no concerns with the websites of service providers, 23.5% of respondents noted that the websites of service providers are either incomplete or not working, while 30.7% were indifferent. Again, 33.5% of the respondents noted that the procedures and conditions for service accessibility provided by service providers were not clear. Older respondents exhibited significant agreement with the assertion, indicating the difficulties they go through in navigating the procedures and conditions before accessing the services. Similarly, urban dwellers significantly agreed with the assertion. 50.5% of respondents agreed that the conditions and procedures for service accessibility present several difficulties. This was a general assertion and independent of gender. However, it is particularly pronounced among the older age groups of 50 years and above. Additionally, 43.1% of respondents were of the view that the service providers have no knowledge of their needs, indicating gaps in service delivery. The place of residence was found to have a significant influence on this assertion. A higher proportion of urban than rural dwellers share this view.

Furthermore, the majority (59.3%) of respondents believe the services provided require some level of improvement in order to meet the needs of PWDs. More males than females share this opinion (p-value = 0.049) at a 0.05 significance level. Older respondents also call for the improvement of the services. In addition, 37.2% of respondents believe the current terms do not adequately reflect the emerging socio-economic contexts (see Figure 4), with the influence of gender on this assertion being statistically insignificant (p-value = 0.264).

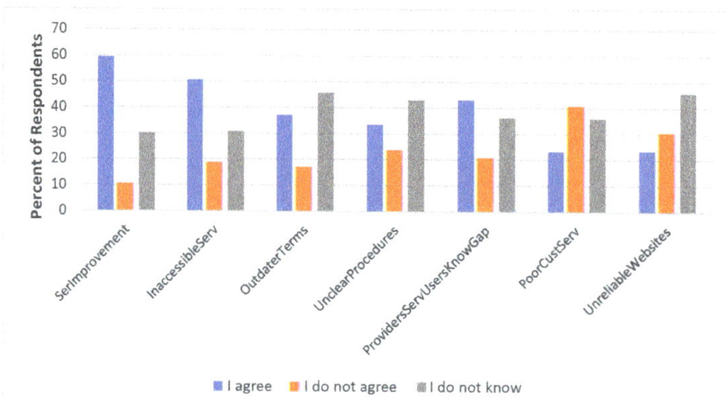

Figure 4. Perception of service quality.

3.2. Factor Analysis and Measurement Model Development

To explore the underlying dimensions of caregivers' perceptions regarding access to services for persons with disabilities (PWDs), an exploratory factor analysis (EFA) was conducted using SPSS (version 26.0). Principal Component Analysis (PCA) with Promax rotation was employed to extract latent constructs from the attitudinal items. This analytical strategy aligns with the Andersen Behavioural Model of Health Services Use [5], which organises determinants of service utilisation into predisposing factors, enabling resources, and perceived or evaluated needs. The extracted components reflect this structure, capturing both barriers and facilitators relevant to caregivers' service experiences.

Table 2 presents the results of the exploratory factor analysis (EFA). The EFA yielded a four-factor solution that accounted for 50.27% of the total variance, indicating a moderate but interpretable model fit [8]. The Kaiser-Meyer-Olkin (KMO) measure of sampling adequacy (value = 0.812) and Bartlett's Test of Sphericity ($\chi^2(153) = 1342.56$, $p < 0.001$) confirmed the suitability of the data for factor analysis. Although the overall explained variance (50.27%) is below the ideal threshold of 60%, it remains within the acceptable range for social science research [44]. Given the conceptual coherence of the constructs and alignment with the Andersen model, the factor solution is retained for subsequent structural analysis. The four extracted factors are discussed below:

Table 2. F ctor Loadings, Reliability and Validity Indicators of the Extracted Constructs.

Construct	Code	Variable *	Item Loading	Cronbach's Alpha (α)	Composite Reliability (CR)	Average Variance Extracted (AVE)
			>0.5	>0.7	>0.6	>0.5
Awareness (Awareness of Services)	SS1	Fajr Program	0.770	0.902	0.895	0.379
	SS2	Housing Support	0.730			
	SS3	Kanaf Funding	0.680			
	SS4	PWD Discounts	0.530			
	SS5	Employment Integration	0.620			
	SS6	Comprehensive Rehab Centre	0.540			
	SS7	Higher Education Access	0.710			
	SS8	Vocational Rehab Centres	0.620			
	SS9	Sign Language Support	0.730			
	SS10	Abuse Protection	0.562			
	SS11	Specialised Care	0.520			
	SS12	Diagnostics Services	0.720			
	SS13	Home Visit Service	0.580			
	SS14	Education Vouchers	0.520			
ServBarrier	SB1	Unclear Procedures	0.840	0.835	0.826	0.425
	SB2	Outdated Service Terms	0.791			
	SB3	Knowledge Gap in Service Use	0.723			
	SB4	Poor Customer Service	0.663			
	SB5	Physical Inaccessibility	0.647			
	SB6	Unreliable Websites	0.643			
	SB7	Lack of Service Improvement	0.630			
ServAcc	SA1	Health Services Quality	0.750	0.82	0.824	0.540
	SA2	Economic Support Services Quality	0.825			
	SA3	Social/Legal Services Quality	0.820			
	SA4	Educational Services Quality	0.778			

Table 2. *Cont.*

Construct	Code	Variable *	Item Loading	Cronbach's Alpha (α)	Composite Reliability (CR)	Average Variance Extracted (AVE)
			>0.5	>0.7	>0.6	>0.5
UserBarrier	UB1	Comfort with Modern Technology	0.710	0.624	0.638	3427
	UB2	Limited Transport Availability	0.672			
	UB3	Limited Service Centres Nearby	0.570			

* We recommend that future studies carefully identify and select constructs that not only meet statistical thresholds but are also appropriately aligned with the evolving service landscape and conceptual relevance to the local context. As service delivery systems mature and caregiver awareness improves, these constructs may yield stronger psychometric properties and offer deeper insight into access-related challenges for persons with disabilities.

Awareness of Services (Awareness): Reflects the caregivers' knowledge, understanding, and recognition of available social, financial, and support services provided for persons with disabilities (PWDs). These include government programs such as Kanaf funding, housing support, rehabilitation centres, and educational vouchers. Within the Andersen Behavioural Model, this factor aligns with "enabling resources", which influence an individual's ability to access health and social care [5]. Awareness is a prerequisite for effective access, as caregivers must first know what services exist before they can pursue or utilise them.

Service Barriers (ServBarrier): Refers to systemic and structural obstacles in service provision, such as unclear procedures, outdated regulations, or inefficient customer service, that hinder effective utilisation. These barriers reflect external environmental factors in Andersen's model and the environmental context domain of the WHO ICF framework [5,6].

User Barriers (UserBarrier): Captures individual-level limitations that impede caregivers' ability to seek or access services, including limited service knowledge, low digital literacy, or transportation difficulties. This aligns with predisposing and personal characteristics in Andersen's framework and contextual and personal factors in the ICF.

Service Accessibility (ServAcc): Reflects caregivers' perceived ease, availability, and quality of services across health, social, economic, and educational domains. This construct corresponds to evaluated need and enabling access in Andersen's model and represents accessibility and acceptability within the WHO ICF framework.

Factor loadings for each variable and the Cronbach's alpha values for each extracted construct are reported in Table 2. Discriminant and convergent validity were further examined using SPSS AMOS 23.0 to assess the robustness of extracted constructs (refer to 3.3). The reliability of the extracted constructs was established using Cronbach's alpha values exceeding the 0.70 threshold [7] and Composite Reliability (CR) values above 0.60 [8]. Average Variance Extracted (AVE) of some of the constructs (e.g., Awareness, UserBarrier) was below the threshold of 0.50. However, as noted by [23], if CR exceeds 0.60, convergent validity can still be considered acceptable despite low AVE.

3.3. Measurement Model Reliability and Validity

A four-factor measurement model (Figure 5) was assessed for their validity by conducting a confirmatory factor analysis (CFA) to test the measurement model using SPSS AMOS 23.0. The model fitness was evaluated based on the indices and thresholds presented in Table 3 [8].

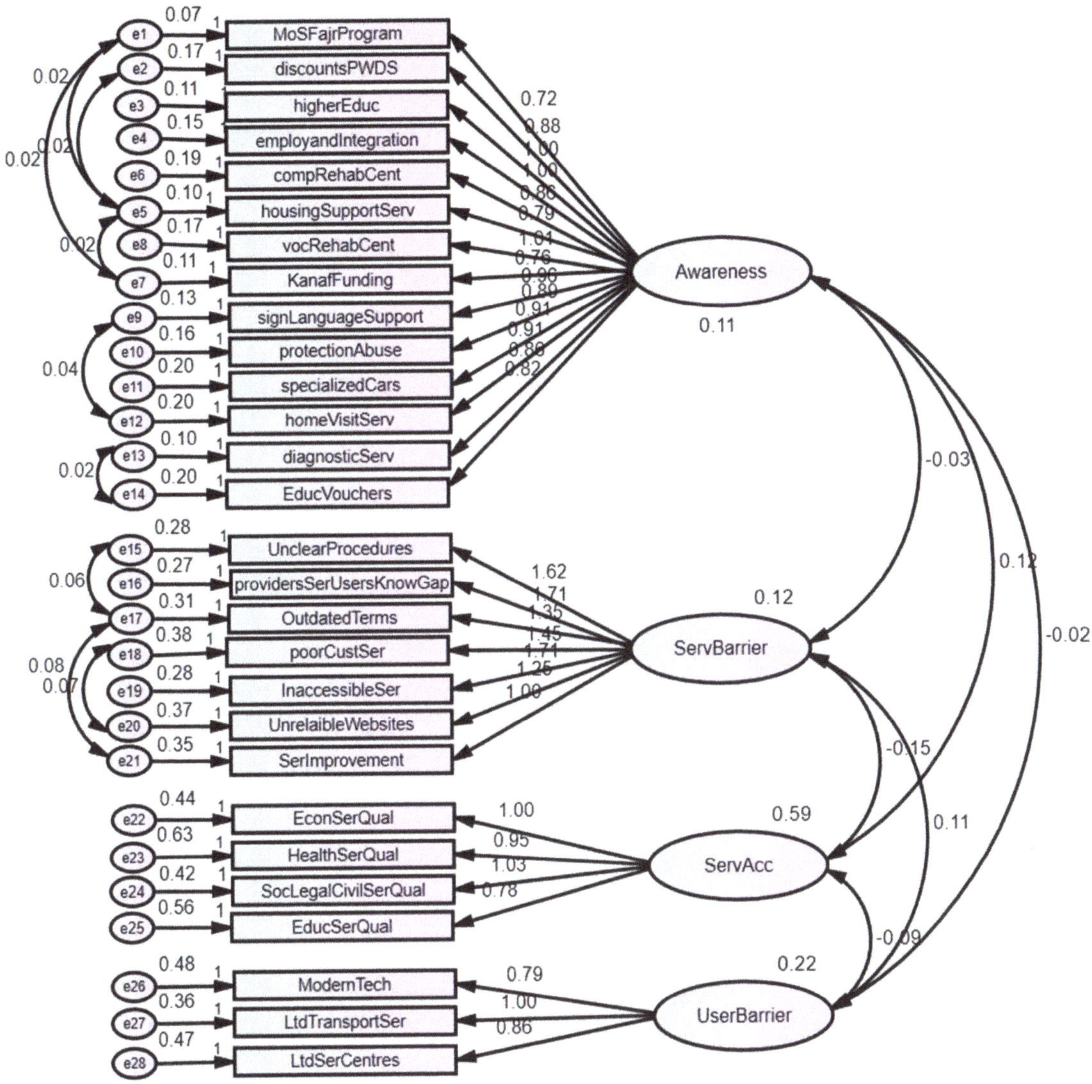

Figure 5. Measurement Model.

Table 3. Measurement Model Fit.

Model Fitness	Chi-Square Group			Absolute Fit		Incremental Fit		Standard RMR
Fitness Indexes	C_{min}	*df*	C_{min}/df	*CFI*	*RMSEA*	*GFI*	*TLI*	*SRMR*
Threshold	>0.05		<5	>0.90	<0.08	>0.90	>0.90	<0.08
This model	1504.150	335	4.490	0.964	0.032	0.968	0.959	0.027

In addition to model fit indices in Table 3 above, other psychometric properties of the scales, such as composite reliability and validity, were examined. As shown in Table 2 above, in terms of composite reliability (CR), the scales exceed the recommended cutoff value of 0.60; thus, it is reasonable to conclude that the scales are reliable [24]. However, the Average Variance Extracted (AVE) values for the constructs were all less than the required threshold of 0.5 except Service Accessibility "ServAcc", which had an AVE of 0.540. However, [23] argue that due to the strictness of the AVE, reliability can often be established on the basis of the CR alone. Furthermore, Table 2 shows that each of the item loadings is greater than 0.50. Therefore, on the basis of the recommendation of [23], the authors assumed good model fit, reliability, convergent validity, and discriminant validity for the measurement model.

3.4. Structural Model

Based on theoretical considerations, we hypothesised that Service accessibility (SerAcc) will be influenced by service awareness (Awareness), service barriers (ServBarrier) and user barriers (userBarrier). Hence, we model service accessibility (SerAcc) with service awareness (Awareness), service barriers (ServBarrier) and user barrier (userBarrier). The results of the analysis are also shown in Figure 6 below. The proposed model was found to fit the data satisfactorily. The fitness indices shown in Table 4 below are all within acceptable limits [23].

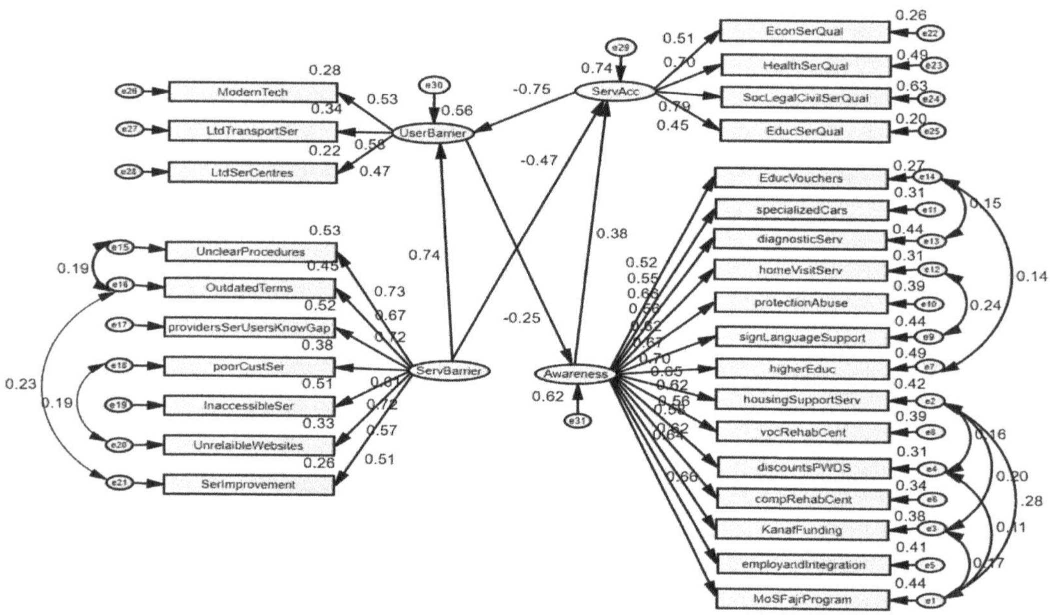

Figure 6. Structural Model (standardised Estimates).

Table 4. Model Fit Indices for the Structural Equation Model.

Model Fitness	Chi-Square Group			Absolute Fit		Incremental Fit		Standard RMR
Fitness Indexes	C_{min}	*df*	C_{min}/df	CFI	RMSEA	GFI	TLI	SRMR
Threshold	>0.05		<5.0	>0.90	<0.08	>0.90	>0.90	<0.08
This model	1449.036	334	4.338	0.965	0.032	0.969	0.961	0.030

The squared multiple correlations were seen to have good values for the three endogenous constructs of User Barriers, Service Accessibility and Social Services in the first-order SEM.

The structural equation model demonstrated strong overall fit, as shown in Table 4, with a chi-square/df ratio of 4.338, which falls within the commonly accepted threshold of less than 5.0 for complex models [23,24,44–46]. Although the chi-square test can be sensitive to large sample sizes and may overestimate lack of fit, additional indices confirm the model's robustness. Specifically, the model achieved excellent values across several criteria: CFI = 0.964, RMSEA = 0.032, GFI = 0.969, TLI = 0.961, and SRMR = 0.030, indicating good absolute and incremental fit. The model also demonstrated strong explanatory power, with squared multiple correlations (R^2) of 0.74 for Service Accessibility, 0.56 for User Barriers, and 0.62 for Service Awareness, as shown in Table 4. These values indicate that the model explained 74%, 56%, and 62% of the variance in these constructs, respectively.

Table 5 presents the final unstandardised regression weights and associated *p*-values, confirming that all structural relationships among the latent constructs were statistically significant ($p < 0.05$). These findings support the model's validity in capturing the factors that influence service awareness and accessibility among caregivers of persons with disabilities in Saudi Arabia.

Table 5. Structural Equation Model Estimates for Path Relationships Among 4, Accessibility, User Barriers, and Awareness.

			Unstandardised Estimate	*SE*	*CR*	*p*-Value
ServAcc	<---	ServBarrier	−0.939	0.046	−20.222	***
UserBarrier	<---	ServBarrier	0.992	0.051	19.599	***
UserBarrier	<---	ServAcc	0.127	0.020	6.279	***
Awareness	<---	UserBarrier	−0.155	0.016	−9.776	***
ServAcc	<---	Awareness	0.919	0.050	18.372	***

*** $p < 0.001$.

Theoretical and Contextual Interpretation of Key Paths:

Service Barriers → Service Accessibility ($\beta = -0.939$):

As expected, systemic obstacles such as poor service coordination, bureaucratic delays, and inaccessible websites severely impair individuals' perception of service accessibility. This aligns with the Andersen Behavioural Model, which classifies enabling resources (or lack thereof) as critical determinants of access. In the ICF framework, these reflect environmental barriers that constrain participation.

Service Barriers → User Barriers ($\beta = +0.992$):

Institutional inefficiencies directly contribute to individual-level challenges—such as difficulty reaching service centres or using digital tools—emphasising a spillover effect from system to user level. This supports the Social Ecological Model logic, which sees personal barriers as shaped by broader institutional and structural contexts.

Service Accessibility → User Barriers ($\beta = +0.127$):

Interestingly, this small but positive path suggests that even when services are more accessible, user-level barriers (e.g., limited awareness or technology discomfort) may persist. In the Saudi context, this could reflect a lag between service provision and user capability, indicating the need for user support and education to match service expansion.

User Barriers → Awareness of Services ($\beta = -0.155$):

This negative association implies that greater personal barriers correlate with reduced awareness of available services. Rather than compensatory behaviour (i.e., seeking more information when challenged), this finding likely reflects information exclusion—where individuals facing transportation, literacy, or digital access barriers are less likely to encounter or comprehend service information. This underscores a crucial access-to-information gap.

Awareness → Service Accessibility (β = +0.919):

Awareness emerged as a strong positive predictor of perceived accessibility, reinforcing the notion that information is a powerful enabler. According to Andersen's model, awareness is a form of enabling resource, while in the ICF framework, it relates to personal factors that facilitate engagement with the environment.

4. Discussion

According to the model, Awareness significantly improves Service Accessibility ($\beta = 0.919$, $p = 0.000$) and is strongly undermined by user barriers ($\beta = -0.155$, $p < 0.000$), suggesting improving awareness alone is not adequate unless service barriers are addressed.

The findings reveal a widespread knowledge gap regarding available services for persons with disabilities (PWDs) across educational, health, and social domains, a trend further supported by the structural model. Specifically, the model showed that user barriers significantly predict awareness of social services ($\beta = -0.155$, $p < 0.001$). This indicates that individuals who face challenges such as unfamiliarity with modern technology or limited access to transportation are less likely to be aware of the social and financial services available to them or their dependents. A lack of awareness acts as a critical obstacle, preventing PWDs and their families from utilising potentially life-enhancing support systems.

One of the most pronounced findings was the low level of awareness regarding educational services for PWDs. For instance, 74.7% of caretakers surveyed reported being unaware of the provision of educational vouchers in cooperation with private education providers, with only 3.3% stating that they had ever accessed such services. Older respondents exhibited significantly lower levels of awareness, highlighting the need for targeted information campaigns that address the needs of different age groups, potentially through in-person channels. Similarly, 73.1% of respondents indicated they were unaware of higher education or scholarship opportunities for PWDs. While this may not seem urgent given that most PWDs in the study were below the age of eligibility for higher education, the lack of future planning is problematic and suggests a broader issue of unpreparedness among families. These gaps present a clear challenge to the realisation of Saudi Arabia's Vision 2030, which pledges to support the educational and employment integration of individuals with disabilities to ensure their independence and full participation in society. This finding is consistent with studies such as [43,47,48], which stress the need for improved communication strategies and user support mechanisms.

The study also found alarmingly low awareness of social and health services critical to the development and inclusion of PWDs. For example, 83% of participants were unaware of diagnostic and measurement services, 56.9% were unfamiliar with comprehensive rehabilitation centre services, and 70.2% had no knowledge of vocational rehabilitation centres. Awareness of employment support programmes, such as those integrating PWDs into the labour market, was also limited, with 61.5% reporting unfamiliarity. This lack of awareness undermines access to vital support systems and perpetuates social exclusion and economic vulnerability. The poor understanding of programmes aimed at employment inclusion is particularly concerning given the disproportionately high unemployment rate among PWDs in Saudi Arabia [49].

The survey further revealed that 56% of respondents were unfamiliar with subsidy applications for assistive medical devices. Notably, usage rates were higher among females and university-educated individuals, suggesting that educational attainment plays a critical role in navigating and accessing support services. Other important services were similarly under-recognised: 85% of respondents were unaware of Kanaf funding for PWDs;

64.6% had not heard of protection from abuse services; 76.8% were unaware of digital autism certification services; 83.8% had no knowledge of housing support services; and 89.1% were unfamiliar with the Ministry of Sports' Fajr Program for sports rehabilitation. Moreover, 80.1% of respondents were unaware of special offers and discounts available to PWDs, with rural residents reporting particularly low levels of awareness. These findings point to an urgent need for wide-reaching and inclusive information campaigns that educate the public about available services and ensure that support reaches the most vulnerable populations.

Technological barriers also emerged as a major concern. The study found that 29.8% of respondents perceived modern technology as a barrier to service access, and 31.5% were indifferent, suggesting a general lack of familiarity or confidence with digital platforms. These findings align with previous studies indicating that assistive technologies often create additional obstacles due to poor design or complexity. To overcome this, the literature recommends a range of strategies, such as short training courses, interactive demonstrations, community-based support networks, and the identification of "super-users" who can offer ongoing mentorship. Notably, older individuals and those with lower education levels faced greater difficulties using technology, reinforcing the need for age-friendly solutions and alternative non-digital service pathways.

Transportation access also remains a significant structural barrier, with 36.7% of respondents reporting difficulty reaching service providers. Those with a university education were less likely to face such issues, possibly due to greater employment and mobility resources. Additionally, 46.9% of respondents cited the limited availability or remote locations of service centres as a major hindrance. Rural residents were particularly affected, underscoring the need for decentralised service delivery and mobile outreach initiatives that can bring services directly to underserved communities.

Service-level barriers, such as unclear and outdated service procedures, are strong determinants of service accessibility, exerting a significant negative impact on access ($\beta = -0.939$, $p < 0.001$). As presented earlier, approximately 50.5% of respondents agreed that the existing conditions and procedures for accessing services present considerable challenges. This perception was generally consistent across gender groups but was notably pronounced among respondents aged 50 years and above. Furthermore, 43.1% of participants believed that service providers lack an understanding of their specific needs, highlighting critical gaps in service delivery. The detrimental impact of service-level barriers on service accessibility or social and economic inclusion of PWDs reinforces conclusions from [11,14], which argue for stronger policy interventions and advocacy efforts.

Overall, the structural model and survey findings provide strong evidence that both service-level and personal-level barriers are restricting access to critical services for PWDs and their caretakers. These challenges, particularly low awareness and accessibility, undermine the progress toward inclusion, independence, and equality envisioned in national development goals. To address this, a dual approach is required: one that improves the availability and accessibility of services while also enhancing public awareness through inclusive, targeted campaigns tailored to users' age, education, and geographic location. Equipping service centres to offer guidance, maintain helplines, and disseminate accurate information can serve as an immediate step toward bridging the current knowledge gap and fostering a more inclusive and equitable society.

5. Conclusions and Policy Recommendations

5.1. Conclusions

This study provides compelling evidence that both systemic and personal barriers significantly hinder the ability of caregivers to access essential services for persons with disabilities (PWDs) in Saudi Arabia. Applying Andersen's Behavioural Model, the structural model confirms that while awareness strongly predicts service accessibility ($\beta = 0.919$, $p = 0.000$), it is substantially influenced by user-level barriers ($\beta = -0.155$, $p < 0.001$) and service-level obstacles ($\beta = -0.939$, $p < 0.001$). These findings underscore the urgent need to address not only information gaps but also structural and procedural inefficiencies that restrict meaningful access to services.

The results show that digital literacy remains a major barrier, with 29.8% of respondents identifying modern technology as an obstacle and 31.5% remaining indifferent, indicating limited engagement with digital platforms. These findings are consistent with the existing literature, highlighting usability challenges, poor interface design, and lack of training as obstacles to effective adoption of assistive technologies [3,36]. Addressing this requires inclusive digital strategies such as workshops, tutorials, post-implementation support networks, and the designation of "super-users" who can mentor others [37–41]. The digital divide was particularly apparent among older and less-educated caregivers, as similarly documented in [41–45,50,51].

Transportation and geographic access also pose critical challenges. With 36.7% of participants reporting difficulty reaching service providers and 46.9% citing distant or limited service centres, particularly in rural areas, there is a clear need for decentralised service delivery and mobile outreach strategies. These findings reinforce calls from [9,15] for flexible and community-based access solutions to reduce spatial inequalities in service provision.

Service-level issues such as outdated procedures, poor customer service, and unclear eligibility criteria further exacerbate exclusion. Nearly half of the respondents (50.5%) agreed that service conditions made access difficult, while 43.1% felt that service providers did not understand their needs. These results echo previous conclusions in [11,14], which emphasise the necessity of stronger policy interventions and user-informed service frameworks. The dissatisfaction expressed, especially by older individuals and males, highlights the importance of incorporating user feedback into ongoing service reform efforts.

While 40.8% of participants described service providers as cooperative, the remaining majority were either dissatisfied or neutral, particularly among university-educated respondents. This finding underscores the disconnect between service users' expectations and actual service performance, further validating the call for service models that are inclusive, culturally sensitive, and family-centred [6,7].

Ultimately, this study confirms that lack of awareness, compounded by personal and systemic barriers, undermines national goals of inclusion and independence for PWDs as articulated in Vision 2030. The Vision pledges to empower PWDs with access to education, employment, and community participation: "We will also enable those of our people with disabilities to receive the education and job opportunities that will ensure their independence and integration as effective members of society. They will be provided with all the facilities and tools required to put them on the path to commercial success" [34,35].

To realise this vision, national-level action is required. This includes a coordinated awareness campaign, the redesign of service portals for user-friendliness, equipping service centres to act as information hubs, and the simplification of procedures. The recommendations in this study align with those made by [12,13], which advocate for responsive, user-informed service models designed to meet the diverse and evolving needs of PWDs and their caregivers. By integrating inclusive strategies across all service levels, policymakers and providers can bridge the current accessibility gaps and move toward a truly equitable, responsive, and empowering service ecosystem for PWDs and their families in Saudi Arabia.

Moreover, this study offers a novel empirical contribution within the Gulf region by systematically examining the intersection of caregiver characteristics, service awareness, and structural barriers in shaping access to disability services in Saudi Arabia. While the global literature has examined similar dynamics, few studies in the Gulf context have employed quantitative methods such as SEM to translate subjective caregiver experiences into validated, measurable constructs. By linking these constructs to broader system-level challenges, including digital inaccessibility, procedural opacity, and limited outreach, our findings not only address a significant research gap but also inform policy development in alignment with Saudi Arabia's Vision 2030. These insights are equally relevant for neighbouring Gulf states undergoing social service reforms, offering evidence-based direction for designing inclusive service delivery models that respond to both user-level and structural constraints [40–42,50]. These region-specific studies provide critical insights into the lived experiences, emotional burdens, and systemic challenges faced by caregivers of persons with disabilities in Gulf countries. For example, research from Saudi Arabia and the UAE highlights the cultural expectations surrounding family caregiving, limited access to formal support services, and the psychological strain on parents, particularly mothers, of children with disabilities. By incorporating these perspectives, our study's discussion on service gaps, caregiver support needs, and policy recommendations becomes more contextually grounded. These findings reinforce our call for culturally responsive interventions and caregiver-inclusive policies aligned with national development goals such as Saudi Arabia's Vision 2030. By integrating these insights, our study contributes valuable knowledge to the existing literature and provides a comprehensive understanding of the challenges faced by caregivers of PWDs in Saudi Arabia.

Finally, it should be noted that while Structural Equation Modelling (SEM) provides robust insights into the relationships between awareness, barriers, and service utilisation, the findings are correlational rather than causal. This limitation stems from the cross-sectional nature of the data, which captures a single point in time. Furthermore, no experimental intervention was implemented in this study; the term "experiment" used earlier refers solely to the statistical modelling of survey data. Future longitudinal or experimental research designs could help establish causality and further validate these relationships.

5.2. Policy Recommendations

Access to inclusive services is a cornerstone of social equity and national development, particularly under Saudi Arabia's Vision 2030. This study highlights the significant barriers caregivers of PWDs face in accessing social and financial services. Findings underscore that user-related challenges (e.g., limited digital literacy), service-level barriers (e.g., complex procedures, unresponsive providers), and broader accessibility issues negatively impact awareness and service utilisation. These results align with prior studies [11–13,41] that highlight institutional and perceptual barriers to disability services. To support inclusive service access, the following policy recommendations are suggested:

- Launch culturally sensitive awareness campaigns via mosques, public schools, and healthcare centres. Establish caregiver helplines and mobile service units in underserved areas.
- Offer orientation workshops at hospitals and rehabilitation centres at the point of diagnosis to familiarise caregivers with available support options.
- Streamline the national Disability Registry and integrate it with service provider portals to reduce administrative burdens.
- Embed disability education into school curricula and develop community-based anti-stigma initiatives to change public perceptions and normalise service use.

These actions not only support caregivers but also contribute to the well-being of PWDs by promoting a more responsive and accessible service system. Further research should focus on improving service quality and user satisfaction, exploring comparative studies across Gulf and international contexts, and identifying best practices to inform policy development and cross-sectoral collaboration.

6. Limitations and Directions for Future Research

This study offers valuable insights into the experiences of caregivers of persons with disabilities (PWDs) in Saudi Arabia, particularly regarding access to social and financial services. However, several limitations should be acknowledged.

First, the sample is limited to familial caregivers of PWDs attending specialised day schools, excluding those caring for PWDs in home settings, mainstream education, rural areas, or institutional facilities. This narrow sampling frame inherently limits the external validity of the study, as it does not capture the full diversity of caregiving contexts across the country. This restricts the generalizability of findings to the broader population of caregivers in the Kingdom. Notably, migrant domestic caregivers—who constitute a large portion of daily care providers in Saudi Arabia—were not included, despite their central role in caregiving. Their exclusion presents a significant gap, as their service access challenges and awareness levels may differ substantially. Second, although the study reveals that 70.7% of caregivers were unaware of available services and only 2.3% had used them, it does not explore the underlying reasons for these low levels. Factors such as geographic disparities, digital exclusion, socio-economic status, cultural stigma, and limited outreach efforts remain underexplored. Future research should address these dimensions through qualitative interviews and targeted surveys. Specifically, we recommend:

- Including caregivers from home-based and rural settings, as well as migrant care workers, for broader representation.
- Conducting in-depth qualitative studies to understand why caregivers lack awareness or face difficulties utilising services.
- Investigating how caregivers receive information and assessing the effectiveness of current communication strategies.
- Exploring the influence of socio-economic, cultural, and regional contexts on service access and perceptions.
- Examining psychosocial factors, such as stigma, caregiver burden, and family dynamics, that influence service utilisation.

Author Contributions: Methodology, W.S. and G.A.; Software, G.A. and A.A.-D.; Validation, H.A. and A.A.-D.; Formal analysis, W.S. and A.A.-D.; Investigation, W.S. and A.A.-D.; Resources, G.A. and H.A.; Data curation, G.A. and H.A.; Writing, W.S. and A.A.-D.; Review and editing, G.A. and H.A. All authors have read and agreed to the published version of the manuscript.

Funding: The authors extend their appreciation to Princess Nourah bint Abdulrahman University Researchers Supporting Project number (PNURSP2025R705), Princess Nourah bint Abdulrahman University, Riyadh, Saudi Arabia.

Institutional Review Board Statement: The IRB (Institutional Review Board of Princess Nourah bin Abdulrahman University) has determined that the proposed project poses no more than minimal risk to the participants. Therefore, the proposal has been deemed EXEMPT from IRB review.

Informed Consent Statement: Informed consent was obtained from all subjects involved in the study.

Data Availability Statement: The data presented in this study are available on request from the corresponding author. (The data are not publicly available due to privacy or ethical restrictions).

Conflicts of Interest: The authors declare no conflict of interest.

References

1. United Nations. Convention on the Rights of Persons with Disabilities. 2006. Available online: https://www.un.org/disabilities/documents/convention/convoptprot-e.pdf (accessed on 12 February 2025).
2. World Health Organization. Disability and Health. 2021. Available online: https://www.who.int/news-room/fact-sheets/detail/disability-and-health (accessed on 12 February 2025).
3. Abed, M.G.; Abed, L.G.; Shackelford, T.K. A Qualitative, Small-Sample Study of Employment Challenges for People with Disabilities in Saudi Arabia. *Healthcare* **2024**, *12*, 346. [CrossRef] [PubMed]
4. Khamis, V. Psychological distress among parents of children with mental retardation in the United Arab Emirates. *Soc. Sci. Med.* **2007**, *64*, 850–857. [CrossRef]
5. Andersen, R.M. Revisiting the behavioral model and access to medical care: Does it matter? *J. Health Soc. Behav.* **1995**, *36*, 1–10. [CrossRef]
6. World Health Organization. *International Classification of Functioning, Disability and Health (ICF)*; WHO: Geneva, Switzerland, 2001.
7. Cronbach, L.J. Coefficient alpha and the internal structure of tests. *Psychometrika* **1951**, *16*, 297–334. [CrossRef]
8. Kline, R.B. *Principles and Practice of Structural Equation Modeling*, 3rd ed.; Guilford Press: New York, NY, USA, 2011.
9. Turnbull, A.P.; Turnbull, H.R. *Families, Professionals, and Exceptionality: Collaborating for Empowerment*; Merrill: Columbus, OH, USA, 2001.
10. Dunst, C.J.; Trivette, C.M.; Deal, A.G. *Supporting and Strengthening Families*; Brookline Books: Cambridge, MA, USA, 1994.
11. Scherer, M.J. *Living in the State of Stuck: How Assistive Technology Impacts the Lives of People with Disabilities*, 3rd ed.; Brookline Books: Brookline, MA, USA, 2025.
12. Hashemi, G.; Wickenden, M.; Bright, T.; Kuper, H. Barriers to Accessing Primary Healthcare Services for People With Disabilities in Low and Middle-Income Countries, a Me-Ta-Synthesis of Qualitative Studies. *Disabil Rehabil.* **2022**, *44*, 1207–1220. [CrossRef]
13. Mitra, S.; Yap, J.; Hervé, J.; Chen, W. Inclusive statistics: A disaggregation of indicators by disability status and its implications for policy. *Glob. Soc. Policy* **2022**, *23*, 39–66. [CrossRef]
14. Puli, L.; Layton, N.; Bell, D.; Shahriar, A.Z. Financial Inclusion for People with Disability: A Scoping Review. *Glob Health Action.* **2024**, *17*, 2342634. [CrossRef] [PubMed] [PubMed Central]
15. Houtenville, A.; Kalargyrou, V. People with Disabilities: Employers' Perspectives on Recruitment Practices, Strategies, and Challenges in Leisure and Hospitality. *CORNELL HOSP Q.* **2012**, *53*, 40–52. [CrossRef]
16. Social inclusion of persons with Disabilities in the Arab Region, United Nations, Department of Economic and Social Affairs, SDGs Action. Available online: https://sdgs.un.org/partnerships/social-inclusion-persons-disabilities-arab-region-accelerated-inclusion-millions (accessed on 31 July 2025).
17. Alshammari, S.H.; Alshammari, M.H. Modelling the effects of perceived system quality and personal innovativeness on the intention to use metaverse: A structural equation modelling approach. *PeerJ Comput. Sci.* **2024**, *10*, e2331. [CrossRef]
18. Clutterbuck, D.; Ramasawmy, M.; Pantelic, M.; Hayer, J.; Begum, F.; Faghy, M.; Nasir, N.; Causer, B.; Heightman, M.; Allsopp, G.; et al. Barriers to healthcare access and experiences of stigma: Findings from a coproduced Long Covid case-finding study. *Health Expect.* **2024**, *27*, e14037. [CrossRef] [PubMed]
19. Medabesh, A.M.; Malik, N.; Shafi, M.; Rashid, J. Employment Scenario for People with Disabilities (PWDs) in Saudi Arabia: Challenges and Opportunities. *JDR* **2024**, *3*. [CrossRef]
20. Kingdom of Saudi Arabia. Vision 2030. 2016. Available online: https://www.vision2030.gov.sa/media/rc0b5oy1/saudi_vision203.pdf (accessed on 12 February 2025).
21. General Authority for Statistics. Disability Survey 2017. 2017. Available online: https://www.stats.gov.sa/en/w/disability-survey-2017 (accessed on 14 February 2025).
22. Malhotra, N.K. *Marketing Research: An Applied Orientation*, 7th ed.; Pearson Education: Upper Saddle River, NJ, USA, 2021.
23. Fornell, C.; Larcker, D.F. Evaluating structural equation models with unobservable variables and measurement error. *J. Mark. Res.* **1981**, *18*, 39–50. [CrossRef]
24. Creswell, J.W.; Creswell, J.D. *Research Design: Qualitative, Quantitative, and Mixed Methods Approaches*; SAGE Publications: Thousand Oaks, CA, USA, 2018; Available online: https://books.google.com.eg/books?id=s4ViswEACAAJ (accessed on 14 February 2025).
25. Lazarus, R.S.; Folkman, S. *Stress, Appraisal, and Coping*; Springer Publishing Company: New York, NY, USA, 1984.
26. Frydenberg, E.; Lewis, R. *Adolescent Coping Scale: Research and Administration Manual*; Australian Council for Educational Research: Melbourne, Australia, 1993.
27. Neill, J.T. *The Adolescent Coping Scale: A Review and Critique*; Unpublished manuscript; University of Canberra: Canberra, Australia, 1994.

28. Gaskin, J.; Lim, J.; Master Validity Tool [AMOS Plugin]. Gaskination's StatWiki. 2016. Available online: https://statwiki.gaskination.com/index.php?title=Main_PageGoogleScholar+5content.cld.iop.org+5ymerdigital.com+5 (accessed on 14 February 2025).
29. Schulz, R.; Beach, S.R.; Lind, B.; Martire, L.M.; Zdaniuk, B.; Hirsch, C.; Jackson, S.; Burton, L. Involvement in Caregiving and Adjustment to Death of a Spouse: Findings From the Caregiver Health Effects Study. *JAMA* **2001**, *285*, 3123–3129. [CrossRef]
30. Brodaty, H.; Green, A.; Koschera, A. Meta-analysis of psychosocial interventions for caregivers of people with dementia. *J. Am. Geriatr. Soc.* **2005**, *53*, 657–664. [CrossRef]
31. AlAteeq, D.; AlDaoud, A.; AlHadi, A.; AlKhalaf, H.; Milev, R. The Experience and Impact of Stigma in Saudi People with a Mood Disorder. *Ann Gen Psychiatry* **2018**, *17*, 51. [CrossRef] [PubMed] [PubMed Central]
32. Lim, J.W.; Zebrack, B.; Wang, J. Assessing the feasibility and acceptability of a stress management intervention for caregivers of cancer patients. *Support. Care Cancer* **2012**, *20*, 1435–1444.
33. Phongtankuel, V.; Czaja, S.; Park, T.; Dignam, R.; Adelman, R.; Shah, S.; Vasquez, F.; Reid, M.C. Assessing the Feasibility, Acceptability, and Preliminary Efficacy of a Novel Symptom Management Care Delivery Intervention for Caregivers Receiving Home Hospice Care: The I-HoME Protocol. *Contemp. Clin. Trials.* **2024**, *136*, 107389. [CrossRef] [PubMed] [PubMed Central]
34. Hayes, A.M.; Bulat, J. *Disabilities Inclusive Education Systems and Policies Guide for Low- and Middle-Income Countries*; RTI Press: Research Triangle Park, NC, USA, 2017.
35. Alzahrani, M. *Vision 2030 and Disability Inclusion in Saudi Arabia*; Ministry of Human Resources and Social Development: Riyadh, Saudi Arabia, 2023.
36. Marinaci, T.; Russo, C.; Savarese, G.; Stornaiuolo, G.; Faiella, F.; Carpinelli, L.; Navarra, M.; Marsico, G.; Mollo, M.; Savarese, G.; et al. An Inclusive Workplace Approach to Disability through Assistive Technologies: A Systematic Review and Thematic Analysis of the Literature. *Societies* **2023**, *13*, 231. [CrossRef]
37. McNicholl, A.; Casey, H.; Desmond, D.; Gallagher, P. The impact of assistive technology use for students with disabilities in higher education: A systematic review. *Disabil. Rehabil. Assist. Technol.* **2019**, *16*, 130–143. [CrossRef]
38. Egan, K.J.; Pot, A.M. Encouraging Innovation for Assistive Health Technologies in Dementia: Barriers, Enablers and Next Steps To Be Taken. *J Am Med Dir Assoc.* **2016**, *17*, 357–363. [CrossRef]
39. Robb, N.; Boyle, B.; Politis, Y.; Newbutt, N.; Kuo, H.J.; Sung, C. Participatory Technology Design for Autism and Cognitive Disabilities: A Narrative Overview of Issues and Techniques. In *Recent Advances in Technologies for Inclusive Well-Being. Intelligent Systems Reference Library*; Brooks, A.L., Brahman, S., Kapralos, B., Nakajima, A., Tyerman, J., Jain, L.C., Eds.; Springer: Cham, Switzerland, 2021; Volume 196. [CrossRef]
40. Dugstad, J.; Sundling, V.; Nilsen, E.R.; Eide, H. Nursing staff's evaluation of facilitators and barriers during implementation of wireless nurse call systems in residential care facilities. A cross-sectional study. *BMC Health Serv. Res.* **2020**, *20*, 163. [CrossRef] [PubMed]
41. Øksnebjerg, L.; Janbek, J.; Woods, B.; Waldemar, G. Assistive Technology Designed to Support Self-Management of People with Dementia: User Involvement, Dissemination, and Adoption. A Scoping Review. *Int. Psychogeriatr.* **2020**, *32*, 937–953. [CrossRef]
42. Gitlow, L. Technology Use by Older Adults and Barriers to Using Technology. *Phys. Occup. Ther. Geri.* **2014**, *32*, 271–280. [CrossRef]
43. Turnbull, H.R.; Stowe, M.J.; Huerta, N.E. *Free Appropriate Public Education: The Law and Children with Disabilities*, 7th ed.; Love Publishing Co.: Denver, CO, USA, 2007.
44. Hair, J.F.; Black, W.C.; Babin, B.J.; Anderson, R.E. *Multivariate Data Analysis*, 8th ed.; Cengage Learning: Boston, MA, USA, 2019.
45. Alkhonezan, S.M.; Alkhonezan, M.M.; Alshayea, Y.; Bukhari, H.; Almhizai, R. Factors Influencing the Lives of Parents of Children with Autism Spectrum Disorder in Saudi Arabia: A Comprehensive Review. *Cureus* **2023**, *15*, e48325. [CrossRef] [PubMed] [PubMed Central]
46. Byrne, B.M. *Structural Equation Modeling with AMOS: Basic Concepts, Applications, and Programming*, 2nd ed.; Routledge: New York, NY, USA, 2010.
47. Dunst, C.J.; Trivette, C.M.; Hamby, D.W. *Meta-Analysis of Family-Centered Helpgiving Practices Research*; Winterberry Press: Asheville, NC, USA, 2013.
48. Alhumaidi, K.A.; Alshwameen, M.O.; Alsayed, M.S.; Alqoaer, D.K.; Albalawi, R.S.; Alanzi, S.M.; Alharthe, A.F.; Abdulaziz Subayyil Alanazi, H. Quality of Life of Primary Caregivers of Children with Cerebral Palsy From a Family Perspective. *Cureus* **2023**, *15*, e49378. [CrossRef]
49. El Kahi, H.; Abi Haidar, M.; Haddad, R.; Salameh, P. Caregivers of Lebanese children with chronic illnesses: Psychosocial status, needs, and coping strategies. *J. Pediatr. Nurs.* **2015**, *30*, e29–e38. [CrossRef]

50. Frączkiewicz-Frączkiewicz-Wronka, A.; Zrałek, M.; Ostrowska, S. Digital Exclusion of Seniors as a Barrier to Leading a Productive Life in the Fourth Industrial Revolution. *OSJ* **2023**, *1*, 55–68.
51. Mohamed, A.; Opoku, M.P.; Almarzooqi, S.; Ramadan, R.; Gyimah, E.M. Children with Intellectual Disability: Fathers' Self-Reported Involvement in Rehabilitation in the United Arab Emirates. *BMC Psychol.* **2025**, *13*, 813. [CrossRef] [PubMed]

healthcare

MDPI

Article

Strategies to Prevent Work Ability Decline and Support Retirement Transition in Workers with Intellectual and Developmental Disabilities

Beatriz Sánchez, Francisco de Borja Jordán de Urríes *, Miguel Ángel Verdugo, Carmen de Jesús Abena and Victoria Sanblás

University Institute on Community Integration (INICO), University of Salamanca, 37005 Salamanca, Spain; bea5sh@usal.es (B.S.); verdugo@usal.es (M.Á.V.); picky@usal.es (C.d.J.A.); victoriasanblascapi@hotmail.es (V.S.)
* Correspondence: bjordan@usal.es

Abstract

Background/Objectives: The aging of workers with intellectual and developmental disabilities is an emerging reality attributed to the rise in life expectancy and improved labor market access. In this study, "workers" is used as an inclusive, neutral term covering all individuals engaged in paid labor—whether employees, self-employed, freelancers, or those performing manual or non-manual tasks. It encompasses every form of work. It is crucial to comprehend the reality of aging workers from the perspectives of the primary individuals involved: the workers, their families, and supporting professionals. **Methods**: A qualitative study was developed, involving 12 focus groups and 107 participants, using NVivo 12 Pro for analysis; we used a phenomenological methodology and grounded theory. **Results**: A set of concrete needs was highlighted: among them, 33 were related to declining work ability due to aging and disability (WADAD), and 30 to transition to retirement. These needs were grouped into categories: workplace accommodations, coordination and collaboration, personal and family support, counseling and training, and other types of needs. **Conclusions**: This study establishes an empirical basis tailored to the needs of this group, enabling the development of prevention and intervention protocols that address WADAD and the transition to retirement.

Keywords: active aging; retirement; work ability decline; disability; intellectual and developmental disabilities; transition to retirement

1. Introduction

1.1. Intellectual Disability and Employment

Intellectual and developmental disability is characterized by limitations in intellectual functioning and adaptive behavior, affecting conceptual, social, and practical skills, and manifesting before the age of 22 years [1]. Diagnostic criteria include an IQ at least two standard deviations below the population mean and limitations in adaptive behaviors in at least one of three domains (conceptual, social, practical) or in the global score. In both cases, the standard error of measurement must be taken into account [1].

Employment is considered a universal and fundamental right for all people and represents a key goal in the process of transition to adult life. Article 27 of the Convention on the Rights of Persons with Disabilities [2] states that "States Parties recognize the right of persons with disabilities to work, on an equal basis with others; this includes the right

 https://doi.org/10.3390/healthcare13141766

to the opportunity to gain a living by work freely chosen or accepted in a labor market and work environment that is open, inclusive and accessible to persons with disabilities." This is especially significant for people with intellectual and developmental disabilities, for whom work is the first step toward independent living and full participation in the community [3].

According to data from Spain published in December 2023 [4], the employment rate of people with disabilities in Spain is 27.88%, compared with 68.1% for people without disabilities. The unemployment rate is 21.4% compared with 8.6% among the population without disabilities. Within the working population with disabilities, 64.8% are between 45 and 64 years of age; this figure rises to 67.4% if we consider only those who are employed. Some authors have estimated that employment in Special Employment Centers (sheltered employment) in Spain accounted for 70% of employment contracts for people with disabilities in 2019 [5], and, more recently, 71% in 2022 [6]. However, Spain's public employment service reports lower percentages: for example, in March 2024, out of 9361 contracts for people with disabilities, 5402 were made in Special Employment Centers, accounting for 57.7% [7].

Regarding supported employment in the ordinary (open) labor market, one study [8] made an approximation of the number of people hired in this type of employment in its latest available national report. However, this estimate is not complete as it is based only on data provided by entities that participated in the study. Consequently, Spain lacks reliable data in this regard due to the absence of a state registry.

Finally, with regard to the type of work carried out by people with intellectual disabilities, according to the EDAD 2020 survey [9], there are 20,166 people with intellectual disabilities working in Spain. Of these, 12,527 (62%) are engaged in elementary occupations. Due to sample limitations, it is not possible to provide reliable data on employment or job types by sector.

1.2. Declining Work Ability Through Aging and Disability and Transition to Retirement

Work ability decline through aging and disability (WADAD) is defined as the process of deterioration in work ability resulting from the interaction between disability and aging, which are two different but interrelated conditions [10]. This process carries the risk of a mismatch between a job role and the satisfactory performance of tasks, which may lead to forced retirement for reasons of health or job instability, causing a drastic change in lifestyle [10].

For any individual, the transition from paid employment to retirement is a significant milestone that impacts daily activity, emotional wellbeing, social relationships, and personal identity. Despite its importance, this reality remains under-researched in the context of intellectual and developmental disabilities [11,12]. To prevent retirement from being an abrupt change, workers with disabilities need a progressive and planned transition. This transition is acknowledged as an objective at the international level [13], and it should align with the principles of active aging, which aims to enhance quality of life in later years by optimizing health, participation, and security opportunities [14]. However, the effectiveness of this approach is frequently challenged due to the social exclusion traditionally experienced by people with disabilities [15].

In the European context, there is a dearth of scientific evidence addressing the specific needs of this group in relation to WADAD and the subsequent transition to retirement, primarily because these are emerging realities.

1.3. Active Participation in the Transition to Retirement

In the Spanish legislative framework [16,17], early retirement for people with intellectual disabilities is governed by two regulations and is defined by reduction coefficients and specific age and contribution period requirements. Royal Decree 1539/2003 establishes a minimum age of 52 years for people with a recognized degree of disability equal to or greater than 65%, and Royal Decree 370/2023 establishes a minimum age of 56 years for people with a recognized degree of disability equal to or greater than 45%.

People perceive aging differently, with some viewing it positively and others experiencing a loss of confidence and self-esteem [13]. However, active retirement carries significant benefits, including improved quality of life, enhanced physical and emotional wellbeing, increased motivation, and better self-image [18–20].

Pre-retirement planning, encompassing physical, leisure, and volunteering activities, along with continued support for education on retirement and aging, positively influences satisfaction levels [21–23].

Control over the timing of retirement is also crucial for a fulfilling aging experience [24]. Some people plan proactively and gradually, while others do so abruptly and reactively due to factors such as health concerns or job instability. Some may contemplate delaying retirement for financial reasons or for fear of inactivity, while others may consider partial retirement to combine work with other activities or to enjoy more rest [25]. What is needed are individualized, inclusive, and person-centered programs, as opposed to the many existing group-based and segregated approaches [26].

1.4. Planning the Transition to Retirement

Sometimes, older people with intellectual and developmental disabilities consider delaying retirement or taking partial retirement to combine work with other activities, enjoy more rest, manage finances, or alleviate the fear of inactivity [24].

The lack of access to day programs is a significant barrier for workers who have not previously engaged with such services, particularly for individuals in regular employment, who face inactivity post-retirement and may fear inadequate support [27]. That said, those in regular (open) employment generally have a more positive outlook on retirement, unlike their counterparts in sheltered employment who tend to associate retirement with boredom [28]. Insufficient funding for programs tailored to this group also represents a major barrier, compounded by low incomes resulting from retirement options [21]. As for health, inadequate access to health care and limited support for preventive care can contribute to unhealthy behaviors among people with intellectual and developmental disabilities [29].

Given their limited social networks, these individuals also require support for autonomy, especially after retirement [13]. It is therefore vital to nurture and strengthen these networks, as individuals with intellectual and developmental disabilities often favor work activity over retirement due to the significant value they place on social relationships in the workplace [27]. Although family support is common, it may diminish after retirement due to circumstances such as death, distance, or a lack of family interest [13]. Furthermore, the simultaneous aging of people with intellectual and developmental disabilities and their primary caregivers has an impact on social opportunities [30].

Accommodation post-retirement is also a major concern. The optimal situation would be for individuals to continue living with their family or in assisted housing, but in the medium to long term, nursing homes often become the only viable option, presenting a challenge due to a lack of staff training in disability care [13].

Financial security is key to choosing the appropriate time to retire [22]. Finally, in rural settings, activities and services for older retirees with intellectual and developmental disabilities are limited; however, the strength of the community may facilitate social support when compared with urban settings [31].

1.5. Purpose

The need for this study arises from the emerging and largely unexplored reality of WADAD and the subsequent transition to retirement. This necessity is further underscored by the increasing presence of people with intellectual disabilities in paid employment and nearing retirement age in Spain.

The purpose of this study is to identify a set of needs to effectively extend working life and facilitate the transition to active retirement for individuals with intellectual or developmental disabilities.

The ultimate aim of identifying these needs is to create two protocols: the first focused on prevention and intervention against WADAD, and the second centered on the transition to active retirement. In both protocols, the identified needs are accompanied by a number of action points.

2. Materials and Methods

A qualitative methodology using focus groups was chosen to explore the experiences, opinions, and perspectives of participants on specific issues [32]. Separate groups were formed for people with disabilities, family members, and professionals. This approach aligns with the suggestions of [33], which emphasize the importance of ensuring homogeneity in group profiles. However, the selection of participants may still vary.

The study proposal was approved by the Ethics Committee of the University Institute for Community Integration (INICO) of the University of Salamanca in 2020.

Twelve focus groups were held—six on WADAD prevention and six on retirement transition—with each block comprising two groups of family members, two groups of support professionals, and two groups of workers with intellectual and developmental disabilities.

We employed a process similar to that used in recent research on retirement and intellectual disability [11]. Adopting a phenomenological approach, we analyzed participants' opinions about a specific reality and the needs associated with that reality, adhering to the framework outlined by [34]. We followed the steps of grounded theory [35,36] for data reduction and employed NVivo 12 Pro for data organization and transformation.

2.1. Participants

Participants were recruited by convenience using a nonprobability sampling method. The 12 groups comprised a total of 107 participants selected according to the following criteria:

1. Workers with intellectual and developmental disabilities with a current employment contract, with verbal intelligibility and communication skills (n = 33; 30.84%).
2. Family members of a worker with intellectual and developmental disabilities with a current employment contract (n = 27; 25.23%).
3. Professionals working in aging or employment services (n = 47; 43.93%), comprising psychologists, job coaches, workshop teachers, or similar.

The majority were women (58.88%). Ages ranged from 26 to 81 years. In terms of educational attainment, 46.73% had been educated to university level, primarily consisting of professionals, while 34.58% had completed primary education, mainly comprising workers with intellectual and developmental disabilities. The majority of participants had either a generic intellectual and developmental disability (58.88%) or Down syndrome (36.45%). Finally, 49.53% of participant contributions pertained to regular (open) employment (whether supported or not), and 44.86% to sheltered employment (in Special Employment Centers). Further sociodemographic data are given in Table 1.

Table 1. Participant sociodemographic data.

		Workers * n = 33 (30.84%)	Family Members n = 27 (25.23%)	Professionals n = 47 (43.93%)	Total n = 107	%
Gender	Female	8	18	37	63	58.88
	Male	25	8	10	43	40.19
	Other/Not shared	0	1	0	1	0.93
Age	From	34	32	26	-	-
	To	63	81	58	-	-
Education	Primary	31	6	0	37	34.58
	Secondary	1	2	0	3	2.80
	Higher Secondary	0	5	2	7	6.54
	Vocational	1	4	5	10	9.35
	University	0	10	40	50	46.73
Etiology **	Intellectual and Developmental Disability	21	15	27	63	58.88
	Down Syndrome	11	9	19	39	36.45
	Autism Spectrum Disorder	1	1	1	3	2.80
	Other	0	2	0	2	1.87
Employment **	Open (supported or not)	14	15	24	53	49.53
	Sheltered	19	12	17	48	44.86
	Both	0	0	6	6	5.61

* With intellectual and developmental disabilities. ** Etiology of the intellectual disability of the participating worker, or in the case of family members or professionals, of the worker to whom they refer.

2.2. Procedure

Social organizations were contacted by email to secure their collaboration. They selected participants according to the provided guidelines to ensure diversity in age, years in employment, organization, sex, disability type, and employment type. The research team then reviewed these selections to achieve balance across all sociodemographic factors.

We collected participants' sociodemographic data using a specially designed questionnaire. A checklist, developed based on topics considered relevant by the research team during the literature review, was used to guide the focus groups. The moderator introduced these topics through questions, allowing participants the freedom to share their perspectives openly.

The sessions lasted between 1.5 h and 2 h, and we obtained informed consent from participants beforehand, including permission record and process their data. For the workers with intellectual and developmental disabilities, the process was adapted using an easy-read preparation booklet, which they reviewed in advance with their support professionals. Additionally, we incorporated a break in the middle of the meeting to minimize fatigue, prevent distraction, and address any questions or concerns. Workers with intellectual disabilities and their family members received support from their designated professionals, as needed. Participants with sufficient autonomy joined remotely from home without any issues.

The focus groups addressing needs associated with the prevention of WADAD were conducted between February and March 2022. The focus groups addressing needs associated with the transition to retirement were conducted between February and March 2023.

The videoconference groups were recorded and then transcribed verbatim. Participants' data were anonymized by assigning codes to prevent their identification during the research. The names of organizations, regions, and other individuals mentioned were also anonymized.

2.3. Data Analysis

For data reduction, we utilized codes (analysis categories) and sentiments expressed in the focus groups (whether positive or negative). The coding process, guided by grounded theory and employing three types of coding (open, axial, and selective), followed the constant comparison method [36,37]. This process required several iterations. If a previously unidentified code was deemed relevant, it was added. The team then reviewed earlier coding to determine whether the new code also applied to those segments.

After iterative coding, project maps were developed for each theme (WADAD prevention and retirement transition), merging literature-based and newly identified codes. These codes were defined in a codebook, and, in the final round, each quotation was systematically assigned to its corresponding code to streamline analysis. An interrater approach was used to achieve consensus and reduce subjectivity [38]. Additionally, focus groups with diverse profiles (professionals, family members, and workers with intellectual and developmental disabilities) enabled source triangulation, enhancing result verification and reliability [37].

3. Results

Table 2 depicts the categories that emerged from participants' contributions during the group discussions. These categories are differentiated based on the frequency of their occurrence in relation to WADAD and the transition to retirement groups.

Table 2. Number of quotes for the main topics of the focus group interviews (FGI), disaggregated by participant profile.

FGI	Topics	Workers *	Family Members	Professionals	Total No. of Quotes by Topic
Work Ability Decline through Aging and Disability (WADAD)	Adjustments and supports in the workplace	37 (28.68%)	19 (12.93%)	54 (21.69%)	110
	Coordination—collaboration	8 (6.20%)	19 (12.93%)	60 (24.10%)	87
	Personal and family support	21 (16.28%)	33 (22.45%)	32 (12.85%)	86
	Counseling and training	16 (12.40%)	14 (9.52%)	34 (13.65%)	64
	Legislation on retirement and disability	1 (0.78%)	17 (11.56%)	28 (11.24%)	46
	Preventing dropout, impairments, or dismissal	17 (13.18%)	12 (8.16%)	17 (6.83%)	46
	Needs not perceived	15 (11.63%)	7 (4.76%)	8 (3.21%)	30
	Preventing reduction of social networks	12 (9.30%)	16 (10.88%)	2 (0.80%)	30
	Financial security	2 (1.55%)	10 (6.80%)	14 (5.62%)	26
	No. of quotes by profile	129 (100%)	147 (100%)	249 (100%)	
Transition to retirement	Services for retirement	67 (15.62%)	68 (24.02%)	148 (34.50%)	283
	Active aging	119 (27.74%)	81 (28.62%)	61 (14.22%)	261
	Personal and family support	102 (23.77%)	65 (22.97%)	76 (17.72%)	243
	Counseling and training	76 (17.72%)	25 (8.83%)	60 (13.99%)	161
	Coordination—collaboration	19 (4.43%)	24 (8.48%)	70 (16.32%)	113
	Financial security	46 (10.73%)	20 (7.07%)	14 (3.26%)	80
	No. of quotes by profile	429 (100%)	283 (100%)	429 (100%)	

* With intellectual and developmental disabilities. **Note**: The percentages reflect the proportion of quotes for each topic relative to the total quotes for that participant profile within each thematic block. Therefore, they sum to 100% vertically (by participant profile), but not horizontally (across profiles). This presentation allows for a clearer comparison of the relative importance of topics within each profile, compensating for differences in the total number of quotes.

Additionally, the data are disaggregated for each participant profile, allowing us to observe the most frequently addressed topics overall and their importance within each group profile.

In the thematic area related to WADAD, the most recurrent topics were workplace adjustments and supports, totaling 110 references (37 from workers, 19 from family members, and 54 from professionals). Interinstitutional coordination and collaboration reached 87 references (8 from workers, 19 from family members, and 60 from professionals), while personal and family support accounted for 86 references (21 from workers, 33 from family members, and 32 from professionals). Other notable themes included counseling and training (64 references), legislation on retirement and disability (46 references), and prevention of abandonment, deterioration, or dismissal (46 references). Less frequently addressed topics were a lack of perceived needs (30 references), prevention of social network reduction (30 references), and financial security (26 references).

In the thematic area regarding the transition to retirement, the topics with the highest number of references were specific services for this process, with 283 mentions (67 from workers, 68 from family members, and 148 from professionals), active aging (261 references; 119 from workers, 81 from family members, and 61 from professionals), and personal and family support, with 243 references (102 from workers, 65 from family members, and 76 from professionals). Counseling and training received fewer mentions, totaling 161 references, followed by coordination and collaboration, with 113 references, and finally financial security, with 80 references.

In the context of work ability decline associated with aging and disability (WADAD), workers primarily focus on workplace adjustments and support (28.68%), as well as personal and family support (16.28%), and the prevention of job loss or dismissal (13.18%). Family members prioritize personal and family support (22.45%), coordination and collaboration among stakeholders (12.93%), and workplace adjustments (12.93%), indicating an interest in both close accompaniment and the proper organization and articulation of services. Professionals emphasize coordination and collaboration (24.10%), workplace adjustments (21.69%), and counseling and training (13.65%) reflecting a more structural and regulatory approach. Regarding the transition to retirement, workers highlight active aging (27.74%) and personal and family support (23.77%), along with retirement services (15.62%) and counseling and training (17.72%). Family members particularly emphasize retirement services (24.02%), active aging (28.62%), and personal and family support (22.97%), underscoring the importance of emotional and practical accompaniment. Professionals focus on retirement services (34.50%), personal and family support (17.72%), and coordination and collaboration (16.32%), with less emphasis on active aging, counselling and training, and financial security. Overall, the findings suggest that, while workers demand concrete supports and practical adaptations to maintain work ability, family members prioritize close support and the adequate organization of services, and professionals concentrate on coordination, regulation, and institutional management to facilitate both the extension of working life and a proper transition to retirement.

These results suggest that the effective management of work ability decline and the transition to retirement requires a balance between practical workplace supports, close personal support, and efficient coordination among the various stakeholders, while integrating the needs and perspectives of workers, family members, and professionals.

Delving deeper into the interrelationships across the categories identified in the groups, we can pinpoint a set of needs associated with WADAD (Table 3) and others linked to the transition to retirement (Table 4).

Table 3. Needs identified in the WADAD focus group interviews, categorized by main topic.

	WADAD Prevention and Intervention Needs
Adjustments and supports in the workplace	1. Updating of on-the-job training 2. Creation of prevention services 3. Variation of tasks and positions 4. Ergonomic and technical support 5. Flexible working hours and reduction of working hours 6. Integration of labor and non-labor services 7. Peer support (avoiding overprotective attitudes) 8. Consider barriers such as rigidity of tasks (impossibility of job adaptations) and lack of resources to intensify support
Coordination and collaboration	9. Collaboration with other services of the entity to coordinate support 10. Adaptation of leisure services to work schedules 11. Implementation of mental agility programs, healthy habits, etc. 12. Collaboration with families to identify occupational impairment and extend support outside the workplace 13. Improvement of interprofessional communication with other areas (public and private), especially with the health sector 14. Coordination with social services for legal aspects of retirement, dependency, etc. 15. Collaboration with companies to create environments that are receptive to needs and accept adaptations in a favorable manner
Personal and family support	16. Family cooperation for work adaptations and to avoid overprotection 17. Family support to maintain worker's health and autonomy 18. Financial difficulties to afford private employment services 19. Consideration of parallel aging and its implications 20. Emotional support for coping with the fear of family aging and other emotional support
Counseling and training	21. Advice on retirement legislation (family and professional) 22. Reducing family anxiety through counseling 23. Training professionals for early detection and intervention 24. Creation of forums on aging and disability 25. Psychological preparation of users for the aging process 26. Preparation for retirement, including formalities and financial aspects 27. Sensitization of companions/natural supports in early signs of decline
Other (legislation, financial stability, continuity of employment, etc.)	28. More flexible retirement requirements 29. Public funding for adaptation of positions 30. Prevention of job abandonment, disability, and reactive layoffs 31. Maintenance of social networks after retirement 32. Reducing working hours to balance leisure and work 33. Guarantee of security, financial stability, and housing

Table 4. Needs identified in transition to retirement focus group interviews, categorized by main topic.

	Transition to Retirement Needs
Retirement services	1. Public services adjusted to older people with disabilities (generational and cultural gap due to early aging) 2. Collective programs for transition to retirement 3. Interdisciplinary teams (comprehensive approach to transition to retirement) 4. Support groups among retired and retiring workers 5. Development of programs and services to occupy leisure time with activities that promote physical and mental health 6. Individualized plans for transition to retirement, taking into account the needs, expectations, and fears of the workers

Table 4. *Cont.*

	Transition to Retirement Needs
Coordination and collaboration	7. Support from companies to identify needs for prolonging working life 8. More full-time job offers to increase the possibility of reaching the required number of years of contribution 9. Collaboration between entity, family, and worker in retirement planning 10. Collaboration between entities to share practices and resources, because this is an emerging reality 11. Collaboration between health services and the disability entity to determine the health status of the employee
Personal and family support	12. Support in understanding and accepting the aging process and its consequences, as well as in adjusting to retirement 13. Support to family members in accepting decline and needs 14. Reconciliation between worker's decisions and family's expectations 15. Psychological support (to deal with parallel aging and family losses) 16. Assistance in financial and administrative retirement procedures 17. Autonomy, personal independence, and self-determination to decide 18. Identify community options tailored to individual needs
Counseling and training	19. Research on aging, retirement, and intellectual disability 20. Training for support technicians and family members in detecting signs of decline and legislation on retirement 21. Updating knowledge on aging and disability in the field of public health 22. Counseling and training for workers on retirement options and active aging 23. Training for companies in the recognition of signs of occupational impairment and support in the final phase of employment
Other (legislation, financial stability, active aging, etc.)	24. Reduction in working hours without affecting contributions for transition to retirement 25. Concerns about requirements for access to retirement (low contributions, etc.) 26. Information on compatible benefits and finding other sources of income to guarantee financial stability 27. Re-evaluation of degree of disability (possible increase to retire earlier) 28. Preventing and delaying cognitive decline and maintaining functionality 29. Routines and meaningful activities (leisure and training) after retirement 30. Social activities outside of work and community connection

It is important to clarify the concept of parallel aging, which appears in both thematic blocks (need 19 in Table 3 and need 15 in Table 4). This term refers to the fact that, due to the earlier manifestation of the signs of aging in individuals with intellectual disabilities, a parallel aging process occurs between these individuals and their parents, who begin to experience aging simultaneously. This is due to the difference in the age of onset of aging between people with and without disabilities.

We present the most relevant needs in the following five subsections, illustrating them with representative quotations from participants.

3.1. Workplace Accommodations and Support Needs

To address and prevent WADAD, there is a need to adapt duties and make adjustments to job functions, while also incorporating a variety of tasks and rotations. This need is more achievable in sheltered employment than in regular (open) employment, as one professional explained:

> "I understand that in the setting of a special employment center it's perhaps easier to adapt tasks, to adjust a little, but in the mainstream setting, sometimes in companies, it's more difficult".
>
> (P.2.9)

Another crucial aspect involves shortening the working day and making adjustments related to duration. Through discussions in the focus groups, it became evident that this issue posed a challenge in calculating the required contribution period for early retirement. The challenge is more pronounced when there is an early onset of decline. However, recent legislative changes now permit partial working days to be counted as full contribution days. The contribution base is what decreases as remuneration is reduced. One worker with a disability described their experience:

> In my company they do it bit by bit, they don't go all of a sudden and make you retire, maybe they take away some hours, instead of 8 h they give you 6, then 4, and so on, bit by bit so that retirement is not very bad all of a sudden.
>
> (W.1.2)

Another need involves regulating public financial resources to counteract the decline in productivity. This includes assuming the financial cost of adjustments and supports, enabling individuals to continue working without their employers having to resort to reactive dismissals or permanent incapacity. Even with adjustments, the decline in productivity over time can become unsustainable, to the point that work incapacity is considered a viable way out for the worker, the company, and the family. One of the professionals put it this way:

> In the SEC (special employment center), we're obliged to have people who are employed but who are really doing occupational activities, at an occupational pace and output. Colleagues said that in regular employment this is obviously impossible and in a special employment center it's unsustainable.... We can see that it's not sustainable in the long term.
>
> (P.2.12)

3.2. Coordination and Collaboration Needs

At the internal level of the service provider organizations, there is a need for coordination with other services within the same entity. This collaboration is essential for joint planning with various types of professionals, and for the combination and implementation of other cross-cutting support measures. However, human resource shortages within the organizations and the growing financial burden on families to cover emerging support needs make this possibility difficult to realize. Furthermore, access to subsidized care resources is not permitted if the person has an income, which makes it difficult to combine reduced working hours with access to, for example, an occupational center. In the words of one professional, there is a need for:

> "More flexibility, so that we could do something hybrid between the worker working and being able to use spaces in the occupational center, which isn't legally possible".
>
> (P.1.2)
>
> A family member raised the following question:
>
> It would be interesting to know if her organization does something to prepare them for retirement, but more than that, because she needs to have busy time and schedules, because she needs routine. To be busy doing things is very important,

> logically it's not going to be a job, but you know, activities or things she might like, I don't know if that's offered.
>
> (F.1.1)

At the external level of the service provider organizations, there is a need for coordination with the other social and institutional stakeholders involved in providing workplace supports, whether directly or indirectly.

The life-course transition to retirement necessitates collaboration among support organizations, families, and employers. This collaborative effort enables the adjustment of expectations, the resolution of discrepancies, the identification of needs, the provision of supports, and the effective extension of working life. Moreover, it facilitates a smoother transition into retirement. In this regard, full-time jobs consistently yield more contributions in terms of time, and companies should take this factor into account in their offerings. One of the professionals made the following suggestion:

> "I would train companies about this, about the aging of people with disabilities and the needs that are identified, then raise awareness within both the business and family environments".
>
> (P.1.4)

In addition, fostering collaboration with other organizations within the disability sector and various public sector services is imperative. This involves simplifying procedures and enhancing cognitive accessibility in both employment and social security services. Furthermore, it is crucial to ensure that health services provide relevant information and support, facilitating the development of strategies to preserve the functioning capabilities of individuals with intellectual and developmental disabilities, with a particular emphasis on Down syndrome. This emphasis is essential due to the unique characteristics of aging in individuals with Down syndrome, such as a higher prevalence of Alzheimer's disease and an earlier and more accelerated aging process. One professional shared the following perspective:

> In both retirement and the general aging of people with Down syndrome and intellectual disabilities … in public health, we talk on a general level about a lack of knowledge about the aging processes of people with Down syndrome, and in many sectors they're equated or normalized to the process of any other person, when in fact there are many studies that say it's not the case.… And also there's a lack of knowledge about the processes at a medical level for our users.… When it comes to giving sick leave or work incapacity issues we see that the health system isn't up to date, there's no specific training.
>
> (P.2.12)

3.3. Training and Counseling Needs

Of particular importance are job coaches and coworkers, who must be informed and trained regarding the implications of WADAD. As one professional pointed out, "I would ask for more coordination with public bodies, with community services" (P.1.5). Similarly, a worker had this to say:

> First the organization, family, and coworkers.… You have to go where the informant is and they'll tell you.… Let's go where your coworkers are. We'll get you together with them and you tell them that, OK? Your coworkers will have to know so they get a better idea, OK?
>
> (W.2.1)

This need for specific training extends to other professionals, who should acquire a better understanding of the signs of WADAD, its implications, and the relevant legal framework. Consideration should be given to the creation of participatory spaces for professionals to share experiences and knowledge. One professional made this point:

> We find that when the first symptoms of aging appear, the main challenge is adapting the job to these new needs.... We need a lot of training to be able to adapt so that these people can continue with their working life.
>
> (P.2.10)

It is necessary to educate workers with intellectual and developmental disabilities and their families about retirement requirements, processes, possibilities, and compatibility with other pensions. This will support informed decision making and also alleviate the family's concerns. As one worker requested:

> Yes, I'd like to know about the paperwork to be completed and all that ... that training is provided to everyone who's also going to retire, to know where to find the positives and the negatives ... the fears we have, what worries us and all that.
>
> (W.1.1)

The need for information on retirement extends to professionals, particularly concerning the prerequisites for eligibility and the aging processes in the context of disability. This pertains specifically to aspects such as legislation, tools, and strategies available within support organizations concerning aging, WADAD, and retirement. One professional highlighted the information gap:

> We need research that we can see, to have objective and real data because the problem we're starting with is that we don't have data from earlier, for people who've been in these situations before, but we're now encountering people in their forties and fifties who are working, and we don't know what will happen in the future.
>
> (P.1.11)

3.4. Personal and Family Support Needs

For families, the challenge is to continue supporting their relative while simultaneously minimizing the stress caused by a new situation, even without a clear understanding of what is happening. As families play a key role, the difficulty of accepting aging and retirement in workers with intellectual and developmental disabilities can compromise successful collaboration. One family member had this to say:

> I agree with my colleague, parents or relatives need information, but also training, on how we can help them take that step in life, because we haven't thought about it. So we're lost and so are they. We need someone to guide us so that we can make life easier for them.
>
> (F.1.2)

Another concern is the simultaneous aging of workers and their parents, as expressed by one worker, who worried that:

> "if I'm old, I won't have any family left"
>
> (W.2.4)

Similarly, a family member stated that:

> "He still has some time left before he retires. But it's definitely a concern, especially because we won't be there when he retires. It's better to have things prepared beforehand.
>
> (F.2.1)

When retirement becomes necessary and is feasible, there is a high degree of confusion around accepting it, navigating the associated aspects, and prioritizing a progressive and positive transition. One worker expressed the following concerns:

> It worries me because I had been with my company for 16 years and, of course, I was useful working and so on. But when I'm not working and I'm starting to retire, I'm lost, because you have to do something to know that you're worth something . . . not to say that you're worth nothing. When you're not working, well, I don't know, I'm lost.
>
> (W.2.3)

There is a need for individualized support to help manage finances and to promote autonomy and independence, along with a psychological approach to address feelings of loneliness, while providing support for navigating retirement and other administrative and legal procedures. This need becomes more significant when family support is absent, and particularly so when procedures are carried out online with no guarantee of cognitive accessibility. One family member put it this way:

> I imagine that what they're thinking about and worrying about is the loss of the support they have from their parents.. . . I think that what worries my daughter the most is that her father or mother won't be there, finding themselves alone or finding themselves a bit helpless, right.. . . They're thinking about the loss of their parents and what will happen to them when we're no longer around. I know that my daughter, when my mother died—and she was the grandmother she was closest to—that got her thinking about the situation with that bereavement.. . . What they're thinking about is this, that at some point their parents might not be there, not about retirement itself.
>
> (F.1.4)

When the parents are still around and are also retired, it creates a dual impact. On the one hand, individuals with intellectual and developmental disabilities may be influenced or form expectations by observing their parents. On the other hand, there arises a need for support in managing family dynamics as a result of parents and children aging simultaneously. As one family member commented:

> If they see us enjoying retirement, they'll accept it. My daughter hasn't thought about it.. . . But seeing her father and me enjoying retirement, I mean right now. Now we're there more for her, so I don't think it would be traumatic.
>
> (F.2.6)

3.5. Other Needs

There is a noticeable gap in the public provision of services for retiring individuals with disabilities. For many of them, this transition tends to occur earlier than for the general population, although this is not universally the case. The areas of social participation they once enjoyed are drastically reduced. The activities and resources available to them are not aligned with their actual age or their past life experience of engagement and participation in the community. As one professional urged:

> "We have to offer them other services. Like, maybe going to the movies … meeting in bars for tapas, trips; in short, in my humble opinion I see a culture shock, I think there could be a culture shock".
>
> (P.2.9)

The initial stages of the transition process, involving a reduction in working hours and gradual integration into other services, may be perceived as a threat rather than a support. This is because it can mean reduced contributions, and there are genuine fears about not meeting retirement requirements and the corresponding monetary benefits based on years of contribution. There is often a disconnect between the needs of the worker and the expectations of the family. One family member expressed the following concern:

> I don't really know anything about retirement or how many years they need to have worked or have been paying contributions or how many they have left, I have no idea about any of this really, it's a whole new world.
>
> (F.1.1.)
>
> The majority of the identified needs can be effectively met by creating individualized plans for the transition to retirement. These plans facilitate prior preparation, helping individuals comprehend and contextualize retirement. Additionally, they serve as a means to set expectations and promote self-determined choices. As one worker stated, "I'd like help preparing for … once I'm retired before, you know more or less how it works … what I'll have left and so on, but I'd love help preparing for … not to be caught unawares".
>
> (W.2.6)

The effective development of individual plans involves addressing the following key issues: the inadequate training of professionals and limited resources; low levels of contributions from workers; personal and family reluctance to reduce working hours; challenges in adapting job responsibilities, routines, or schedules, particularly in regular employment; difficulties in accessing and reconciling employment and care resources; workers' reluctance to return to resources they relied on prior to being employed; and workers' rejection of life choices that curtail their present levels of social participation.

4. Discussion

The results section highlighted some differences in the importance that different participant profiles give to the various issues identified. However, what is relevant is the complementarity of their points of view and the set of emerging needs collectively identified.

In this study, general strategies such as varying tasks, incorporating rotations, and shortening working hours were mentioned as potential accommodations. However, focus group data revealed a broader and more diverse range of workplace adjustments, including adaptations to work rhythms, the use of assistive technologies, ergonomic modifications, and the reinforcement of natural supports in the workplace. Likewise, it is important to acknowledge that different types of jobs—such as physically demanding versus sedentary roles—may require distinct types of adjustments. These issues are currently being addressed in the continuation of this research—the PROLAB APOYOS study—which aims to analyze in greater depth the types of supports provided, their sources, and their effectiveness in supporting workers with intellectual and developmental disabilities.

All of these findings are consistent with the literature, as other researchers [21,39] have already demonstrated that individuals who choose part-time work experience increased satisfaction during the transition to retirement and are able to engage in community activities while still being employed. Nevertheless, our study identifies issues concerning adjustments and productivity, which may drive individuals, particularly in mainstream employment, to consider work incapacity as a way out. This observation aligns with the findings of [21], highlighting the increased frequency of forced retirement in regular employment.

It is apparent that individuals with intellectual and developmental disabilities may, at times, want to sustain their working life because of what it brings them and make a gradual transition. Previous research has highlighted the benefits of a progressive transition [29,40] and the benefits of keeping active [41,42] on self-esteem, independence, physical and mental health [43], identity and security [41], community participation and social connectedness [30,40], cognitive decline [44,45], and a positive outlook on aging [40].

This research highlights the importance of coordinating internal and external services to provide comprehensive support for the prevention and management of WADAD, and for the transition to retirement. However, we have also pointed out that access to subsidized care resources is not permitted if the person has an income, which makes it difficult to combine reduced working hours with access to care resources, thus hindering a gradual transition. The family plays a key role, yet insufficient information often leads to resistance and a lack of acceptance. For their part, professionals emphasize the need for specific training. Workers with intellectual and developmental disabilities may experience concerns about retirement and therefore need access to appropriate information and support to better understand and evaluate these fears. Ref. [27] noted that retirement can be disruptive, especially when information about post-retirement activities is lacking. Ref. [42] highlighted that workers with intellectual and developmental disabilities often lack a complete understanding of retirement, resulting in feelings of dissatisfaction and a sense of diminished control. Similar sentiments are experienced by those who do comprehend the situation but cannot make decisions about it, supporting the observations of [28] regarding the insufficient preparation of individuals with disabilities for retirement decision-making processes.

This study addresses various financial issues that, according to the literature, are considered a primary concern. For example, ref. [21] underscores the critical role of financial aspects in retirement decisions, while [46] highlights how financial self-sufficiency enhances resilience against adversities in aging. In addition, the authors of [28] note that the decrease in income upon leaving the workforce is a barrier for people with disabilities when they retire. However, in our research, financial security was among the least frequently mentioned topics across participant groups.

Workers with intellectual and developmental disabilities are sometimes denied financial self-determination in their families, limiting them from pursuing the activities they desire [40]. This represents a challenge because, despite possessing financial resources, they may not have had the opportunity to learn how to manage them in preparation for the next stage of their lives as retirees. While it should be acknowledged that full financial autonomy may not always be achievable, it is crucial to consider who will provide this support once parents are no longer present.

Additionally, middle-aged individuals with disabilities face more limited social networks and fewer opportunities for relationships [40,47,48]. Our study also recognizes this reality as a barrier to be addressed during the transition to retirement.

Our study has revealed that WADAD and reduced productivity can sometimes result in sudden dismissals or recourse to solutions such as work incapacity, without proper transition planning. The transition to retirement can be either proactive and planned or reactive and sudden [49,50]. However, individuals with intellectual disabilities predominantly undergo reactive transitions, occurring abruptly and without sufficient planning [51].

This study underscores the fears and reservations of workers with intellectual and developmental disabilities and their families regarding post-retirement futures potentially filled with meaningless routines and tasks far removed from their employment experiences. These concerns align with findings from previous research [28,31,50].

The need for support both before and after retirement to facilitate a successful transition, alleviating fears and promoting continued social participation, has been demonstrated in other studies [21,27,48]. However, little is known about the types of supports or services needed by people with intellectual and developmental disabilities to foster active aging during the transition process [52].

Early planning is thus key to achieving a meaningful and positive transition. The authors of [30] previously emphasized the importance of promoting active aging through pre-retirement planning and preparation.

Active aging is considered the most effective response to the challenges posed by aging populations. However, there is substantial variation in how public bodies respond to the needs of older adults with intellectual and developmental disabilities. Other studies [12,42] reported that community-based programs were the most beneficial. While individuals with intellectual and developmental disabilities typically receive tailored supports, public initiatives to assist older adults with disabilities in their transition to retirement are limited [52]. Excluded from general social policies for older adults; this group requires specific services tailored to their needs [27]. Our research has identified a sense of dissatisfaction among individuals with intellectual and developmental disabilities and their families regarding general services for older people, which are designed for older people without disabilities. The same is true for residential services, complicating the prospect of aging in place. This difficulty has been reported by other authors [40,46,50], all of whom underscored aging in place as a fundamental pillar for aging individuals with intellectual and developmental disabilities.

4.1. Limitations

Conducting remote focus groups with workers nearing retirement or showing signs of decline presented challenges, as many participants were unfamiliar with the technology, and their support professionals were not present during the sessions. To facilitate participation, support technicians provided assistance before the sessions began. However, to ensure participants' freedom of expression, the research team requested that these professionals leave the virtual room once the connection was established. During the focus groups, the research team provided timely support and, when necessary, contacted the technicians to intervene and assist participants. Additionally, easy-to-read manuals, breaks, and extra assistance were provided whenever possible.

In the family groups, difficulties arose due to a lack of volunteers and the advanced age of the participants, but these were overcome with the help of the collaborating organizations.

Although the wide age range of participants (from 26 to 81 years old) may be considered a limitation—especially given the study's focus on the transition to retirement—this was an intentional decision. The research team chose to include a diverse sample in terms of age and profile in order to capture perspectives from individuals who were already beginning to consider retirement, as well as those who were not yet doing so. This diversity was deemed to enrich the findings by allowing the exploration of a broader variety of experiences, concerns, and needs related to aging in the workplace and preparing for retirement.

The translation of the participants' statements may involve a loss of idiomatic meaning, which we consider acceptable and impossible to eliminate. To mitigate this issue, the translation was performed by a competent professional familiar with the area of study. The full texts of the original-language transcriptions are available in an open repository [53].

Finally, it is important to highlight that participant selection through collaborating organizations may introduce sampling bias. This limits the representativeness of the overall population of workers with intellectual and developmental disabilities and, consequently, the generalizability of the results to other contexts or groups. Additionally, given the qualitative nature and sample size, the findings should be interpreted with caution and considered as an exploratory approach rather than definitive conclusions that are applicable to the entire population.

4.2. Future Research Directions

Future research should focus on refining a robust and evidence-based tool that allows professionals to detect work ability decline, provide support through individualized plans, and progressively plan for the transition to retirement. The qualitative approach employed in this study could prove beneficial for developing protocols applicable to other types of disabilities (and for analyzing differences between groups, such as those in people with Down syndrome versus other intellectual disabilities). It enables the consolidation of knowledge derived from organizations with established practices in this field. Further, there is an opportunity to create a guide outlining common types of supports and adjustments for older workers with intellectual and developmental disabilities, along with guidelines to facilitate decision making.

5. Conclusions

This study aimed to identify the specific needs required to prevent work-related aging and decline among adults with disabilities (WADAD) and to support an active, planned transition to retirement for individuals with intellectual and developmental disabilities.

In this regard, there is a clear need to better understand the decline in work ability and how it progresses among aging individuals with intellectual and developmental disabilities. By conducting a qualitative analysis, this study examined the needs of this group, their families, and the professionals supporting them. The use of specific assessment tools could help professionals in the creation of individualized plans and supports to prevent and effectively manage WADAD, thereby enabling the self-determined extension of working life. Individual plans should be adjusted based on identified needs, encompassing task diversification and the integration of rotations to prevent boredom. Furthermore, these plans should align activities with workers' capabilities, adjusting the pace and redistributing breaks accordingly. Similarly, changes in the job role should be instituted as needed, but in a controlled manner and with support, given the complexities associated with adapting to new responsibilities later in life. Vital aspects encompass ergonomic and technological support, a more flexible workday, and the training of coworkers who serve as natural supports within the workplace.

In this context, it is crucial to establish specialized prevention services. These services should address psychological aspects, offer prevention workshops, assemble interdisciplinary teams, improve the flow of communication between professionals within the organization, and foster connections with other social stakeholders. This comprehensive approach facilitates cohesive care across various areas of the lives of older workers with intellectual and developmental disabilities as they approach retirement. Additionally, training and information options on WADAD should be channeled to all stakeholders involved.

When the time to transition to retirement comes, individualized programs should consider workers' preferences and provide detailed information on potential benefits and income sources. Support groups and programs addressing the pre-retirement stage can prove highly beneficial. Essential elements include providing information on leisure resources, cognitive exercises, and opportunities to enhance mental and physical health. Families also need advice and information to support them throughout the process. Additionally, legislation must be appropriately tailored to the identified needs.

Once the transition process is complete, there is a need for a comprehensive approach in the form of an active aging plan, encompassing health, leisure, social relationships, community participation, and housing options. Specialized training in this domain, along with collaboration between all public and private stakeholders in the areas of work, health, leisure, and independent living, is essential to address the complexities of aging in individuals with intellectual and developmental disabilities. This combination of specialized training and collaboration also serves to detect WADAD and facilitate the necessary adjustments for a fulfilling retirement.

These results offer relevant practical implications for policy design, service planning, and professional intervention. The identification of specific needs related to work ability decline and the transition to retirement provides a foundation for developing individualized, coordinated, and sustainable protocols. These should include workplace accommodations, early retirement planning, accessible training, and the development of community-based support networks. Thus, this study not only contributes empirical knowledge but also provides specific guidance to transform practice and improve the quality of life of people with intellectual and developmental disabilities as they age.

Author Contributions: All authors contributed to all phases of the research and preparation of the manuscript: conceptualization, review of bibliographic resources, data collection and analysis, writing, revision, and editing. As Principal Investigators, F.d.B.J.d.U. and M.Á.V. were responsible for directing the project in which this work is framed and for obtaining and administering funds. B.S. was primarily responsible for supervising the qualitative methodology applied. All authors have read and agreed to the published version of the manuscript.

Funding: This study was funded by Plena Inclusión España, Fundación Once, Asociación Española de Empleo con Apoyo, and Down España.

Institutional Review Board Statement: The study was conducted in accordance with the Declaration of Helsinki and approved by the Ethics Committee of the University Institute for Community Integration [INICO] of the University of Salamanca (protocol code CEI-INICO/2021-01 and 15 January 2021).

Informed Consent Statement: Informed consent was obtained from all subjects involved in the study.

Data Availability Statement: The transcript data are available in the University of Salamanca repository: Sánchez Herráez, B.; Jordán de Urríes Vega, F.B.; Verdugo Alonso, M.A.; Abena Abang, C.J.; Sanblás Capote, V. Transcripts from the Focus Groups of the PROLAB Project Research (Dataset); Gredos Repository, University of Salamanca: Salamanca, Spain, 2025. https://doi.org/10.71636/3j5p-9z03.

Acknowledgments: We would like to express our heartfelt gratitude to all the individuals who participated in the focus groups, as well as to the collaborating organizations in the field of disability at the national level, including Plena Inclusión, the Spanish Association for Supported Employment, Down España, and Fundación ONCE. Their generous collaboration and commitment were essential to the development of this research. Without their participation, this work would not have been possible.

Conflicts of Interest: The authors declare no conflicts of interest.

Abbreviations

INICO	University Institute for Community Integration
WADAD	Work Ability Decline through Aging and Disability
IQ	Intellectual Quotient
P	Professional

W	Worker with disability
F	Family member
SEC	Special Employment Center

References

1. Schalock, R.L.; Luckasson, R.; Tassé, M.J. An Overview of Intellectual Disability: Definition, Diagnosis, Classification, and Systems of Supports (12th ed.). *Am. J. Intellect. Dev. Disabil.* **2021**, *126*, 439–442. [CrossRef] [PubMed]
2. United Nations. Convention on the Rights of Persons with Disability. 2006. Available online: https://social.desa.un.org/issues/disability/crpd/convention-on-the-rights-of-persons-with-disabilities-crpd (accessed on 15 May 2024).
3. Laborda Molla, C.; Jariot García, M.; González Fernández, H. Calidad de vida y competencias de empleabilidad en personas trabajadoras en centros especiales de empleo. *Educación XX1* **2021**, *24*, 117–139. [CrossRef]
4. Instituto Nacional de Estadística. El Empleo de las Personas con Discapacidad (EPD) Año 2022 (Internet). 2023. Available online: https://www.ine.es/prensa/epd_2022.pdf (accessed on 15 May 2024).
5. Ortega-Camarero, M.T.; Cuesta-Gómez, J.L.; de la Fuente-Anuncibay, R. Intellectual Disability, Employment and Aging: Intervention Measures. *Int. J. Environ. Res. Public Health* **2021**, *18*, 2984. [CrossRef] [PubMed]
6. Observatorio Sobre Discapacidad y Mercado de Trabajo en España O. Fundación ONCE. 2023. Informe 8. Available online: https://odismet.es/sites/default/files/2023-05/INFORME%208.v2_0.pdf (accessed on 15 May 2024).
7. Servicio Público de Empleo Estatal S. Servicio Público de Empleo Estatal. Datos Estadísiticos de Contratos. 2024. Available online: https://www.sepe.es/HomeSepe/es/que-es-el-sepe/estadisticas/contratos/estadisticas-nuevas/2024/enero.html (accessed on 15 May 2024).
8. Observatorio Estatal de la Discapacidad. Realidad, Situación, Dimensión y Tendencias del Empleo con Apoyo en España en el Horizonte del año 2020 (Internet). 2017. Available online: https://www.observatoriodeladiscapacidad.info/wp-content/uploads/2018/05/Informe-OED-ECA-v3.pdf (accessed on 15 May 2024).
9. INE—Instituto Nacional de Estadística. *Encuesta de Discapacidad, Autonomía Personal y Situaciones de Dependencia 2020 (EDAD2020)*; Instituto Nacional de Estadística: Madrid, Spain, 2022.
10. Jordán de Urríes Fde, B.; Sánchez, B.; Verdugo, M.Á. Assessment of work ability decline in workers with intellectual and developmental disabilities. *J. Vocat. Rehabil.* **2022**, *57*, 187–195. [CrossRef]
11. Anderson, L.L.; Hall, S.; Kramme, J.E.D.; Stancliffe, R. Transition to retirement: The lived experiences of adults with intellectual disabilities. *J. Appl. Res. Intellect. Disabil.* **2023**, *36*, 547–557. [CrossRef]
12. Bigby, C. Comparative Program Options for Aging People with Intellectual Disabilities. *J. Policy Pract. Intellect. Disabil.* **2005**, *2*, 75–85. [CrossRef]
13. Buys, L.; Aird, R.; Miller, E. Service providers' perceptions of active ageing among older adults with lifelong intellectual disabilities. *J. Intellect. Disabil. Res.* **2012**, *56*, 1133–1147. [CrossRef]
14. World Health Organization. Active Ageing: A Policy Framework. 2002. Available online: https://apps.who.int/iris/bitstream/handle/10665/67215/WH0?sequence=1 (accessed on 15 May 2024).
15. Foster, L.; Boxall, K. People with learning disabilities and 'active ageing'. *Br. J. Learn. Disabil.* **2015**, *43*, 270–276. [CrossRef]
16. España. Real Decreto 1539/2003. de 5 de diciembre, por el que se establecen coeficientes reductores de la edad de jubilación a favor de los trabajadores que acreditan un grado importante de minusvalía. *Boletín Oficial del Estado*, 20 December 2003; pp. 45343–45345.
17. España. Real decreto 370/2023. de 16 de mayo, por el que se modifica el Real Decreto 1851/2009, de 4 de diciembre, por el que se desarrolla el artículo 161.bis de la Ley General de la Seguridad Social en cuanto a la anticipación de la jubilación de los trabajadores con discapacidad en grado igual o superior al 45 por ciento. *Boletín Oficial del Estado*, 17 May 2023; pp. 68237–68242.
18. Chng, J.P.L.; Stancliffe, R.J.; Wilson, N.J.; Anderson, K. Engagement in retirement: An evaluation of the effect of Active Mentoring on engagement of older adults with intellectual disability in mainstream community groups. *J. Intellect. Disabil. Res.* **2013**, *57*, 1130–1142. [CrossRef]
19. Miller, S.M.; Chan, F. Predictors of life satisfaction in individuals with intellectual disabilities. *J. Intellect. Disabil. Res.* **2008**, *52*, 1039–1047. [CrossRef]
20. Miller, E.; Cooper, S.; Cook, A.; Petch, A. Outcomes Important to People with Intellectual Disabilities. *J. Policy Pract. Intellect. Disabil.* **2008**, *5*, 150–158. [CrossRef]
21. Brotherton, M.; Stancliffe, R.J.; Wilson, N.J.; O'Loughlin, K. Supporting workers with intellectual disability in mainstream employment to transition to a socially inclusive retirement. *J. Intellect. Dev. Disabil.* **2016**, *41*, 75–80. [CrossRef]
22. Noone, J.; O'Loughlin, K.; Kendig, H. Australian baby boomers retiring 'early': Understanding the benefits of retirement preparation for involuntary and voluntary retirees. *J. Aging Stud.* **2013**, *27*, 207–217. [CrossRef] [PubMed]
23. Schellenberg, G.; Turcotte, M.; Ram, B. Preparing for retirement. *Can. Soc. Trends.* 2005. 8–11. Available online: https://www150.statcan.gc.ca/n1/en/pub/11-008-x/2005002/article/8452-eng.pdf?st=zt51VaqY (accessed on 15 May 2024).

24. De Vaus, D.; Wells, Y.; Kendig, H.; Quine, S. Does gradual retirement have better outcomes than abrupt retirement? Results from an Australian panel study. *Ageing Soc.* **2007**, *27*, 667–682. [CrossRef]
25. Buys, L.; Boulton-Lewis, G.; Tedman-Jones, J.; Edwards, H.; Knox, M.; Bigby, C. Research: Issues of active ageing: Perceptions of older people with lifelong intellectual disability. *Australas. J. Ageing* **2008**, *27*, 67–71. [CrossRef] [PubMed]
26. Bigby, C.; Wilson, N.J.; Stancliffe, R.J.; Balandin, S.; Craig, D.; Gambin, N. An Effective Program Design to Support Older Workers with Intellectual Disability to Participate Individually in Community Groups. *J. Policy Pract. Intellect. Disabil.* **2014**, *11*, 117–127. [CrossRef]
27. Bigby, C.; Wilson, N.J.; Balandin, S.; Stancliffe, R.J. Disconnected expectations: Staff, family, and supported employee perspectives about retirement. *J. Intellect. Dev. Disabil.* **2011**, *36*, 167–174. [CrossRef]
28. McDermott, S.; Edwards, R. Enabling Self-determination for Older Workers with Intellectual Disabilities in Supported Employment in Australia. *J. Appl. Res. Intellect. Disabil.* **2012**, *25*, 423–432. [CrossRef]
29. Fesko, S.L.; Hall, A.C.; Quinlan, J.; Jockell, C. Active Aging for Individuals with Intellectual Disability: Meaningful Community Participation Through Employment, Retirement, Service, and Volunteerism. *Am. J. Intellect. Dev. Disabil.* **2012**, *117*, 497–508. [CrossRef]
30. Llewellyn, G.; Balandin, S.; Dew, A.; McConnell, D. Promoting healthy, productive ageing: Plan early, plan well. *J. Intellect. Dev. Disabil.* **2004**, *29*, 366–369. [CrossRef]
31. Wark, S.; Canon-Vanry, M.; Ryan, P.; Hussain, R.; Knox, M.; Edwards, M.; Parmenter, M.; Parmenter, T.; Janicki, M.; Leggatt-Cook, C. Ageing-related experiences of adults with learning disability resident in rural areas: One Australian perspective. *Br. J. Learn. Disabil.* **2015**, *43*, 293–301. [CrossRef]
32. Sánchez-Gómez, M.C.; Martín-Cilleros, M.V. Implementation of Focus Group in Health Research. In *Computer Supported Qualitative Research*; Costa, A., Reis, L., Neri de Sousa, F., Moreira, A., Lamas, D., Eds.; Studies in Systems, Decision and Control; Springer: Cham, Switzerland, 2017; Volume 71, pp. 67–78. [CrossRef]
33. Costa, A.P.; de Sousa, F.N.; Moreira, A.; de Souza, D.N. Research through Design: Qualitative Analysis to Evaluate the Usability. In *Computer Supported Qualitative Research Studies in Systems, Decision and Control*; Costa, A., Reis, L., Neri de Sousa, F., Moreira, A., Lamas, D., Eds.; Springer: Cham, Switzerland, 2017; pp. 1–12.
34. Miles, M.B.; Huberman, A.M. *Qualitative Data Analysis: An Expanded Sourcebook*, 2nd ed.; Sage Publications Inc.: Thousand Oaks, CA, USA, 1994.
35. Glaser, B.; Strauss, A. *The Discovery of Grounded Theory: Strategies for Qualitative Research*; Sociology Press: Mill Valley, CA, USA, 1967.
36. Corbin, J.; Strauss, A. *Basics of Qualitative Research, Techniques and Procedures for Developing Grounded Theory*, 4th ed.; Sage Publications Inc.: Thousand Oaks, CA, USA, 2015.
37. Creswell, J.W.; Poth, C.N. *Qualitative Inquiry and Research Design: Choosing Among Five Approaches*, 4th ed.; Sage Publications Inc.: Thousand Oaks, CA, USA, 2017.
38. Brantlinger, E.; Jimenez, R.; Klingner, J.; Pugach, M.; Richardson, V. Qualitative Studies in Special Education. *Except. Child.* **2005**, *71*, 195–207. [CrossRef]
39. Engeland, J.; Kittelsaa, A.; Langballe, E.M. How do People with Intellectual Disabilities in Norway Experience the Transition to Retirement and Life as Retirees? *Scand. J. Disabil. Res.* **2018**, *20*, 72–81. [CrossRef]
40. Mee Kim, K.; Shin, Y.R.; Hwang, S. Psychosocial experiences of the ageing of middle-aged people with intellectual disabilities in South Korea. *Int. J. Dev. Disabil.* **2020**, *66*, 196–203. [CrossRef]
41. David, N.; Duvdevani, I.; Doron, I. Older Women with Intellectual Disability and the Meaning of Aging. *J. Women Aging* **2015**, *27*, 216–236. [CrossRef] [PubMed]
42. Judge, J.; Walley, R.; Anderson, B.; Young, R. Activity, Aging, and Retirement: The Views of a Group of Scottish People with Intellectual Disabilities. *J. Policy Pract. Intellect. Disabil.* **2010**, *7*, 295–301. [CrossRef]
43. McGlinchey, E.; McCallion, P.; Burke, E.; Carroll, R.; McCarron, M. Exploring the Issue of Employment for Adults with an Intellectual Disability in Ireland. *J. Appl. Res. Intellect. Disabil.* **2013**, *26*, 335–343. [CrossRef]
44. Signo, S. *El Proceso de Envejecimiento en las Personas con Síndrome de Down: Estudio Multicéntrico para la Detección de los Cambios Neuropsicológicos*; Universitat Ramon Llull: Barcelona, Spain, 2016.
45. Su, C.Y.; Lin, Y.H.; Wu, Y.Y.; Chen, C.C. The role of cognition and adaptive behavior in employment of people with mental retardation. *Res. Dev. Disabil.* **2008**, *29*, 83–95. [CrossRef]
46. Dew, A.; Llewellyn, G.; Gorman, J. "Having the Time of My Life": An Exploratory Study of Women with Intellectual Disability Growing Older. *Health Care Women Int.* **2006**, *27*, 908–929. [CrossRef]
47. Wilson, N.J.; Bigby, C.; Stancliffe, R.J.; Balandin, S.; Craig, D.; Anderson, K. Mentors' experiences of using the Active Mentoring model to support older adults with intellectual disability to participate in community groups. *J. Intellect. Dev. Disabil.* **2013**, *38*, 344–355. [CrossRef]

48. Newberry, G.; Martin, C.; Robbins, L. How do people with learning disabilities experience and make sense of the ageing process? *Br. J. Learn. Disabil.* **2015**, *43*, 285–292. [CrossRef]
49. Stancliffe, R.J.; Brotherton, M.; O'Loughlin, K.; Wilson, N. Retirement. In *Handbook of Positive Psychology in Intellectual and Developmental Disabilities*; Springer International Publishing: Cham, Switzerland, 2017; pp. 339–355.
50. Strnadová, I. Transitions in the Lives of Older Adults with Intellectual Disabilities: "Having a Sense of Dignity and Independence". *J. Policy Pract. Intellect. Disabil.* **2019**, *16*, 58–66. [CrossRef]
51. Taggart, L.; Truesdale-Kennedy, M.; Ryan, A.; McConkey, R. Examining the support needs of ageing family carers in developing future plans for a relative with an intellectual disability. *J. Intellect. Disabil.* **2012**, *16*, 217–234. [CrossRef]
52. Wilson, N.J.; Stancliffe, R.J.; Bigby, C.; Balandin, S.; Craig, D. The potential for active mentoring to support the transition into retirement for older adults with a lifelong disability. *J. Intellect. Dev. Disabil.* **2010**, *35*, 211–214. [CrossRef]
53. Sánchez Herráez, B.; Jordán de Urríes Vega, F.B.; Verdugo Alonso, M.A.; Abena Abang, C.J.; Sanblás Capote, V. *Transcripts from the Focus Groups of the PROLAB Project Research (Dataset)*; Repositorio Gredos; Universidad de Salamanca: Salamanca, Spain, 2025. [CrossRef]

healthcare

MDPI

Review

Inclusion in Neglected Tropical Disease Programmes: A Review of Inclusive Approaches for Control and Elimination

Ismat Zehra Juma *, Opeoluwa Oguntoye, Girija Sankar, Joerg Weber, Babar Qureshi and Juliana Amanyi-Enegela

Christian Blind Mission, 64625 Bensheim, Germany; opeoluwa.oguntoye@cbm.org (O.O.); girija.sankar@cbm.org (G.S.); joerg.weber@cbm.org (J.W.); babar.qureshi@cbm.org (B.Q.); juliana.amanyi-enegela@cbm.org (J.A.-E.)

* Correspondence: ismat.juma@cbm.org

Abstract

Neglected Tropical Diseases (NTDs) disproportionately affect the world's most marginalised populations, yet programmes aiming to control and eliminate NTDs often fail to fully address the structural, social, and political dimensions of exclusion. This narrative review examines the concept of inclusion within NTD programming, with a particular focus on intersecting forms of marginalisation, including poverty, gender, disability, and displacement. Drawing on studies from 2010 to 2025, from various databases such as google scholar, PubMed and PLOS, this review synthesises evidence on barriers to equitable healthcare access, the role of community-driven approaches, and the integration of inclusive strategies within NTD programming and broader health systems. Key themes include the impact of structural inequalities such as racism and poverty, the need for gender-responsive services, the marginalisation of displaced communities, and the critical role of community empowerment through mechanisms like peer support and community drug distribution of NTD medicines. The review proposes a working definition of inclusion in NTDs as the intentional integration of underserved groups into all levels of programming, policy, and service delivery. It highlights the urgency of reframing NTDs not just as biomedical challenges but as deeply embedded social justice issues. By embedding inclusion into programme design, implementation, and evaluation, stakeholders can better align NTD responses with global equity goals and the Sustainable Development Goals.

Keywords: neglected tropical diseases; NTDs; disability inclusion; elimination; control; gender inclusion; health systems strengthening; DMDI; MMDP; IDM; healthcare

1. Introduction

Neglected tropical diseases (NTDs) encompass a diverse group of 21 diseases, including trachoma, onchocerciasis, lymphatic filariasis, soil-transmitted worm infections, and schistosomiasis, among others, that disproportionately affect vulnerable communities in tropical and subtropical regions, inflicting a significant burden on health and well-being [1,2]. Globally, over one billion individuals require prevention or treatment services for at least one NTD, thus accounting for approximately 19 million disability-adjusted life years (DALYs) annually [3].

These conditions have earned the label **"neglected"** because, despite inflicting profound physical and social suffering, they have historically received scant attention in global health. This neglect has manifested across multiple levels: within communities, where fear and stigma discourage diagnosis and care-seeking; within national systems, where health authorities deprioritise remote rural regions lacking NTD support services; and on the global stage, where investments in NTDs are overshadowed by other attention to other infectious diseases [1,2,4,5].

The impact of NTDs extends far beyond acute infection. They are embedded in environmental and socioeconomic deprivation, including inadequate sanitation, poor access to healthcare, and limited educational opportunities, all of which sustain a destructive cycle of poverty and disease transmission [4]. When coupled with ongoing malnutrition, inadequate housing, climate events, conflict, and economic vulnerability, these conditions create fertile ground for NTD epidemics [6].

Additionally, many NTDs result in long-term impairments such as blindness (e.g., trachoma, onchocerciasis), lymphedema (lymphatic filariasis), and physical disfigurement (leprosy). These impairments significantly restrict daily functioning and social participation [7,8]. Compounding these issues, stigma and social exclusion frequently produce adverse mental health outcomes among affected individuals [8,9]. Despite this clear evidence, disability and mental health dimensions remain clearly under-addressed in NTD programmes, which typically emphasise infection control metrics rather than functional outcomes or social inclusion strategies [10].

Recognising this gap, the concept of disability inclusion in NTDs has evolved to encompass broader frameworks for health and social engagement. Rather than merely providing chemotherapeutic medicines, inclusive approaches advocate for equitable access to healthcare and social services, meaningful representation in programme design and decisions, and supportive structures that empower individuals and communities to manage their health and well-being [11]. Hence, this review aims to explore disability inclusion within the context of NTD programmes.

In the context of NTD programming, *inclusion* refers to the intentional integration of historically excluded populations—such as persons with disabilities, women, and displaced people—into all phases of programme design, implementation, and evaluation. This framing is informed by WHO guidance on people-centred health systems and disability equity [12,13]. This framing also aligns with Kuper's conceptualization of disability inclusion as ensuring that people with disabilities can equitably access and participate in NTD programmes by addressing structural barriers such as physical inaccessibility, financial constraints, stigma, and lack of representation and by involving disability-led organisations in programme planning and delivery [8].

Inclusion is distinct yet interrelated with concepts such as equity and participation:

- **Equity** refers to the fair distribution of resources and outcomes, particularly addressing structural disadvantages [14].
- **Participation** denotes meaningful involvement of affected groups in planning, decision-making, and implementation, but does not always ensure equity or empowerment [15].

Inclusion integrates both dimensions with a particular emphasis on recognising and removing barriers for historically excluded groups. In this review, we look at inclusion as encompassing four interlinked domains, access, participation, empowerment, and governance, each essential for building equitable NTD programmes.

1.1. Objective

The primary objective of this review is to explore the multidimensional concept of inclusion in the context of NTDs. Specifically, this review aims to:

- **Define the Concept:** To provide a clear and comprehensive definition of inclusion as it relates to NTDs, considering the various components and dimensions of the

https://doi.org/10.3390/healthcare14010027

concept. Additionally, consider the cross sections of disability inclusion within NTD programming as well as the intersectionality between disability inclusion and NTDs.

- **Explore the Dimensions:** Examine the different dimensions of inclusion, including but not limited to access to healthcare, social participation, gender equity, and their interplay in the context of NTDs.
- **Identify Research Gaps:** Identify gaps in the existing literature, highlighting areas where further research is needed to advance the understanding of inclusion in NTD programmes and policies.

Based on the objectives outlined above, the paper will address the following research question:

How is the concept of inclusion defined and operationalized within NTD programming, and what are the key dimensions and gaps that shape inclusive NTD interventions and policies?

This current paper aims to review existing literature and develop a concept on inclusion within NTDs, specifically focusing on gender and disability.

1.2. Significance

Addressing inclusion within NTD programmes is essential for several reasons. First, NTDs are inextricably tied to poverty and inequity, affecting over one billion people living in 149 countries, making inclusion a matter of social justice and human rights [12,16,17]. Second, inclusive NTD services can be contextual, community-driven, and sustainable. Recent estimates indicate that around 1.62 billion people required NTD interventions in 2022, a 26% decrease since 2010, highlighting how tailored programme strategies can successfully increase treatment uptake [18,19]. Additionally, inclusion aligns with broader global health and development agendas, including the Sustainable Development Goals (SDGs), which emphasise the importance of leaving no one behind [20].

On the other hand, approximately 15% of the global population has a disability [21–23], and this large group must be considered when designing NTD programmes. Improving the inclusion of people with disabilities may require adaptations to NTD programmes, such as making them physically accessible or training staff about disability awareness. Without incorporating disability within NTD programmes, the quality of life of people with NTDs will suffer, and global targets for elimination and management of NTDs will not be met [7].

This review fills a significant gap in the existing literature by consolidating current knowledge and conceptual frameworks in relation to inclusion in NTDs. Synthesising evidence from diverse contexts and disease-specific studies provides policymakers, researchers, and practitioners with a resource for designing more inclusive and practical strategies to combat NTDs. Ultimately, this review contributes to the broader discourse on global health equity and underscores the imperative of inclusion as a central tenet in the fight against NTDs.

2. Methodology

This review employed a narrative synthesis, allowing for an in-depth and interpretive examination of the literature on disability inclusion in neglected tropical disease (NTD) programming. Compared to systematic reviews, narrative reviews offer flexibility that accommodates diverse study designs and methodologies, allowing nuanced thematic exploration [24].

2.1. Search Strategy

A comprehensive search was conducted across PubMed, Scopus, and Web of Science, covering the period from January 2010 to April 2025. Medical Subject Headings (MeSH)

https://doi.org/10.3390/healthcare14010027

and free-text search strings, including terms such as *"neglected tropical diseases"*, *"disability inclusion"*, *"equity"*, *"community participation"*, *"stigma"*, and *"rehabilitation"* were used. These were combined using Boolean operators (AND/OR), and search terms were iteratively refined according to guidelines by Sukhera [24].

2.2. Screening and Eligibility

We followed the SALSA framework (Search, Appraisal, Synthesis, Analysis) to guide selection [25]. Two reviewers conducted an initial screening of titles and abstracts independently, followed by a full-text assessment. Eligibility criteria, as shown in Table 1, included: (1) English-language publications from 2010 to 2025 focusing on disability inclusion within NTD programming; (2) primary empirical studies (quantitative, qualitative, mixed methods), programme evaluations, or policy analyses explicitly addressing disability adaptations, data systems, or community participation; (3) policy or grey literature with relevant insights. Exclusion criteria encompassed laboratory-only articles, clinical trials without disability focus, grey literature lacking sufficient methodological detail, and non-NTD studies. Figure 1 shows the PRISMA flow for screening and selection of articles.

Table 1. Eligibility Criteria.

Eligibility Criteria	
Inclusion Criteria	**Exclusion Criteria**
Studies published in English	Studies published in languages other than English
Studies published from 2010–2025	Studies published before 2010
Primary research studies, including quantitative, qualitative, and mixed-methods studies	Review articles, commentaries, and editorials.
Studies focusing on NTDs and the concept of inclusion, covering various dimensions of inclusion such as access to healthcare, social participation, and empowerment. Additionally, other public health interventions and how they look at inclusion to plan their projects was also looked at.	Studies not directly related to NTDs or the concept of inclusion within public health
Studies that provide clear definitions, frameworks, or models related to inclusion in the context of NTDs.	Studies lacking relevant data or clear definitions of inclusion

2.3. Data Extraction and Synthesis

From included studies, we extracted data on how disability inclusion was defined, integrated into NTD service delivery, and evaluated; types of programme adaptations; reported outcomes; enabling conditions; and implementation obstacles. Dual independent screening and data extraction were used, with disagreements resolved through discussion. Although we did not apply a formal risk-of-bias tool—consistent with narrative review conventions—we conducted an informal critical appraisal based on the Mixed Methods Appraisal Tool (MMAT), focusing on methods clarity and contextual framing.

Thematic content analysis was performed iteratively, with emerging themes organised around our three review questions: conceptualization, practical strategies, and barriers to inclusive implementation.

https://doi.org/10.3390/healthcare14010027

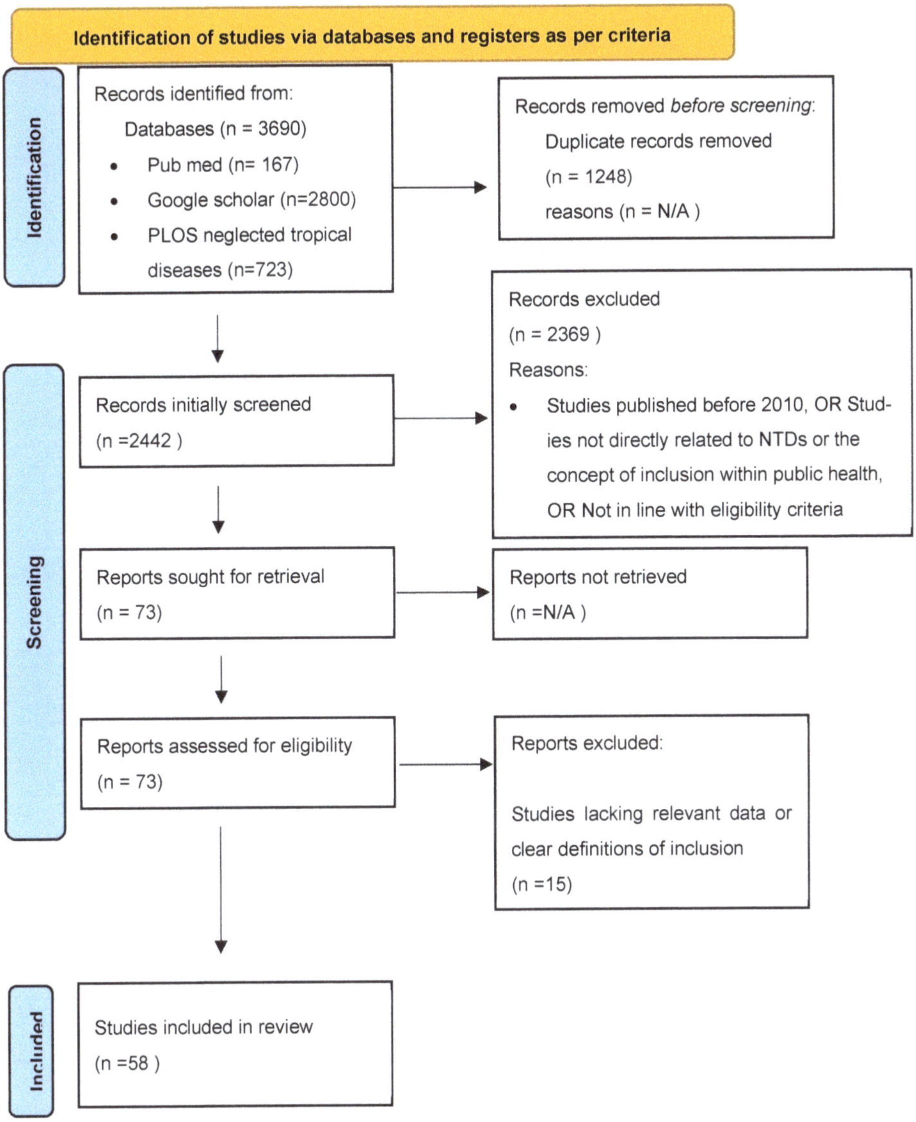

Figure 1. PRISMA Flow Chart.

2.4. Ethical Considerations

This review was based entirely on secondary information, which is publicly available literature and did not involve primary data collection; hence, no formal ethical approval was required [24]. Nonetheless, ethical standards were upheld by ensuring the accurate representation of prior research, giving proper credit to original authors, avoiding any distortion of their findings, and selecting sources based on their relevance, credibility, and methodological quality [26]. Sources were selected based on relevance, credibility, and methodological rigour to ensure the integrity of the synthesis [27].

https://doi.org/10.3390/healthcare14010027

3. Results and Findings

This narrative review included studies comprising primary research articles and systematic reviews published between 2010 and 2025 that met our inclusion criteria. The selected literature encompassed qualitative, quantitative, and mixed methods designs, with a predominant focus on sub-Saharan Africa (Nigeria, Uganda, Kenya, Cameroon, Ethiopia, and Liberia) and Latin America (Brazil). Several studies also addressed transnational and global health policy contexts related to disability inclusion in NTD programming. Drawing from this rich corpus, we distilled key thematic insights, clarified emerging concepts, and identified critical research gaps. It is essential to note that, although comprehensive in scope, this review does not exhaustively cover disability inclusion theories; thus, it limits its focus to studies most relevant to our research questions.

As shown in Table 2, the synthesis of the eligible studies highlights five overarching themes, each examined through specific methodologies, in targeted geographies, and with distinct populations, offering essential insights into the current landscape of disability inclusion within NTD programmes.

Table 2. Summary of Findings.

Theme	Key Method	Geographic Focus	Population Targeted	Main Findings	Publication Year	Sample Type	Study Count
1. Social and Economic Inequalities	Qualitative, Mixed-Methods, Systematic Review	Brazil, Sub-Saharan Africa	Racial minorities, Poor, Displaced	- Social and economic inequalities, including poverty, racism, gender discrimination, and displacement, significantly increase vulnerability to NTDs and limit access to care, especially among marginalised and underserved populations. - To eliminate NTDs effectively, programmes must adopt inclusive, equity-focused approaches that address structural barriers, ensure representation in data systems, and tailor services to meet the diverse needs of affected communities.	2018–2025	Mixed: affected populations, national data	22
2. Gender Equity	Qualitative, Gender Frameworks (Women's Empowerment Framework (WEF), Socio Ecological Model (SEM).	Uganda, Ethiopia, Benin	Women (esp. pregnant/lactating), Men	- Gender norms, power dynamics, and lack of sex-disaggregated data shape access. - Gender-related barriers, worsened by factors like poverty and disability, limit women's access to NTD treatment and reduce programme effectiveness. - Adopting gender-responsive strategies improves equity, increases treatment coverage, and supports progress toward universal health goals.	2011–2023	Women, Men, Programme implementers	11
3. Inclusive Delivery and Intervention	Participatory Action Research, Case Studies	Multi-Country	Migrant workers, Women, Out-of-school youth	- Rigid models miss marginalised groups; inclusive design improves equity - Effective NTD treatment delivery is hindered by weak health systems and lack of community engagement, but participatory, locally driven approaches and strong health-system integration improve coverage, trust, and sustainability. - Empowering communities, integrating NTD services with broader healthcare, and using disaggregated data to identify and reach underserved groups are essential to closing equity gaps and achieving elimination goals.	2021–2024	Community members, CDDs, Health workers	9
4. Health Systems Inclusion	Systematic Review, Policy Case Study	Liberia, Global Review	Women, Children, Persons with Disabilities	- Integrated, equity-driven systems are needed but are underdeveloped - NTD programmes are moving toward integrated, people-centred models embedded in national health systems, which improve coverage and cost-effectiveness when supported by strong governance, stable financing, and community participation. - Achieving sustainable and equitable NTD care requires embedding intersectional, gender-sensitive planning, reducing donor dependence through domestic resource mobilisation, and centring local civil society in micro-planning and accountability.	2019–2025	Health system actors, Policy documents	8

https://doi.org/10.3390/healthcare14010027

Table 2. *Cont.*

Theme	Key Method	Geographic Focus	Population Targeted	Main Findings	Publication Year	Sample Type	Study Count
5. Inclusion of Community Members in NTD Programmes	Community-Based Participatory Research (CBPR), Programme Evaluation	Multi-country Africa	Affected persons, Community volunteers	- Peer-led groups and Community Directed Distributors (CDDs) empower communities and improve outcomes - Inclusive community engagement with trained, diverse distributors and peer support boosts treatment adherence and participation for marginalised groups in NTD programmes. - Formalising distributor roles, providing disability-focused training, and using detailed data monitoring are essential to prevent exclusion and improve care equity.	2017–2025	Persons with disabilities, CDDs, Peer groups	10

Below, each theme is explored in-depth based on the findings of the review.

3.1. Social and Economic Inequalities in NTD Programmes

A substantial body of evidence underscores how social and economic determinants profoundly influence both the burden of NTDs and individuals' ability to access care. Factors such as poverty, geographic marginalisation, displacement, systemic racism, and inadequate infrastructure consistently emerge as barriers to equitable treatment in endemic regions [28–31]. People with disabilities are disproportionately impacted by systemic poverty and social exclusion, especially when combined with low-income or rural settings. Disability often intersects with racial and economic marginalisation, leading to multi-layered vulnerabilities [28]. While gender itself is a pivotal axis of social exclusion, it has been intentionally examined as a distinct theme in this review to fully highlight its unique and intersecting impacts on disability and inclusion within NTD programming.

3.1.1. Racism

Research in Brazil has revealed a clear link between systemic racism and the disproportionate impact of NTDs on black and marginalised communities [28]. In Brazil, Black Brazilians with disabilities are largely invisible in health systems due to a lack of disaggregated data, making it difficult to ensure they benefit from NTD programmes [28]. Historical and structural inequities have limited access to healthcare, education, and economic opportunities, exacerbating disease burden among these groups. One study emphasises that such communities are routinely denied "decent living conditions, health, and social justice stemming from institutional racism," a dynamic that reinforces their invisibility in health systems and research agendas [28].

The authors further argue that insufficient investment in research and development for NTD prevention and treatment deepens this inequity, underscoring the need for inclusive public health approaches that address both medical and social determinants of health. Additionally, black individuals with disabilities in Brazil remain largely invisible in health systems due to a lack of disaggregated data by race and disability, making it difficult to assess their healthcare engagement or advocate for targeted interventions [32]. This invisibility perpetuates inequities and policy neglect. Moreover, systemic intersectional discrimination severely increases their vulnerability: they are overrepresented among the homeless, institutionalised, and incarcerated populations, and are disproportionately exposed to violence, including police brutality and gender-based abuse [33].

3.1.2. Poverty

Poverty is a fundamental driver of both the persistence and spread of NTDs, disproportionately impacting populations with limited financial resources, inadequate access to healthcare, and scarce prevention and treatment options [28,34]. This vulnerability is compounded by socioeconomic factors such as gender inequality, unemployment, illiteracy,

https://doi.org/10.3390/healthcare14010027

malnutrition, political instability, and poor sanitation and education systems, which collectively increase exposure risk and constrain the effectiveness of disease control strategies like mass drug administration (MDA) [28,35].

In Brazil, economically disadvantaged regions bear the highest NTD burdens, including those caused by schistosomiasis, leprosy, and chagas disease, highlighting the necessity of health interventions that go beyond biomedical solutions and emphasise social justice, improved living conditions, and inclusive health frameworks [3,28]. Across marginalised communities, lack of essential services like clean water and sanitation further impedes NTD prevention, underscoring the urgent need for universal health coverage and equitable access to treatment [3,28].

Research further demonstrates the strong correlation between socioeconomic status and the prevalence of NTDs. A systematic review analysing over 5500 studies indicated that lower socioeconomic status correlates closely with elevated risk of NTDs, some twice as high, illustrating a clear social gradient in disease prevalence [36]. This inequality is particularly evident in diseases such as soil-transmitted helminth infections (STH), visceral leishmaniasis (VL), and schistosomiasis. While wealthier individuals in endemic areas may also be affected, the broader trend reflects a social gradient in disease burden, underscoring the urgent need for equity-focused interventions in NTD surveillance and monitoring systems [36]. To address this, equity-focused interventions must integrate socioeconomic indicators into surveillance systems, ensuring the most vulnerable are reached.

Even though MDA remains central to NTD control, significant gaps persist in treatment access and surveillance, particularly among marginalised groups. Individuals excluded from these programmes often remain invisible in the data, artificially inflating reported programme success. Modelling studies, such as those by Clark et al. [34], reveal that overlooking these excluded groups diminishes the likelihood of achieving elimination goals. This disconnect between treatment and surveillance data highlights the crucial need to engage these populations to ensure accurate monitoring, effective evaluation, and ultimately, the elimination of NTDs [29,33].

3.1.3. Displacement

Displacement presents substantial and intersecting challenges to embedding disability-inclusive approaches within NTD programmes. Roughly one in six forcibly displaced people worldwide lives with a disability, yet they commonly encounter inaccessible facilities, shortages of assistive devices, a dearth of sensory-adapted information, and exclusion from registration databases, factors that collectively restrict their access to NTD services in camps and other humanitarian settings [37,38]. Furthermore, disability prevalence is higher among the forcibly displaced and economically disadvantaged populations, yet they often remain excluded from NTD surveillance and drug distribution systems due to inaccessibility and stigma [39,40]. The Ascend programme in Niger demonstrates how these gaps can be narrowed by linking UNHCR registration with disability identifiers, overlaying treatment maps with camp-level inclusion data, and recruiting caregivers with lived experience as community drug distributors who use context-appropriate communication modes. As a result, the Ascend programme has shown that equitable coverage is achievable [41]. Nevertheless, such practices remain exceptions; most routine operations in fragile settings continue to omit persons with disabilities because of structural inaccessibility and limited planning [42].

Intersectional analysis further reveals that disability, displacement, gender, and poverty compound marginalisation. UNHCR's Working with Persons with Disabilities in Forced Displacement toolkit urges agencies to capture disaggregated data, guarantee accessible emergency messaging, and involve persons with disabilities in decision-making,

https://doi.org/10.3390/healthcare14010027

yet these recommendations are rarely implemented in NTD campaigns [37,43]. Displaced people with disabilities are also at heightened risk of violence, homelessness, and service loss from theft of wheelchairs to gaps in psychosocial support undermining trust in health providers and reducing treatment uptake [44].

Delivering disability-inclusive NTD programmes hinges on four mutually reinforcing measures: first, ensuring that both UNHCR and national NTD databases systematically capture disability status using tools such as the Washington Group questions to make people with disabilities visible in planning and resource allocation [41,45]. Additionally, redesigning service delivery so that treatment sites are accessible, and informational materials are designed to meet diverse physical, sensory and communication needs [46]; furthermore, meaningfully engaging displaced persons with disabilities by training them to serve as peer educators and community drug distributors, thereby increasing trust and contextual relevance [47]. Incorporating disability-sensitive indicators into routine monitoring so coverage gaps and access barriers can be identified and addressed through adaptive management is also critical [12,39]. Without this integrated approach, even programmes that incorporate a "leave no one behind" approach would risk systematically overlooking displaced persons with disabilities, deepening health inequities and undermining global NTD-elimination targets [48,49].

3.2. Gender Equity in NTD Programmes

Gender remains a critical yet persistently undervalued determinant of success in NTD control and elimination. Biological sex alone does not explain differential risk; rather, exposure, treatment access and long-term disability are mediated by intersecting inequities such as poverty, geographic isolation and disability status [50]. Programmes that fail to integrate gender analysis run the risk of reinforcing these power imbalances, under-serving large segments of the population and, ultimately, missing elimination targets [50].

Evidence from 16 African and Asian countries shows that coverage data disaggregated by gender routinely uncover hidden gaps; in 3% of districts male uptake exceeded female uptake by $\geq$10 percentage points, signalling structural barriers for women and girls [51]. Uganda's National NTD Control Programme illustrates these barriers in practice: men were more likely to miss treatment because of labour migration, whereas community drug distributors lacked guidance on treating pregnant or breastfeeding women, leading to systematic under-treatment of this group [52]. In Ulanga, Tanzania, coverage gaps in mass drug administration were exacerbated by gender-related dynamics, including women's higher participation in ivermectin distribution compared to men, and greater community trust in female distributors. However, structural issues such as poor timing of campaigns during farming seasons and absence of tailored guidance for gender-sensitive delivery continued to affect overall coverage [53].

While gender-informed approaches may increase short-term costs, they ultimately lead to more sustainable and inclusive outcomes, enabling NTD programmes to contribute meaningfully to the goal of universal health coverage without reinforcing existing inequalities [50]. Gender-responsive frameworks, such as those proposed by Theobald and colleagues, advocate three core actions: (i) sex and age-disaggregated monitoring; (ii) community dialogues that address household power dynamics; and (iii) explicit budgeting for gender-sensitive delivery (e.g., women CDDs, pregnancy-safe guidelines) [50]. Where implemented, these measures have yielded measurable gains. For example, programmes that recruited women as CDDs in Malawi and Nigeria reported higher trust among female beneficiaries and increases of 6 to 12 percentage points in female coverage [54].

Importantly, gender intersects with disability, and women with disabilities face amplified stigma, mobility constraints and heightened exposure to gender-based violence, all of

https://doi.org/10.3390/healthcare14010027

which deter health-seeking and limit participation in NTD campaigns [55]. Yet disability-sex disaggregation is virtually absent from routine surveillance, obscuring inequities and hampering corrective action [4].

Expanding on existing frameworks, Figure 2 in the study highlights the central role of community attitudes and distribution strategies, illustrating that a more comprehensive understanding of the complexities of community-based treatment programmes is essential. Gender-related obstacles, such as social norms and unequal power dynamics, must be addressed to ensure the future success of these programmes, particularly in contexts where community attitudes and distribution methods play a pivotal role in treatment access and adherence [52].

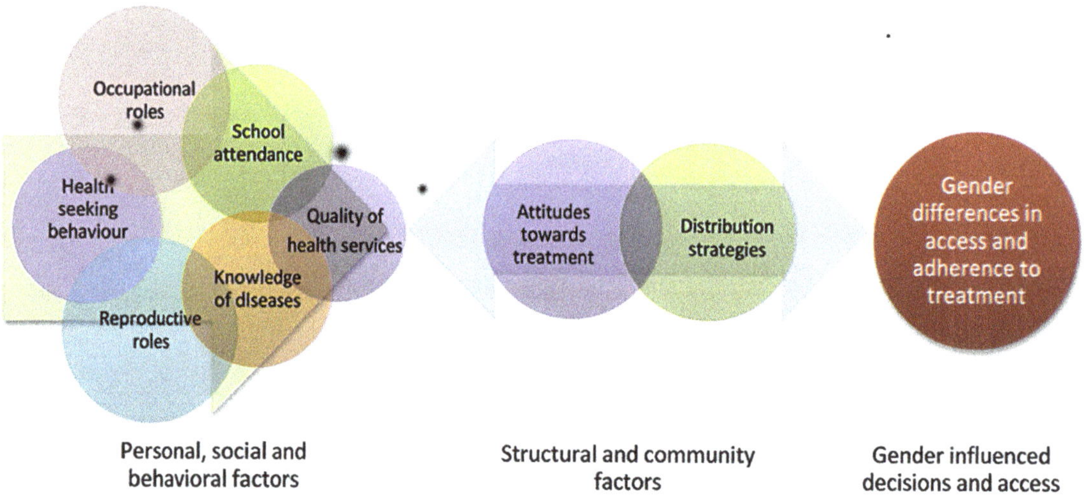

Figure 2. Framework for gendered differences in access and adherence to NTD treatment programmes [52].

Gender exerts a decisive influence on how people experience and seek care for NTDs in Ethiopia. Qualitative work across five endemic diseases including lymphatic filariasis, podoconiosis, schistosomiasis, soil-transmitted helminth infections and trachoma shows that restrictive social norms, unequal household power and stigma surrounding genitourinary symptoms delay or prevent women from presenting for treatment, problems compounded by low community awareness and discomfort discussing "private" complaints [56]. Wharton-Smith and colleagues therefore argue that national NTD strategies must move beyond binary sex categories and adopt intersectional gender analyses that consider disability, poverty, and geography to achieve universal coverage [56].

Comparable patterns emerge in West Africa. In Comé, Benin, focus-group research revealed that both men and women valued the economic benefits of soil-transmitted helminth MDA. Yet, women were sceptical after previously disorganised campaigns and demanded a voice in planning, safer timing, and door-to-door delivery to increase control over household decision-making [52,57,58]. Men, by contrast, downplayed their risk of infection and were less concerned about the delivery mode [57]. Applying the Welfare, Access, Conscientisation, Mobilisation, and Control (WEF) framework, together with the Social-Ecological Model (SEM), shown in Figure 3, Geyer et al. demonstrated that gender-tailored MDA, mainly when led by female community drug distributors (CDDs), improved coverage and equity at every societal level [57].

https://doi.org/10.3390/healthcare14010027

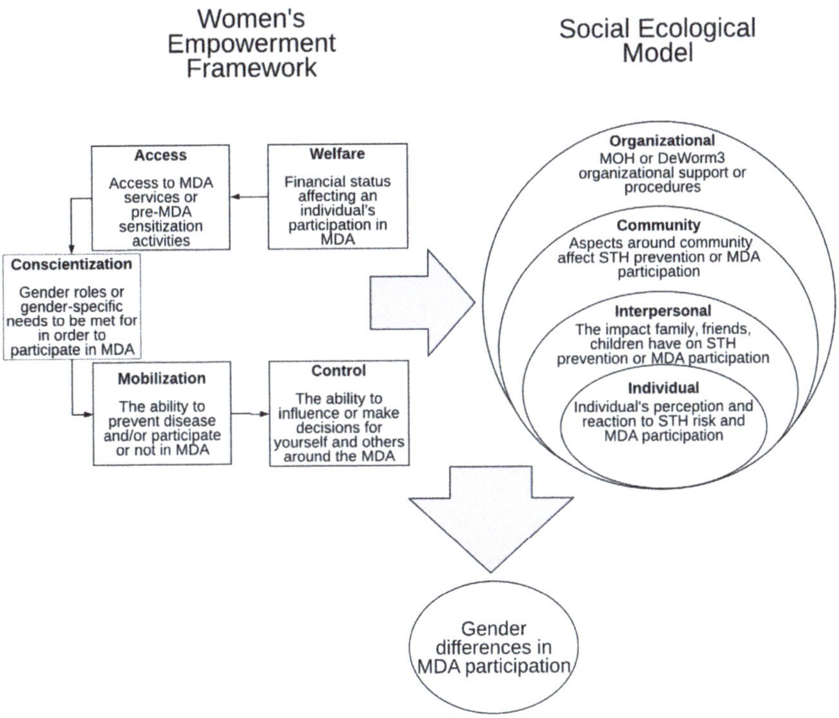

Figure 3. Welfare, Access, Conscientization, Mobilization, and Control (WEF) framework and the Social-Ecological Model (SEM) [57].

These findings echo cross-country evidence from Ethiopia and Tanzania, where routine NTD surveillance systems lacked sex- and disability-disaggregated indicators, making women with disabilities nearly invisible in programme planning. The study also highlighted critical gaps in pregnancy-specific treatment guidance and emphasised that meaningful involvement of women with disabilities in programme design is essential for inclusive NTD interventions [51]. While gender-responsive approaches may incur initial costs, they lay the foundation for more equitable and sustainable progress toward universal health coverage [51].

Ultimately, gender equity should be a central focus in NTD programmes. This includes allocating time for community sensitization and developing educational messaging that addresses women's specific concerns, especially regarding fertility and treatment safety. Collaborative, multisectoral approaches, especially those involving reproductive and maternal health professionals, are crucial for addressing NTDs such as female genital schistosomiasis. Achieving the Sustainable Development Goals (SDGs), which focus on reducing health disparities and expanding access to healthcare, will significantly contribute to the elimination of NTDs. Progress in these areas will depend on strong, coordinated efforts from governments, civil society, researchers, funders, and communities [59].

3.3. Inclusion in Intervention Delivery and Health System Integration

Inclusive delivery and strong health-system integration remain the decisive bottlenecks for taking proven NTD treatments to the people who need them most. Evidence from multiple settings indicates that weak primary-care platforms, shortages of trained staff, and sporadic community engagement systematically undermine the impact of MDA campaigns and case-management services [60,61]. Scholars therefore emphasise inter-sectoral

https://doi.org/10.3390/healthcare14010027

collaboration, enforceable reporting rules, and genuinely "bottom-up" approaches that give communities power to diagnose their own priorities and co-create solutions [62].

In western Kenya, Ochola, Karanja, and Elliott utilised Sen's capability lens to demonstrate that when villages define success in their own terms, such as determining safe water points, locally chosen drug distribution sites, and establishing transparent feedback loops, MDA coverage rises, and social trust deepens [60]. Their findings underline that national strategies will only be sustainable when local capability and national priorities are aligned.

Nigeria's Equity-PAR project demonstrates how this can be implemented at scale. Piotrowski et al. [61] identified nine iterative steps, from participatory mapping and cross-sector working groups to routine "learning health-system" reviews, that increased ivermectin coverage in two states and embedded continuous reflection into district plans [61]. Similar participatory micro-planning tools have since been piloted in Ghana and Sierra Leone with promising early results [48].

Yet significant gaps persist. Rigid distribution timetables, myths about infertility, and the absence of pregnancy-safe guidelines all decreased uptake, while school-based models missed pupils in private, informal, or Quranic schools [62]. Modelled data from Mali, meanwhile, show that leaving "never-treated" mobile households out of surveillance reduces the likelihood of reaching elimination thresholds by up to 30% [48].

Liberia's Disease Management, Disability, and Inclusion (DMDI) platform demonstrates the potential of health-system integration, as it links case management with rehabilitation and psychosocial services. As a result, Liberia cut the average travel time in half and improved treatment completion by a quarter [62]. WHO now encourages such cross-programme collaboration as part of its 2030 road map targets [63].

CDDs, often women, remain the "foot-soldiers" of MDA. Where they receive disability and gender training, trust rises and coverage gaps narrow; where they do not, fear and misinformation flourish [64]. Mobile migrant reviews confirm that mixed-gender CDD teams are more successful in reaching herders, artisanal miners, and displaced households than male-only teams [40,42].

Collectively, these studies demonstrate that re-centring equity necessitates three reinforcing steps: empowering communities through participatory planning, integrating NTD services with broader, people-centred health functions, and monitoring who remains missing using sex-, age-, and disability-disaggregated metrics. Without this triad, programmes risk perpetuating the very inequities they seek to solve. Recent WHO guidance calls for programmes to collect and act on disability-disaggregated data, yet most countries lack such metrics, making it harder to identify exclusion patterns [12].

3.4. *Inclusion in Health Systems to Combat NTDs*

NTD programmes are shifting from vertical, drug-centric campaigns toward integrated, people-centred delivery models that can be sustained by national systems. Liberia's Disease Management, Disability, and Inclusion (DMDI) platform illustrates this evolution: the strategy bundles case management, rehabilitation, and psychosocial services for five skin-NTDs and is now embedded in county health plans, although donor dependence and fiscal shortfalls still threaten scale-up [62]. Experience elsewhere echoes Liberia's lesson. A systematic scoping review of found that integrating NTD activities into primary health services improves coverage and cost-effectiveness, provided there is strong governance, stable financing, and active community participation [65]. Yet many health systems continue to overlook equity: women, children, and persons with disabilities are under-represented in registers and often absent from decision-making bodies. Intersectional, gender-sensitive planning, as recommended by global analyses that frame NTDs as a "litmus test" for universal health coverage, must therefore be embedded from the outset [13].

https://doi.org/10.3390/healthcare14010027

Recent evidence from Nigeria confirms the value of participatory action research: nine iterative steps, ranging from community mapping to inter-ministerial working groups, have improved ivermectin coverage and normalised continuous learning across sectors [61]. Similar gaps have been documented among mobile agricultural workers in Mali and artisanal miners in Ghana, where failure to adapt MDA schedules to labour patterns reduced projected elimination probabilities by up to 30% [63]. International funding volatility compounds these risks: recent cuts to a significant bilateral NTD portfolio may leave 100 million people without treatment and strand nearly US $1 billion in donated medicines [66].

To make integrated care durable, countries must align with the WHO 2030 road-map pillars, change operating models and culture to facilitate country ownership, which highlights people-centred delivery, cross-programme collaboration, and country ownership [1,67] while mobilising domestic resources to reduce donor dependence [68]. Emerging models place local civil-society organisations at the centre of micro planning and accountability, arguing that "last-mile" equity hinges on grassroots legitimacy and social capital [68]. Sustainability research further emphasises the need for explicit metrics that capture equity, financing, and community empowerment, in addition to disease prevalence [66].

3.5. Inclusion of Community Members in NTD Programmes

NTD programmes have long relied on community mobilisation, yet many still focus narrowly on biomedical endpoints, overlooking the psychosocial realities and disability-specific barriers that shape uptake and long-term well-being [69,70]. High levels of depression and anxiety were found among people affected by skin NTDs, especially women, with stigma and disability as key predictors. Community-based responses, including peer support, are urgently needed to reduce psychological distress and improve treatment outcomes [71,72]. When such groups are co-designed with individuals with disabilities, they generate accessible meeting formats, tactile or pictorial health education, and caregiver accompaniment, thereby increasing participation among people with visual, hearing, or mobility impairments [70].

Community-directed distributors (CDDs) remain pivotal for last-mile service delivery, having treated more than about 200 million people annually across 27 countries; yet disability training is rarely part of their curriculum [64]. Studies from countries such as Cameroon and Uganda reveal that CDDs often exclude pregnant women, persons with mobility limitations, and the deaf community, mainly because they lack guidance on pregnancy-safe regimens or sign-language skills [58,73]. Inclusive refresher training covering accessible communication, stigma reduction, and safe drug protocols for pregnant and breastfeeding women has raised female and disability-specific coverage by 8 to 12 percentage points in pilot districts [58,73].

Systematic reviews indicate that CDD motivation is contingent upon social recognition and modest financial or in-kind incentives; when these incentives are absent, attrition rates increase and coverage among hard-to-reach groups declines [74]. Policy briefs now recommend formalising CDD roles within national community-health strategies and integrating disability indicators into routine supervision tools, aligning with the WHO's 2030 Road Map commitment to people-centred care [1].

Ultimately, inclusive community engagement must combine three elements: (i) peer support groups that tackle psychosocial and livelihood needs; (ii) disability-trained, gender-balanced CDD cadres; and (iii) monitoring systems that disaggregate data by sex, age, and disability. Without these, programmes risk perpetuating the very exclusions that drive NTD transmission and disability in the first place [74–76].

https://doi.org/10.3390/healthcare14010027

4. Discussion

NTD control cannot be judged a success until programmes reach and empower the communities that carry the heaviest burden. Evidence synthesised in this review shows that inclusion is not a "value-add" but a pre-condition for effective, equitable and sustainable NTD elimination. Yet blind spots remain pervasive: the poorest rural households, displaced communities, women, and persons with disabilities continue to fall through the cracks of surveillance, drug distribution, and policy design.

For example, in their study, Clark et al. show that untreated and unobserved groups (those excluded from drug distribution) also tend to be excluded from surveillance, leading to bias in what is observed vs. what is happening in the full eligible population, impacting the implementation of NTD programmes as well as their evaluation [34].

Systemic poverty, gender inequality, racial discrimination, and forced displacement continue to shape who is infected, who receives care, and who is left behind. Importantly, people with disabilities represent a sizeable and routinely invisible segment of every one of those vulnerable groups.

Our synthesis demonstrates that social and economic inequalities remain deeply embedded in the persistence and spread of NTDs. The disproportionate burden borne by Black communities in Brazil and marginalised groups in sub-Saharan Africa illustrates how systemic racism and poverty intersect to deepen exclusion from healthcare access and surveillance systems [28,59]. These findings align with Houweling et al.'s [36] review, which showed that NTD prevalence strongly correlates with low socioeconomic status, making equity-focused interventions an imperative rather than a luxury.

Gender emerged as another critical but under-addressed axis of exclusion. Multiple studies highlighted the gendered barriers to NTD treatment access, including power imbalances, lack of sex-disaggregated data, and inadequate training for treating pregnant or lactating women [50,52]. These gaps point to the urgent need for intersectional and gender-responsive strategies that address not only health access but also broader social determinants of health, such as decision-making authority and caregiving roles [56,57].

The review also underscores that displacement due to conflict, climate change, or economic instability exacerbates invisibility in NTD programming. As Harvey et al. [41] discuss, displaced populations often fall through the cracks of national health systems, highlighting the need for multisectoral collaboration and data innovation to fully implement the "Leave No One Behind" (LNOB) principle in practice.

Encouragingly, several studies demonstrate how inclusive intervention models can help bridge these divides. Participatory action research (PAR) approaches and community-driven planning processes, such as those trialled in Nigeria and Kenya, show promise in realigning programmatic priorities with local needs [60,61]. These approaches not only increase treatment uptake but also foster trust and long-term engagement, crucial for the sustainability of NTD efforts.

The role of community-led initiatives, particularly peer support groups and CDDs, emerged as vital for delivering integrated and person-centred care. While such models are cost-effective and highly adaptable, they remain undervalued within national health systems, often lacking proper incentives, training, or recognition [71,75]. Systemic support for these grassroots actors is key to realising inclusive health outcomes and building resilience against future public health threats.

Finally, the integration of inclusion into health systems rather than isolated programmes is a consistent recommendation across the literature. Liberia's DMDI model [62] and systematic evidence from Branda et al. [3] emphasise that mainstreaming disability, equity, and gender considerations into national health policies leads to more efficient and

https://doi.org/10.3390/healthcare14010027

impactful outcomes. However, barriers such as fragmented funding and weak governance structures continue to hinder progress.

Based on the analysis above, we would also like to put forth a definition of inclusion within NTDs:

Inclusion in NTDs refers to the intentional integration of marginalized, underserved, and affected populations, such as people living in poverty, women, displaced persons, and people with disabilities, into all aspects of NTD programming, policymaking, and service delivery. It emphasizes equitable access to healthcare, meaningful participation in decision-making, and the removal of social, economic, and structural barriers that hinder full engagement in prevention, treatment, and support services. Inclusion goes beyond clinical access to encompass empowerment, representation, and the recognition of intersecting forms of exclusion that perpetuate health inequities.

Figure 4 shows how inclusion is interlinked across four domains, access, participation, empowerment, and governance, necessary for building equitable NTD programmes.

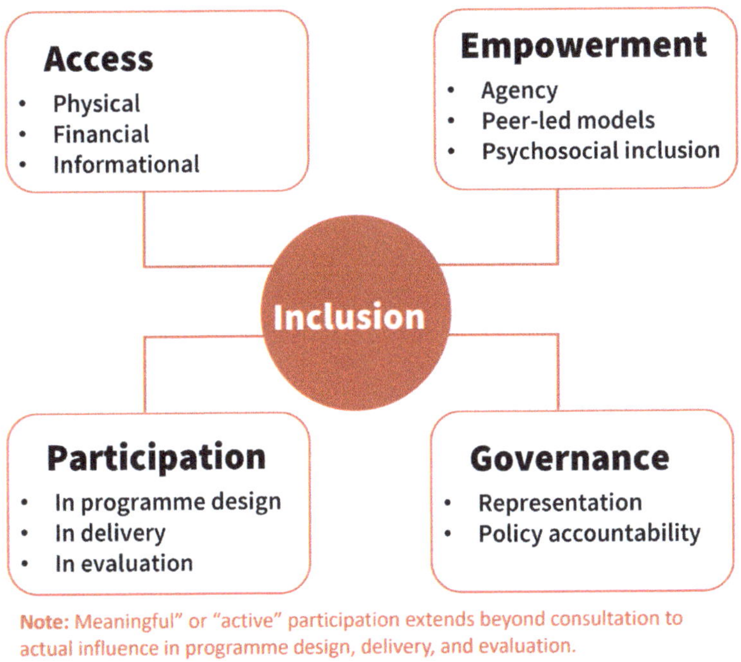

Figure 4. Definition of Inclusion in NTDs developed by CBM based on the findings.

This definition aligns with the themes in our review, including the intersection of disability and gender, systemic exclusion, and the role of community empowerment in NTD responses [7,59,60].

Taken together, this review calls for a paradigm shift: from treating NTDs solely as biomedical issues to addressing them as deeply social, structural, and political problems. Inclusion must be embedded across all levels of NTD programming, from community engagement to policy design and implementation, if global health equity goals are to be realised.

Practical Implementation of Inclusion in NTD Programming

Operationalising inclusion in NTD programming can be facilitated practically through initiatives such as the NTD Inclusion Score Card (NISC), which serves as a tool for NTD organisations to assess and enhance their inclusivity practices by identifying gaps and fostering accountability, aiming to improve the effectiveness and relevance of NTD interventions [77,78].

Additionally, research has highlighted the importance of community-based groups (CBGs) and initiatives, as well as centring OPDs and persons affected in all stages of programming to support inclusion. In their paper, Hotopf et al. map out evidence on existing CBG models for skin-NTDs and lay out a best-practice framework across domains such as self-care, mental health, livelihoods, governance, and advocacy. This model has been designed to include people affected by NTDs in planning, delivery, and evaluation of services, embedding inclusion into the programme [79].

The NISC, on the one hand, is a tool for measuring and improving inclusion in NTD organisations, while the community-based models presented by Hotopf et al. demonstrate how inclusion can be implemented on the ground [78,79].

Similarly, Zongo et al. argue that despite advances in NTD control and elimination programmes, many affected communities remain excluded due to social, economic, and geographic barriers. They explore how civil society organisations (CSOs) play a critical role in advancing equity and inclusion in NTD programmes by acting as trusted community intermediaries, advocating for marginalised groups, enhancing accountability, and ensuring that NTD services reach the most underserved and hard-to-reach populations, thereby strengthening the sustainability and impact of global health efforts [68].

Another aspect that should be a focus for inclusion in NTD programmes is data. Kuper (suggests that Disability and morbidity have not been routinely measured in NTD programmes, and this lack of data hinders advocacy efforts, impedes effective planning and implementation of interventions, and limits the ability to monitor, evaluate programme impact, and secure funding. Collecting such data and utilising it supports more effective planning, enhances advocacy and resource mobilisation, and ensures that interventions are inclusive and responsive to the needs of affected populations [7,8].

From these, we can highlight that although there is still a long way to go when it comes to the concept of inclusion in NTD programming, the area is being advanced through tools like the NTD Inclusion Score Card, community-based models, and stronger data-driven practices. These approaches emphasise the involvement of affected persons in planning and service delivery, with civil society organisations playing a crucial role in reaching marginalised groups. Additionally, better data on disability and morbidity are essential for effective planning, advocacy, and inclusive impact.

5. Limitations

As a narrative review, the methodology of this paper prioritises depth and thematic synthesis over exhaustive or systematic coverage, which may introduce selection bias. Although rigorous inclusion and exclusion criteria were applied, relevant studies may have been inadvertently omitted due to publication language (English-only) or date restrictions (2010–2023). While narrative reviews provide a broad and flexible overview of a topic, they are subject to several limitations that can affect the validity and reproducibility of their conclusions. One major limitation is the potential for selection bias, as the inclusion of studies is often based on the authors' subjective judgement rather than a systematic process [80]. This can lead to incomplete coverage of the literature and an overemphasis on particular viewpoints or findings [26]. Additionally, narrative reviews often lack a standardised methodological framework, which can lead to inconsistencies in how evidence is synthesised and interpreted [77].

Secondly, the heterogeneity in the methodological quality and design of the included studies, ranging from qualitative case studies to mixed-methods research, limits direct comparison and generalizability of findings. Another limitation of this study could be the

https://doi.org/10.3390/healthcare14010027

lack of use of quantitative synthesis or risk-of-bias scoring that would be part of different research methods. Additionally, the review primarily draws from studies based in sub-Saharan Africa and Latin America, which, while highly relevant, may not fully reflect regional dynamics in Asia or the Middle East. Finally, the evolving and context-specific nature of "inclusion" itself means that interpretations may vary across disciplines and cultural settings, affecting the consistency of its conceptualization and operationalization across studies.

Recommendations for Future Research

While this review highlights strategies for embedding inclusion into NTD programming, it also reveals critical gaps that warrant further investigation. Future research should focus on operationalizing inclusion through concrete programmatic interventions and measurable indicators. There is a pressing need for studies that test the effectiveness of inclusive approaches in practice, particularly in health systems, community engagement, and mass drug administration efforts, and how they impact health outcomes for marginalised groups.

Additionally, there is a limited understanding of how intersecting forms of exclusion (e.g., gender, disability, displacement, and socioeconomic status) combine to hinder access to care. Research should employ intersectional frameworks to explore these dynamics more deeply and guide the design of responsive, context-specific interventions. Finally, more evidence is needed from underrepresented regions, such as Asia and the Middle East, as well as on financing models that support equity-driven programming. Strengthening monitoring and evaluation systems with disaggregated data and participatory feedback loops will be key to advancing the inclusive NTD agenda.

6. Conclusions

Inclusion is not peripheral but foundational to the success of NTD programmes. This review highlights the multifaceted nature of exclusion rooted in socioeconomic disparities, gender dynamics, displacement, disability, and systemic neglect and demonstrates how such exclusion undermines progress toward disease control and elimination. Yet, the literature also provides a hopeful trajectory: inclusive, community-driven, and gender-responsive interventions show significant promise in increasing coverage, equity, and sustainability. Achieving the targets outlined in the WHO NTD 2030 Roadmap and the SDGs requires reframing inclusion not just as a principle but as a strategic priority. Moving forward, national governments, implementing partners, and donors must embed inclusion into health systems planning, allocate resources for community empowerment, and institutionalise equity-based monitoring and evaluation frameworks. Only by doing so can we ensure that the fight against NTDs leaves no one behind.

Author Contributions: Conceptualization, G.S., J.W., B.Q. and J.A.-E.; Methodology, I.Z.J., O.O., G.S. and J.A.-E.; analysis, I.Z.J., O.O. and J.A.-E.; writing—original draft preparation, I.Z.J., O.O. and J.A.-E.; writing—review and editing, I.Z.J., O.O., J.A.-E., G.S. and J.W.; visualisation, I.Z.J. and O.O.; project administration, J.A.-E. All authors have read and agreed to the published version of the manuscript.

Funding: This research received no external funding.

Institutional Review Board Statement: Not applicable.

Informed Consent Statement: Not applicable.

Data Availability Statement: No new data were gathered or developed; the findings are based on reviews of currently existing research.

Conflicts of Interest: The authors declare no conflicts of interest.

https://doi.org/10.3390/healthcare14010027

Abbreviations

The following abbreviations are used in this manuscript:

CDD	Community Directed Distributers
CSO	Civil Society Organization
DMDI	Disease Management, Disability, and Inclusion
MDA	Mass Drug Administration
NTDs	Neglected Tropical Diseases
SDGs	Sustainable Development Goals

References

1. World Health Organization. *A Road Map for Neglected Tropical Diseases 2021–2030*; WHO: Geneva, Switzerland, 2021; Available online: https://www.who.int/publications/i/item/9789240010352 (accessed on 9 June 2025).
2. Hotez, P.J. What Constitutes a Neglected Tropical Disease? *PLoS Neglected Trop. Dis.* **2020**, *14*, e0008001. [CrossRef] [PubMed]
3. Branda, F.; Ali, A.Y.; Ceccarelli, G.; Albanese, M.; Binetti, E.; Giovanetti, M.; Ciccozzi, M.; Scarpa, F. Assessing the Burden of Neglected Tropical Diseases in Low-Income Communities: Challenges and Solutions. *Viruses* **2025**, *17*, 29. [CrossRef]
4. World Health Organization. *Neglected Tropical Diseases—Key Facts*; WHO: Geneva, Switzerland, 2024; Available online: https://www.who.int/health-topics/neglected-tropical-diseases#tab=tab_1 (accessed on 9 June 2025).
5. Reed, S.L.; McKerrow, J.H. Why Funding for Neglected Tropical Diseases Should Be a Global Priority. *Clin. Infect. Dis.* **2018**, *67*, 323–326. [CrossRef]
6. Houweling, T.A.; Karim-Kos, H.E.; Kulik, M.C.; Stolk, W.A.; Haagsma, J.A.; Lenk, E.J.; Richardus, J.H.; de Vlas, S.J. Socioeconomic Inequalities in Neglected Tropical Diseases: A Systematic Review. *PLoS Neglected Trop. Dis.* **2016**, *10*, e0004546. [CrossRef] [PubMed]
7. Kuper, H. Neglected tropical diseases and disability-what is the link? *Trans. R. Soc. Trop. Med. Hyg.* **2019**, *113*, 839–844. [CrossRef] [PubMed]
8. Kuper, H. Disability, mental health, stigma and discrimination, and neglected tropical diseases. *Trans. R. Soc. Trop. Med. Hyg.* **2020**, *115*, 145–146. [CrossRef]
9. Koschorke, M.; Al-Haboubi, Y.H.; Tseng, P.-C.; Semrau, M.; Eaton, J. Mental health, stigma, and neglected tropical diseases: A review and systematic mapping of the evidence. *Front. Trop. Dis.* **2022**, *3*, 808955. [CrossRef]
10. Kollmann, K.M.; Abrahamsson, S.; Jesudason, T. Why disability inclusion is essential for trachoma elimination. *Community Eye Health J.* **2020**, *33*, 10–11.
11. Ochola, E.A.; Karanja, D.M.S.; Elliott, S.J. The impact of Neglected Tropical Diseases (NTDs) on health and wellbeing in sub-Saharan Africa (SSA): A case study of Kenya. *PLoS Neglected Trop. Dis.* **2021**, *15*, e0009131. [CrossRef]
12. World Health Organization. *Global Report on Health Equity for Persons with Disabilities*; World Health Organization: Geneva, Switzerland, 2022; Available online: https://www.who.int/publications/i/item/9789240063600 (accessed on 9 June 2025).
13. Dean, L.; Ozano, K.; Adekeye, O.; Dixon, R.; Fung, E.G.; Gyapong, M.; Isiyaku, S.; Kollie, K.; Kukula, V.; Lar, L.; et al. Neglected Tropical Diseases as a 'litmus test' for Universal Health Coverage? Understanding who is left behind and why in Mass Drug Administration: Lessons from four country contexts. *PLoS Neglected Trop. Dis.* **2019**, *13*, e0007847. [CrossRef]
14. Braveman, P.; Gruskin, S. Defining equity in health. *J. Epidemiol. Community Health* **2003**, *57*, 254–258. [CrossRef]
15. Cornwall, A. Unpacking 'Participation': Models, meanings and practices. *Community Dev. J.* **2008**, *43*, 269–283. [CrossRef]
16. World Health Organization. *Disability and Health Fact Sheet*; World Health Organization: Geneva, Switzerland, 2023; Available online: https://www.who.int/news-room/fact-sheets/detail/disability-and-health (accessed on 9 June 2025).
17. Sun, N.; Amon, J.J. Addressing Inequity: Neglected Tropical Diseases and Human Rights. *Health Hum. Rights* **2018**, *20*, 11–25. Available online: https://pubmed.ncbi.nlm.nih.gov/30008549/ (accessed on 9 June 2025).
18. Trachoma Coalition. *Reaching the Furthest Behind First: Disability Inclusion Essential to Universal Trachoma Programmes*; Trachoma Coalition: London, UK, 2020.
19. CBM Global. *Mental Health of People with NTDs: Towards a Person-Centred Approach*; CBM Global: Hamburg, Germany, 2022.
20. United Nations. *Leave No One Behind: Inclusion of Persons with Disabilities in the 2030 Agenda for Sustainable Development*; UN Department of Economic and Social Affairs: New York, NY, USA, 2019; Available online: https://www.un.org/development/desa/disabilities/ (accessed on 9 June 2025).
21. World Bank. *Disability Inclusion Overview*; World Bank: Washington, DC, USA, 2024; Available online: https://www.worldbank.org/en/topic/disability (accessed on 10 June 2025).

https://doi.org/10.3390/healthcare14010027

22. United Nations Enable. *Factsheet on Persons with Disabilities*; United Nations: New York, NY, USA, 2021. Available online: https://www.un.org/development/desa/disabilities/resources/factsheet-on-persons-with-disabilities.html (accessed on 10 June 2025).
23. UN Sustainable Development Group. *Leave no One Behind: A UN Framework for the 2030 Agenda*; United Nations: New York, NY, USA, 2016.
24. Sukhera, J. Narrative Reviews: Flexible, Rigorous, and Practical. *J. Grad. Med. Educ.* **2022**, *14*, 414–419. [CrossRef]
25. Kaushik, P.; Pati, P.K.; Khan, M.L.; Khare, P.K. Flow Diagram for Systematic Literature Review Using SALSA Framework. *Environ. Sci. Policy* **2022**, *130*, 55–64.
26. Greenhalgh, T.; Thorne, S.; Malterud, K. Time to challenge the spurious hierarchy of systematic over narrative reviews? *Eur. J. Clin. Investig.* **2018**, *48*, e12931. [CrossRef] [PubMed]
27. Ferrari, R. Writing narrative-style literature reviews. *Med. Writ.* **2015**, *24*, 230–235. [CrossRef]
28. da Conceição, J.R.; Lopes, C.P.G.; Ferreira, E.I.; Epiphanio, S.; Giarolla, J. Neglected Tropical Diseases and Systemic Racism, Especially in Brazil: From Socio-Economic Aspects to the Development of New Drugs. *Acta Trop.* **2022**, *235*, 106654. [CrossRef]
29. Simionato de Assis, I.; Arcoverde, M.A.M.; Ramos, A.C.V.; Alves, L.S.; Berra, T.Z.; Arroyo, L.H.; Queiroz, A.A.R.D.; Santos, D.T.D.; Belchior, A.D.S.; Alves, J.D.; et al. Social Determinants, Their Relationship with Leprosy Risk and Temporal Trends in a Tri-Border Region in Latin America. *PLoS Neglected Trop. Dis.* **2018**, *12*, e0006407. [CrossRef]
30. Dyal, J.W.; Grant, M.P.; Broadwater, K.; Bjork, A.; Waltenburg, M.A.; Gibbins, J.D.; Hale, C.; Silver, M.; Fischer, M.; Steinberg, J.; et al. COVID-19 Among Workers in Meat and Poultry Processing Facilities—19 States, April 2020. *MMWR Morb. Mortal. Wkly. Rep.* **2020**, *69*, 557–561. [CrossRef] [PubMed]
31. Mackey, T.K.; Ayers, C.K.; Kondo, K.K.; Saha, S.; Advani, S.M.; Young, S.D.; Spencer, H.; Rusek, M.; Anderson, J.; Veazie, S.; et al. Racial and Ethnic Disparities in COVID-19-Related Infections, Hospitalizations, and Deaths: A Systematic Review. *Ann. Intern. Med.* **2021**, *174*, 362–373. [CrossRef] [PubMed]
32. Minority Rights Group; Vidas Negras com Deficiência Importam. *The Situation of Black People with Disabilities in Brazil*; Minority Rights Group: London, UK; VNDI: São Paulo, Brazil, 2022.
33. Polack, S.; Delgado Ramos, V.; Sepúlveda Köptcke, L.; de Araujo Morais, I.; Reichenberger, V.; Scherer, N.; Veloso de Albuquerque, M.D.S.; Kuper, H.; Lyra, T.M.; Moran de Brito, C.M. Disability Inclusion in the Brazilian Health System: Results of a Health System Assessment. *Glob. Health Action* **2025**, *18*, 2550793. [CrossRef] [PubMed]
34. Clark, J.; Davis, E.L.; Prada, J.M.; Gass, K.; Krentel, A.; Hollingsworth, T.D. How Correlations Between Treatment Access and Surveillance Inclusion Impact Neglected Tropical Disease Monitoring and Evaluation—A Simulated Study. *PLoS Neglected Trop. Dis.* **2023**, *17*, e0011582. [CrossRef] [PubMed]
35. Magalhães, A.R.; Codeço, C.T.; Svenning, J.-C.; Escobar, L.E.; Van de Vuurst, P.; Gonçalves-Souza, T. Neglected Tropical Diseases Risk Correlates with Poverty and Early Ecosystem Destruction. *Infect. Dis. Poverty* **2023**, *12*, 32. [CrossRef]
36. Houweling, T.A.J.; Kristensen, T.K.; Dada, N.; D'Amico, G. Socio-Economic Inequality in Neglected Tropical Disease Risk. *Trans. R. Soc. Trop. Med. Hyg.* **2016**, *110*, 79–82.
37. United Nations High Commissioner for Refugees. *Working with Persons with Disabilities in Forced Displacement*; UNHCR: Geneva, Switzerland, 2019.
38. UNHCR. *Guidance: Identification of Persons with Disabilities at Registration Using the Washington Group Questions*; UNHCR: Geneva, Switzerland, 2022.
39. Elmukashfi ShamsEldin Elobied, H.; Bushra Masaad Ahmed, M.; Balla Ahmed, A.M.; Abdelrahman Hassan Salih, R.; Mohammed Mokhtar Ahmed, S.; Mahgoub, A.M.A.; Hashim Abdelmagid Mohamed, A.; Hamid Abdallah Elamin, E.; Osman Khalafalla El-Haj, A.-R.M.; Hamed Abd-Allah, M.A.-H.; et al. Healthcare Accessibility, Utilisation and Quality of Life among Internally Displaced Persons in Somalia: A Cross-Sectional Study. *Confl. Health* **2025**, *19*, 11. [CrossRef]
40. Kelley-Hope, L.; Harding-Esch, E.M.; Willems, J.; Ahmed, F.; Sanders, A.M. Conflict–Climate–Displacement: A Cross-Sectional Ecological Study Determining the Burden, Risk and Need for Strategies for Neglected Tropical Disease Programmes in Africa. *BMJ Open* **2023**, *13*, e071557. [CrossRef]
41. Harvey, D.; Shu'aibu, J.; Debam, M.T.; Aba, A.K.; Torres-Vitolas, C.A. How can the neglected tropical disease community be inclusive and equitable in programme delivery? Reaching refugees and internally displaced persons through integrating a 'leave no one behind' approach. *Int. Health* **2022**, *14*, ii33–ii37. [CrossRef]
42. Adams, M.W.; Sutherland, E.G.; Eckert, E.L.; Saalim, K.; Reithinger, R. Leaving no one behind: Targeting mobile and migrant populations with health interventions for disease elimination—A descriptive systematic review. *BMC Med.* **2022**, *20*, 172. [CrossRef]
43. International Disability Alliance. *Advancing Disability-Inclusive Strategies at the Global Refugee Forum*; IDA: New York, NY, USA, 2023.
44. Women's Refugee Commission; UNHCR. *Translating Disability-Inclusive Policy into Practice in Humanitarian Settings*; WRC: New York, NY, USA, 2020; Available online: https://www.womensrefugeecommission.org/wp-content/uploads/2020/04/Disability-Inclusion-Translating-Policy-into-Practice-in-Humanitarian-Action.pdf (accessed on 9 June 2025).

45. Rust, J.; Clark, A.; Woodgate, M.; Koch, C.; Mohammed, T.; Steinmann, P.; Krentel, A.; Torres-Vitolas, C.A.; Carlin, A.; Pavluck, A. Innovate to eliminate: A prerequisite in NTD programmes. *Int. Health* **2022**, *14*, ii20–ii24. [CrossRef]
46. Elrha. *Investing in Inclusive WASH: Examining Barriers and Value in Humanitarian Response*; Elrha: London, UK, 2023.
47. United Nations Children's Fund (UNICEF). *Including Children with Disabilities in Humanitarian Action: WASH*; UNICEF: New York, NY, USA, 2022.
48. Sangare, M.; Diabate, A.F.; Coulibaly, Y.I.; Tanapo, D.; Thera, S.O.; Dolo, H.; Dicko, I.; Coulibaly, O.; Sall, B.; Traore, F.; et al. Understanding the barriers and facilitators related to never treatment during mass drug administration among mobile and migrant populations in Mali: A qualitative exploratory study. *BMJ Glob. Health* **2024**, *9*, e015671. [CrossRef]
49. Obani, P. Inclusiveness in Humanitarian Action: Access to Water, Sanitation and Hygiene for People with Disabilities. *Int. J. Disaster Risk Reduct.* **2023**, *96*, 104937. [CrossRef]
50. Theobald, S.; MacPherson, E.E.; Dean, L.; Jacobson, J.; Ducker, C.; Gyapong, M.; Hawkins, K.; Elphick-Pooley, T.; MacKenzie, C.; Kelly-Hope, L.; et al. 20 years of gender mainstreaming in health: Lessons and reflections for the neglected tropical diseases community. *BMJ Glob. Health* **2017**, *2*, e000512. [CrossRef]
51. Cohn, D.A.; Kelly, M.P.; Bhandari, K.; Zoerhoff, K.L.; Batcho, W.E.; Drabo, F.; Negussu, N.; Marfo, B.; Goepogui, A.; Lemoine, J.F.; et al. Gender equity in mass drug administration for neglected tropical diseases: Data from 16 countries. *Int. Health* **2019**, *11*, 370–378. [CrossRef] [PubMed]
52. Rilkoff, H.; Tukahebwa, E.M.; Fleming, F.M.; Leslie, J.; Cole, D.C. Exploring Gender Dimensions of Treatment Programmes for Neglected Tropical Diseases in Uganda. *PLoS Neglected Trop. Dis.* **2013**, *7*, e2312. [CrossRef]
53. Mushi, V. Implementation challenges of community directed treatment with ivermectin program for control of onchocerciasis in Ulanga, Tanzania. *East Afr. Health Res. J.* **2021**, *5*, 123–128. [CrossRef] [PubMed]
54. University of Washington START Center. *Neglected Tropical Diseases: Women and Girls in Focus*; START Center: Seattle, WA, USA, 2021; Available online: http://uwstartcenter.org/projects/ntdwomenandgirls/ (accessed on 9 June 2025).
55. World Health Organization. World Bank. In *World Report on Disability*; WHO: Geneva, Switzerland, 2011; Available online: https://www.who.int/teams/noncommunicable-diseases/sensory-functions-disability-and-rehabilitation/world-report-on-disability (accessed on 11 June 2025).
56. Wharton-Smith, A.; Rassi, C.; Batisso, E.; Ortu, G.; King, R.; Endriyas, M.; Counihan, H.; Hamade, P.; Getachew, D. Gender-Related Factors Affecting Health Seeking for Neglected Tropical Diseases: Findings from a Qualitative Study in Ethiopia. *PLoS Neglected Trop. Dis.* **2019**, *13*, e0007840. [CrossRef]
57. Geyer, R.E.; Ibikounlé, M.; Emmanuel-Fabula, M.; Roll, A.; Avokpaho, E.; Elijan, A.; Wèkè, L.C.; Togbevi, C.I.; Chabi, F.; Houngbégnon, P.; et al. Gender norms and mass deworming program access in Comé, Benin: A qualitative assessment of gender-associated opportunities and challenges to achieving high mass drug administration coverage. *PLOS Neglected Trop. Dis.* **2020**, *14*, e0008153. [CrossRef]
58. Arney, J.K.; Headland, M.K.; Bertone, A.M.; Meite, A.; Ettiegne-Traore, V.; Asemanyi-Mensah, K.; Dede Teiko Dzathor, I.; Kargbo-Labour, I.; Jalloh, U.; Houck, P.; et al. Synthesis of findings from the literature and a qualitative research study on the impacts of gender, disability, and ethnicity in Neglected Tropical Diseases programs. *PLoS Neglected Trop. Dis.* **2023**, *17*, e0011782. [CrossRef]
59. George, N.S.; David, S.C.; Nabiryo, M.; Sunday, B.A.; Olanrewaju, O.F.; Yangaza, Y.; Shomuyiwa, D.O. Addressing neglected tropical diseases in Africa: A health equity perspective. *Glob. Health Res. Policy* **2023**, *8*, 30. [CrossRef]
60. Ochola, E.; Karanja, S.; Elliott, S. Local tips, global impact: Community-driven measures as avenues of inclusion for NTD control in western Kenya. *Infect. Dis. Poverty* **2022**, *11*, 65. [CrossRef]
61. Piotrowski, H.; Gwani, N.; Yashiyi, J.; Oluwole, A.; Ayuba, S.; Surakat, M.; Adekeye, O.; Lar, L.; Kevin, D.G.; Lawong, B.D.; et al. Promoting equity through inclusive learning, planning and implementation of mass drug administration in Nigeria. *Int. Health* **2023**, *15*, i63–i74. [CrossRef]
62. Dean, L.; Tolhurst, R.; Nallo, G.; Kollie, K.; Bettee, A.; Theobald, S. A health-systems journey towards more people-centred care: Lessons from neglected tropical disease programme integration in Liberia. *Health Policy Plan.* **2023**, *38*, 420–430. [CrossRef]
63. World Health Organization. Collaboration for the Control of Neglected Tropical Diseases. 2024. Available online: https://www.who.int/teams/control-of-neglected-tropical-diseases/collaboration (accessed on 11 June 2025).
64. Amazigo, U.; Leak, S.G.; Zoure, H.G.; Okoronkwo, C.; Diop Ly, M.; Isiyaku, S.; Crump, A.; Okeibunor, J.C.; Boatin, B. Community-directed distributors—The "foot soldiers" in the fight to end NTDs. *PLoS Neglected Trop. Dis.* **2021**, *15*, e0009588. [CrossRef] [PubMed]
65. Banda, G.T.; Deribe, K.; Davey, G. How can we better integrate the prevention, treatment, control and elimination of neglected tropical diseases with other health interventions? A systematic review. *BMJ Glob. Health* **2021**, *6*, e006968. [CrossRef]
66. World Health Organization. *Ending NTDs Together Towards 2030: Progress Report*; World Health Organization: Geneva, Switzerland, 2024.

https://doi.org/10.3390/healthcare14010027

67. Research for Development (R4D). *Mobilising Domestic Financing for Neglected Tropical Diseases: Five Lessons for Policy-Makers*; R4D Policy Brief: Washington, DC, USA, 2022; Available online: https://r4d.org/blog/5-lessons-in-mobilizing-domestic-financing-for-ntds/ (accessed on 9 June 2025).
68. Zongo, K.; Mberu, M.; Assefa, L.; Kucera, T.; Pappa, S.; Amin, A.; Sankar, G. Bridging the last mile: The critical role of local civil society in advancing equity and inclusion for neglected tropical diseases. *Int. J. Infect. Dis.* **2025**, *152*, 107789. [CrossRef]
69. Alderton, D.L.; Ackley, C.; Trueba, M.L. The Psychosocial Impact of Skin-Neglected Tropical Diseases: A Scoping Review. *Front. Trop. Dis.* **2024**, *5*, 1421522. [CrossRef]
70. CBM Global Disability Inclusion. *Community-Based Peer Groups and Psychosocial Support in Humanitarian Settings*; CBM Global: Bensheim, Germany, 2023; Available online: https://cbm-global.org/resource/community-mental-health-good-practice-guide-inclusive-mhpss-in-humanitarian-emergencies? (accessed on 11 June 2025).
71. Seekles, M.L.; Kadima, J.K.; Ding, Y.; Bulambo, C.B.; Kim, J.J.; Kukola, J.K.; Omumbu, P.O.; Mulamba, R.M.; Nganda, M.; Ngenyibungi, S.M.; et al. Mental health, stigma and the quality of life of people affected by neglected tropical diseases of the skin in Kasai Province, Democratic Republic of the Congo: A sex-disaggregated analysis. *Int. Health* **2023**, *15*, iii28–iii36. [CrossRef]
72. Nayak, P.K.; Mackenzie, C.D.; Agarwal, A.; van Wijk, R.; Mol, M.M.; Eaton, J.; Semrau, M.; Valle-Trabadelo, C.; Kaloiya, G.S.; Pratap, A.; et al. A new guide for basic psychological support for persons affected by neglected tropical diseases: A peer support tool suitable for persons with a diagnosis of leprosy and lymphatic filariasis. *PLOS Neglected Trop. Dis.* **2025**, *19*, e0011945. [CrossRef] [PubMed]
73. Badu, E.; Murphy, R.; Agyemang, D.; Jolley, E. *Ghana Disability Data Disaggregation Pilot Project: Results of Integrating Disability into Routine Data Collection Systems*; Sightsavers: Mumbai, India, 2018. [CrossRef]
74. Krentel, A.; Gyapong, M.; Mallya, S.; Boadu, N.Y.; Amuyunzu-Nyamongo, M.; Stephens, M.; McFarland, D.A. Review of the factors influencing the motivation of community drug distributors towards the control and elimination of neglected tropical diseases (NTDs). *PLoS Neglected Trop. Dis.* **2017**, *11*, e0006065. [CrossRef] [PubMed]
75. Worrell, C.M.; Brant, T.A.; Javel, A.; Denis, E.; Fayette, C.; Monestime, F.; Knowles, E.; Bennett, C.; Utzinger, J.; Odermatt, P.; et al. Microplanning improves stakeholders' perceived capacity and engagement to implement lymphatic filariasis mass drug administration. *PLoS Neglected Trop. Dis.* **2025**, *19*, e0012105. [CrossRef]
76. The Guardian. 'Some of These Diseases Are in the Bible': Despair as Cuts Halt Progress on Neglected Tropical Diseases. 9 April 2025. Available online: https://www.theguardian.com/global-development/2025/apr/09/despair-as-cuts-halt-progress-on-neglected-tropical-diseases-usaid (accessed on 11 June 2025).
77. Baethge, C.; Goldbeck-Wood, S.; Mert95ens, S. SANRA—A scale for the quality assessment of narrative review articles. *Res. Integr. Peer Rev.* **2019**, *4*, 5. [CrossRef] [PubMed]
78. van Wijk, R.; Baudoin, S.J.M.; Ejiogu, B.; Regmi, U.; Duck, M.; Rabiu, I.; Vettel, C.; Broekkamp, H.; Geutjes, R.; Peters, R.M.H.; et al. From words to action: The development of the Neglected Tropical Disease Inclusion Score Card (NISC). *Infect. Dis. Poverty* **2025**, *14*, 80. [CrossRef] [PubMed]
79. Hotopf, I.; Chowdhury, S.; Robert, G.; Sellers, M.E.; Phillip, M.; Fastenau, A.; del Mar Marais, M.; Vettel, C.; Rahman, M.; Singh, R.K.; et al. Community-based models for neglected tropical diseases affecting the skin: A scoping review. *Front. Trop. Dis.* **2025**, *6*, 1544842. [CrossRef]
80. Grant, M.J.; Booth, A. A typology of reviews: An analysis of 14 review types and associated methodologies. *Health Inf. Libr. J.* **2009**, *26*, 91–108. [CrossRef]

https://doi.org/10.3390/healthcare14010027

healthcare

MDPI

Review

Inclusive Healthcare System for Children with Disabilities: A Bibliometric Analysis and Visualization

Erkan Gulgosteren [1], Yavuz Onturk [2], Abdullah Cuhadar [3], Mihaela Zahiu [4], Monica Stanescu [5,*] and Rares Stanescu [4]

1 Faculty of Sports Sciences, Mersin University, Mersin 33010, Türkiye; egulgosteren@mersin.edu.tr
2 Faculty of Sports Sciences, Yalova University, Yalova 77400, Türkiye; yavuzonturk@hotmail.com
3 Faculty of Applied Sciences, Karamanoğlu Mehmetbey University, Karaman 70100, Türkiye; abdullahcuhadar@kmu.edu.tr
4 Faculty of Physical Education and Sports, National University of Physical Education and Sports, 060057 Bucharest, Romania; mihaela.zahiu@gmail.com (M.Z.); raresuniv@yahoo.com (R.S.)
5 Doctoral School, National University of Physical Education and Sports, 060057 Bucharest, Romania
* Correspondence: monica_iulia@yahoo.com

Abstract

Background: Children with disabilities face complex, systemic health access barriers rooted in societal, institutional, and structural inequities, requiring urgent global policy attention. Publications on access to health services for this population category have been found to have a significant growth in both quantity and content. The article aims to examine the structure and evolution of scientific literature in analyzing the healthcare system through the lens of inclusive services. Methods: We present the bibliometric profile of the global literature on access to health services for children with disabilities, the publication trends, the structure of research in this field concerning geographical distribution, methodological approaches, and interdisciplinary collaborations, and the core research topics, conceptual clusters, and future research directions in the field. The publications were screened from Web of Science databases, using PRISMA methodology. Finally, 1100 academic publications published between 1984 and 2025, obtained from a total of 432 different sources, the majority of which were peer-reviewed journals, were screened. Results: The calculated annual publication growth rate of 8.37% and the distinct upward trend observed, especially after 2015. The highest level was reached in 2023, with over 90 publications showing that the topic has become a focus of international academic interest. The USA (33.5%), the United Kingdom (15.7%), Australia (9.5%), and Canada (9.5%) stood out in publications, and there were strong collaborative networks among European nations (8.2%). Conclusions: Although high-income countries still appear to play a dominant role in research production, expanding international collaborations and distributing resources more equitably will contribute to the development of more inclusive solutions on a global scale. Temporal trends show an evolution toward diagnostic processes, family-centered approaches, and psychosocial dimensions. The results draw a clear picture of the current research landscape regarding access to health services for pediatric disability populations and identify potential directions for future research.

Keywords: children with disabilities; healthcare services; bibliometric analysis; special laws

1. Introduction

A significant and long-debated issue in contemporary health policy is the challenge children with disabilities face in accessing health services. Data from the World Health Organization's 2022 "Global Report on Health Equity for Persons with Disabilities" confirms that 1.3 billion people globally experience significant disability, a figure corresponding to 16% of the world's population [1]. Children constitute a substantial portion of this number. As stated in UNICEF's 2021 "Seen, Counted, Included" report, approximately 240 million children live with various forms of disability [2]. Such figures indicate that one in every ten children has a disability, which renders the elimination of health service inequities for this group a key requisite for both fundamental human rights and sustainable development goals. A comprehensive global scoping study demonstrates the multidimensional nature of systemic barriers that individuals with disabilities encounter in accessing healthcare [3] and another one, emphasized, disability during childhood and adolescence stands out as an area that requires greater priority on the global health agenda [4].

The health injustices experienced by pediatric populations with disabilities are too complex to be explained by medical reasons alone, and that complexity is highlighted in the WHO's global report, which documents that individuals with disabilities often face premature death risks of up to 20 years, experience significantly poorer health outcomes, and encounter substantial limitations in daily functioning [1]. Epidemiological evidence shows that children with disabilities have a two-fold higher risk of developing chronic conditions such as asthma, depression, diabetes, obesity, oral diseases, and stroke as compared to their non-disabled peers. UNICEF's analysis corroborates this as it reports that children facing disability-related challenges are 53% more likely to present with acute respiratory tract infection symptoms, 51% more likely to experience unhappiness, and 41% more likely to feel discriminated against [2].

Root causes of those health inequities are not confined to the disability itself but stem from multidimensional factors such as societal prejudice, institutional discrimination, poverty, exclusion from education and employment, and structural problems within the health system. The Levesque's conceptual framework for access to health services offers a valuable theoretical perspective for analyzing this multilayered phenomenon—it considers access to healthcare as a patient-centered process and examines the interaction between five dimensions of accessibility (approachability, acceptability, availability-accommodation, affordability, and appropriateness) and five corresponding population capacities (ability to perceive, seek, reach, pay, and engage) [5]. Applying this theoretical framework specifically to minors with disabilities allows for a thorough analysis of access barriers by integrating both health system and patient perspectives.

Recent large-scale research for the WHO Global Report categorized barriers to healthcare access for people with disabilities under six broad health system components: (1) health and care workforce, (2) health information systems, (3) health system financing, (4) leadership and governance, (5) service delivery, and (6) essential medicines and equipment [1]. This methodical work covers research from 2011 to 2022 and recommendations from WHO consultation meetings involving more than 1250 experts [1]. The study's exhaustive scope discloses the multilayered nature of structural barriers in healthcare access for children with complex health needs.

The original contributions of our study are focused on three main areas. Firstly, from an academic perspective, we systematically identify knowledge gaps, determine research priorities, and define opportunities for interdisciplinary collaboration. Secondly, from a policy development standpoint, we provide an objective assessment of the current situation regarding healthcare access for children with disabilities and contribute to evidence-based policymaking processes. Thirdly, from a methodological viewpoint, our study is the first comprehensive bibliometric analysis conducted in the field of health services for children in this demographic, and it establishes a methodological foundation for future research.

Analyses of the literature show that half (50.6%) of studies on access to healthcare services for individuals with disabilities use qualitative methods, a quarter (25.3%) use mixed methods, 15.7% use a quantitative approach, and 8.4% are systematic reviews. Most studies examined mixed disability types (33.7%), followed by psychosocial (25.3%), physical (16.9%), intellectual (14.5%), and sensory disabilities (9.6%). Nearly half of the studies (54.2%) provide information on specific groups at higher risk of exclusion, with a particular focus on women (19.3%) and children with disabilities (13.3%).

From a geographical perspective, research on healthcare access for individuals with disabilities is largely concentrated in the Americas (28.9%) and the Europe-Western Pacific (19.3%) regions. In the case of Türkiye, the Eastern Mediterranean region was found to be the least studied area (3.6%). It is noteworthy that 66.3% of the studies were carried out in high-income countries, whereas only 3.6% were performed in low-income countries. These findings indicate a substantial research gap in terms of global health equity.

In Türkiye, access to health services for pediatric populations who have disabilities is based on a broad legal and institutional framework coordinated by the Ministry of Family and Social Services. The "Special Needs Assessment Report for Children" (ÇÖZGER) system functions as a national evaluation mechanism to identify the special needs of children aged 0–18 (Ministry of Family and Social Services, 2023) [6]. Within this system, children are assessed in categories such as "Mild Special Needs," "Significant Special Needs," and "Very Profound Special Needs" to determine their rights to education, health, and social services. Individuals with disabilities also have priority status when receiving healthcare in Türkiye. Citizens registered as "priority" with the Ministry of Health can book appointments through special quotas.

However, a 2018 report by UNICEF and the European Disability Forum covering Türkiye points to significant systemic problems, stating that children with disabilities are "excluded from birth" and experience inadequate access to early diagnosis and intervention programs, community support, health services, and genuinely inclusive education [7]. Similar concerns were noted in Türkiye's evaluation by the UN Committee on the Rights of Persons with Disabilities. Although progress in inclusive education policies was acknowledged, the fact that over 30% of children within the disability community do not participate in any level of education is seen as a serious problem [8].

In Romania, the access to healthcare services for children with disabilities is clearly regulated by Law no. 448/2006, Law no. 95/2006, and Law no. 272/2004, and reinforced by the UN Convention on the Rights of Persons with Disabilities [9]. These laws guarantee free, prioritized, and adapted access to medical care and rehabilitation. They impose clear obligations on authorities to ensure nondiscriminatory access, tailored support, and integration into the community. In practice, the authorities are obliged to provide not only treatment but also prevention, early diagnosis, and ongoing support services.

Law no. 448/2006 on the Protection and Promotion of the Rights of Persons with Disabilities is the main law that classifies disabilities and establishes the corresponding rights: children with mild disabilities, children with moderate disabilities, children with severe disabilities, and children with pronounced disabilities. The classification is determined following a medical-psycho-social assessment, carried out by the Child Protection Commission, based on a certificate of disability classification. Also, the inclusion of children with disabilities in Romania continues to face numerous challenges, as reported in both national and international official documents, academic research, and by non-governmental organizations. A national report presents that less than 30% of children with disabilities receive regular rehabilitation services [10].

Bibliometric Analysis of the Topic

Bibliometric analysis is known to be a powerful research technique that provides a systematic and quantitative evaluation of scientific literature in a specific field [10]. As stated in a methodological guide bibliometric analysis is a "popular and rigorous method for exploring and analyzing large volumes of scientific data," and it serves to "unravel the evolutionary nuances of a specific field" and "illuminate its emerging areas" [11]. The methodology is reported to offer unique advantages for the systematic review of large literature collections, mapping of research networks, analysis of interdisciplinary collaborations, and identification of future research priorities.

Bibliometric analysis in health research has become considerably more common in recent decades. Various guides and standards have been developed for its application in the health sector. Some authors reviewed 31 empirical studies and showed that the Levesque's theoretical model has been effectively applied in healthcare access research [12]. Their results show that the model offers researchers a comprehensive perspective to evaluate the complex and dynamic process of access in both health system and community contexts. While bibliometric studies focusing specifically on children with disabilities are limited, they demonstrate that various dimensions of the field have been systematically addressed [13]. A bibliometric review on physical activity in children and adolescents with disabilities comprehensively analyzed publications from the Web of Science Core Collection between 1995 and 2023. [14] The study identified cerebral palsy, developmental coordination disorder, and autism as the most common clinical conditions in the field, also reporting that the USA and Australia are leading countries and that the dominant disciplines are neurosciences and neurology, psychology, rehabilitation, and sports sciences [14].

The impact of the COVID-19 global pandemic on healthcare access for children living with disabilities has attracted significant attention in the literature. A comprehensive review by McBride-Henry et al. (2023), which examined a total of 2201 articles from PubMed, Web of Science, CINAHL, and OVID databases between 2020 and 2023, shows that problems in healthcare access during the pandemic further deepened existing inequities [15]. Of the 81 studies analyzed, 18 specifically addressed experiences of healthcare access, while 63 examined health challenges as a secondary topic [15]. These findings bring to scholarly attention the multidimensional impact of the pandemic on individuals with disabilities.

Integrative review studies on healthcare access for individuals with intellectual and developmental disorders identify six main themes: education, information, and awareness; communication; fear and shame; participation in health decision-making processes; and the time factor [14]. All these themes seem to hinge on the need for greater care, dignity, respect, collaborative relationships, and reasonable accommodations, which brings to the fore the urgent need of a holistic approach to healthcare access for pediatric disability populations.

Our literature review verified the absence of a specialized bibliometric analysis study on healthcare access for children with disabilities, a finding that indicates a critical research gap in the field. As noted in a UNICEF report (2021a), these populations "remain largely invisible in research and in programs aimed at building more equitable, inclusive societies." [2]. This invisibility is considered both a cause and a consequence of their exclusion.

2. Research Methodology

2.1. Research Questions

Against this backdrop, the primary research questions for our study were as follows:

1. What is the bibliometric profile of the global literature on access to health services for children with disabilities, and what are the publication trends?
2. What is the structure of research in this field concerning geographical distribution, methodological approaches, and interdisciplinary collaborations?

3. What are the core research topics, conceptual clusters, and future research directions in the field?

2.2. Research Aim

The main purpose of our study was to examine the international literature on access to health services for children with disabilities via bibliometric analysis and to systematically identify the research trends in the field. The objectives were to (1) determine thematic trends and conceptual evolution in the literature; (2) identify the most influential publications, authors, and institutions; (3) evaluate methodological approaches and research paradigms; (4) analyze international collaboration networks; and (5) forecast future research directions.

2.3. Material

The data forming the basis of the bibliometric analysis in this study were obtained from the Web of Science Core Collection (WoS) database. The scope of the search included publications listed in the Science Citation Index Expanded (SCI-Expanded), Social Sciences Citation Index (SSCI), Arts and Humanities Citation Index (AHCI), and Emerging Sources Citation Index (ESCI). A thorough keyword strategy was developed to analyze trends, collaboration networks, and knowledge production dynamics in the literature on healthcare access for children with disabilities.

The data collection process was performed on 15 June 2025, and no time restrictions were applied. The search was conducted through the "Topic" field (title, abstract, and author keywords) in the WoS database. To retrieve all relevant studies, the search string was structured as follows to encompass children with disabilities, access to health services, and the pediatric context:

"children with disabilities" OR "disabled children" OR "childhood disability" OR "pediatric disability" OR "children with special needs" OR "special needs children" OR "developmental disorders" OR "neurodevelopmental disorders" OR "intellectual disability" OR "learning disability" OR "physical disability" OR "cognitive impairment" OR "autism spectrum disorder" OR "ASD" OR "Down syndrome" OR "cerebral palsy" OR "hearing impaired children" OR "visually impaired children"

AND "health services" OR "healthcare access" OR "access to health care" OR "health service accessibility" OR "barriers to healthcare"

AND child * OR pediatric

The search query yielded a total of 1318 articles. The publications were then filtered to include only those of the "Research Article" and "Early Access" type, which resulted in a total of 1134 articles. Finally, by limiting the selection to English-language publications, we reduced the number of studies included in the analysis to 1100.

2.4. Methods

This study was structured following a quantitative bibliometric analysis approach. As a research method, we adopted the systematic bibliometric analysis framework [16]. In the data collection process, academic publications covering the period 1984–2025 were screened via the Web of Science Core Collection database.

This method serves the aim of the research, to systematically screen the scientific literature focused on healthcare access for children within the disability community, evaluate productivity indicators, and reveal structural patterns in the field. The analysis process was conducted on two fundamental levels: (1) performance analysis evaluated metrics such as publication counts, author productivity, and institutional and geographical distributions; (2) science mapping provided a visualization of the scientific structure through keyword co-occurrence, thematic evolution, collaboration networks, and citation relationships.

Data analysis was performed via Biblioshiny, the graphical user interface for the bibliometrix R-package, which is customized for bibliometric reviews of scientific publications and runs in R version 4.5.0. [16]. Its Bibliometrix package executes the following multidimensional analyses: performance analysis (publication counts, citation analysis, country and institutional productivity); science mapping (co-authorship, co-citation, and bibliographic coupling analyses); thematic analysis (keyword clustering, thematic mapping, and thematic evolution); and trend analysis (time series and burst detection). Through this tool, key indicators were analyzed, including the annual distribution of publications, the most cited studies, the most productive authors and institutions, international collaborations, and networks of co-citation and co-word occurrences, country-based collaboration maps, source utilization, keyword analysis, and citation patterns. The thematic structure and evolution of topics in the field were assessed with strategic mapping and thematic analysis methods.

The literature selection process was conducted transparently and systematically in accordance with the PRISMA 2020 (Preferred Reporting Items for Systematic Reviews and Meta-Analyses) guideline [17,18]. This in-depth methodology ensures a holistic evaluation of both the quantitative and qualitative dimensions of the international literature on healthcare access for pediatric disability populations. The criteria for including and excluding publications, along with the screening process, were visualized by means of a PRISMA flow diagram.

The data selection criteria are defined according to the PICOS (Population, Intervention, Comparison, Outcomes, Study design) framework used as the basis for determining inclusion and exclusion criteria [19]. This method was adapted to the bibliometric analysis format and applied as follows:

- Population: Academic publications concerning health services for children with developmental, intellectual, physical, or sensory disabilities (e.g., autism spectrum disorder, Down syndrome, cerebral palsy, hearing and visual impairments, learning disabilities).
- Intervention: Studies addressing access to health services for children with disabilities in the context of reaching healthcare, barriers within the health system, or service utilization.
- Comparator: As is inherent to the nature of bibliometric analysis, comparisons of productivity and collaboration levels were made between categories such as countries, institutions, authors, and publication years, rather than experimental comparisons.
- Outcomes: Bibliometric outputs such as publication counts, citation levels, collaboration networks, keyword patterns, thematic trends, and keyword relationships were evaluated.
- Study Design: The analysis included only original research articles published in the English language and categorized as "Research Article" or "Early Access."

3. Results

Detailed information regarding the systematic filtering process for the publications selected in this study is visualized in the PRISMA flow diagram presented in Figure 1. Which studies were included in or excluded from the literature search can be transparently traced through this diagram. The publication evaluation and selection processes were structured according to the PICOS framework to ensure relevance to the research question. Application of this framework ensured that the studies included in the analysis were selected with a specific methodological integrity in terms of population, topic scope, comparison level, expected outcomes, and study design.

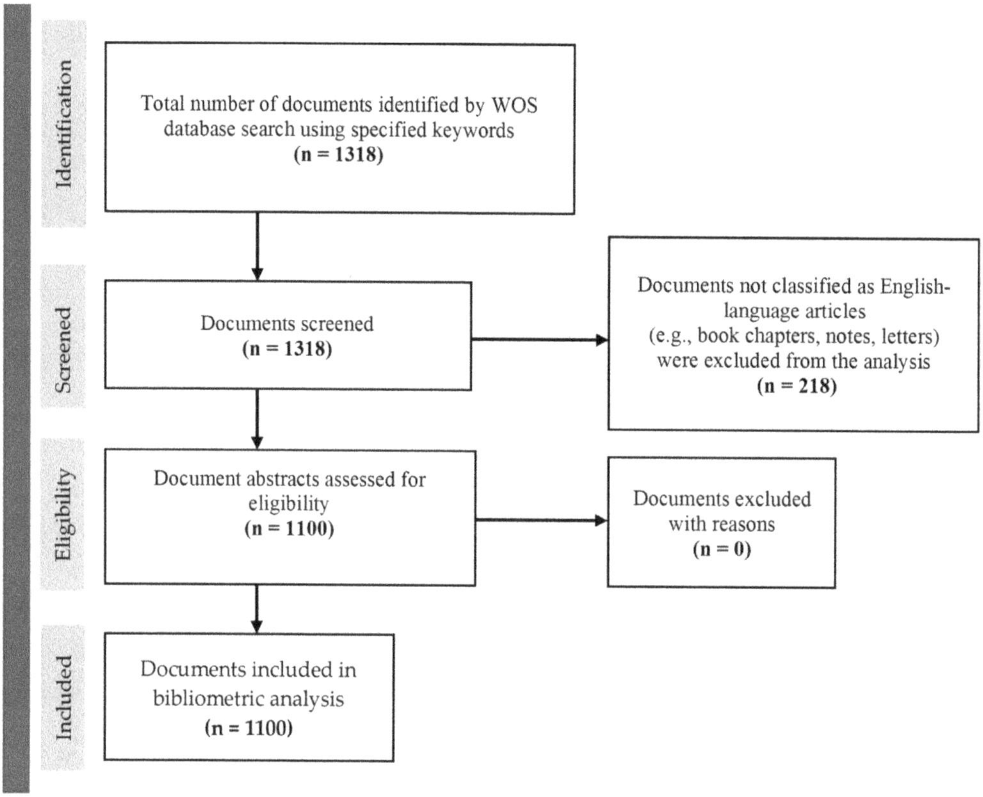

Figure 1. PRISMA flow chart.

Table 1 presents the descriptive characteristics of the bibliometric dataset. The indicators shown in the table were obtained according to standard bibliometric procedures [16]. In the table, the annual growth rate is calculated according to a compound annual growth formula based on the annual distribution of publications, while the average document age is calculated as the average difference between the publication year of the articles and the last year covered by the dataset.

The average number of citations per document is calculated by dividing the total number of citations received by all documents by the total number of documents. References analyzed represent the cumulative number of cited references across the dataset. Keywords Plus (ID) refers to indexing terms generated by the database provided by Web of Science, while authors' keywords (DE) represent words specified by the authors themselves. Total authors represent the number of contributing authors, while single-authored articles represent publications authored by only one author. The average number of co-authors per document represents the average number of authors per article and represents a measure of collaboration intensity. International co-authorships (%) indicate the extent of international scientific collaboration by expressing the proportion of documents co-authored by researchers from different countries. Finally, the distribution by document type (e.g., research article, early access) follows the WOS classification.

The final dataset created for bibliometric analysis, whose descriptive statistics are provided in Table 1, contains a total of 1100 academic publications published between 1984 and 2025. These publications were obtained from a total of 432 different sources, the majority of which were peer-reviewed journals. The annual growth rate of the documents was calculated at 8.37%. The rate shows that studies themed on healthcare access for pediatric disability populations have received increasing academic interest over time. The average publication age of the documents in the dataset stood at 8.07 years; the figure indicates that the literature in the field includes both historical and current contributions, whereas the average number of citations per publication was 25.2, a value that is significant for indicating the academic impact level of the literature.

Table 1. Characteristics of the dataset used for bibliometric analysis.

Description	Value
Publication Years	1984:2025
Publication Sources	432
Documents	1100
Annual Growth Rate (%)	8.37
Average Document Age (Years)	8.07
Average Citations per Document	25.2
References Analyzed	34,984
Keywords Plus (ID) [a]	1712
Author's Keywords (DE) [b]	2357
Total Authors	5719
Single-Authored Documents	46
Average Co-Authors per Document	47
International Co-Authorships (%)	6.12
Publication Years	17.82
Article	1081
Article; Early Access	19

Note. The dataset was compiled from the Web of Science Core Collection. [a] ID refers to "Identification" keywords indexed by the database. [b] DE refers to "Descriptor" keywords provided by the authors.

The studies in the dataset contain a total of 34.984 different references, which reveals that the field is enriched by an interdisciplinary body of knowledge. They contain 1.712 keywords and 2.357 author-specified keywords, a finding that points to the conceptual diversity and thematic richness of the relevant literature. Among the documents contributed by a total of 5.719 different authors, only 47 are single-authored; the proportion of single-authored publications is therefore quite low. This observation shows that the field is largely shaped by multi-authored, interdisciplinary, and collaborative academic production practices. The average number of authors per document, 6.12, also supports this inference. The presence of international collaborations in 17.82% of the studies reveals that the topic attracts global scientific interest and is supported by joint research between countries. As for the distribution of document types in the dataset, 1.081 studies are categorized as "research articles" and 19 as "early access."

The annual publication trend presented in Figure 2 illustrates the development over time in academic literature concerning access to health services for minors with disabilities. Although the first studies in this field date back to 1984, it is noteworthy that a very limited number of publications existed until the mid-2000s. However, a significant increase in the number of publications has been observed since 2015; this upward trend peaked between 2021 and 2023. Reaching the highest level in 2023 with over 90 publications shows that the topic has become a focus of international academic interest. This high level of interest can be associated with the growing importance of themes such as equity in health services, children's rights, inclusive health policies, and the quality of life for individuals with disabilities. The data for 2025 remain partial, as the year had not concluded at the time of data collection.

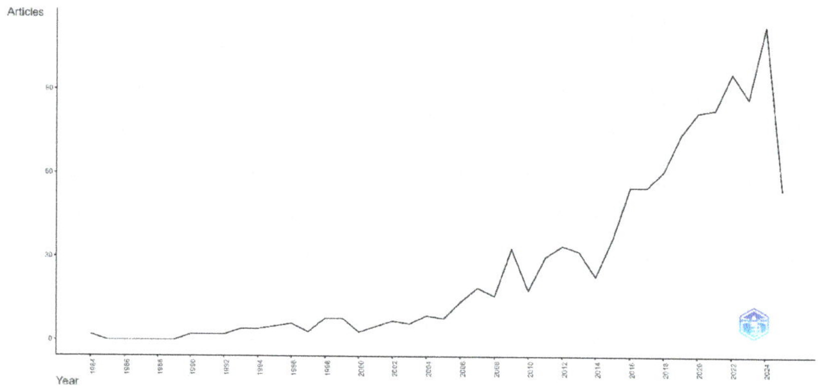

Figure 2. Annual scientific publication output on access to health services for children with disabilities (1984–2025).

The graph in Figure 3 reflects the distribution of corresponding authors by country and the breakdown of this output in terms of single-country (SCP) versus multi-country (MCP) collaborations. With 368 publications, corresponding to 33.5% of the total output, the United States stands out as by far the most productive country. It is followed by the United Kingdom (15.7%), Australia (9.5%), and Canada (9.5%), respectively. Academic interest in health services for children with disabilities is shaped by high-income countries, particularly English-speaking developed nations. Regarding multi-country publication rates, it is seen that only 8.2% (30/368) of the output from the United States, the most prolific country, is based on international collaborations. In contrast, countries such as the United Kingdom (18.5%), Canada (18.3%), and Australia (18.1%) are notable for both high productivity and more intensive international collaborations. The considerably high MCP rates in European countries such as Ireland (36.0%), Spain (36.8%), Germany (33.3%), and France (85.7%) reflect the open nature of these countries' research collaborations.

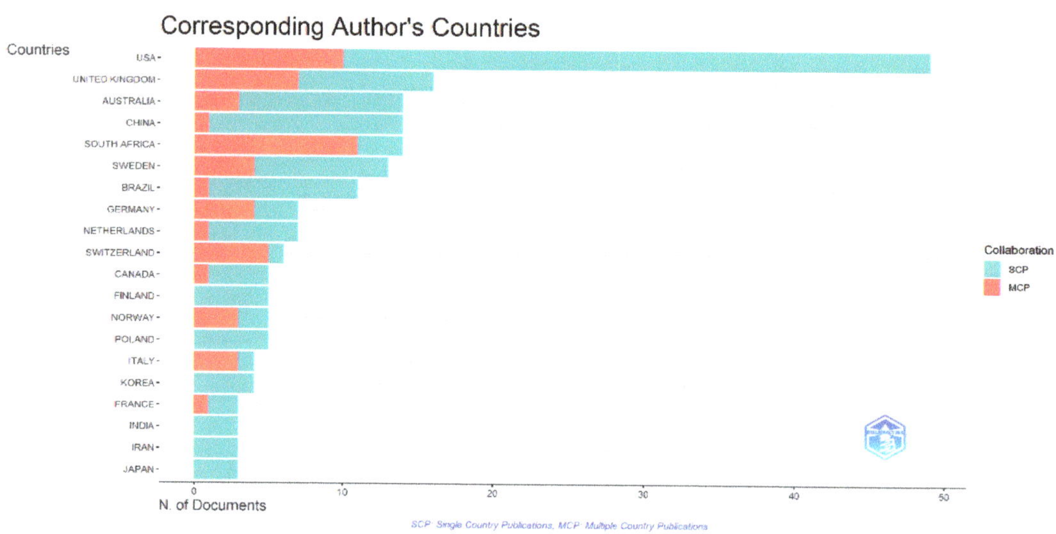

Figure 3. Distribution of corresponding authors by country and types of international collaboration (SCP vs. MCP).

The multi-country collaboration trends outlined above are supported by the country-based co-publication frequencies presented in Table 2. The 19 joint publications between the USA and Canada reveal the scientific integration in North America, whereas the multi-center collaborations conducted by the United Kingdom with numerous countries (Ireland, Italy, Australia, France, Spain, and Denmark) demonstrate its central role in international research networks. The eight joint publications between Australia and New Zealand also imply a strong regional academic interaction. These multifaceted international collaborations show that the field is being addressed on a global scale and is enriched by interdisciplinary approaches.

Table 2. Frequency distribution of inter-country collaborations.

From	To	Frequency
USA	Canada	19
United Kingdom	Ireland	15
USA	United Kingdom	15
United Kingdom	Italy	13
United Kingdom	Australia	10
United Kingdom	France	10
United Kingdom	Spain	10
United Kingdom	Denmark	9
Australia	New Zealand	8
Italy	Germany	8
United Kingdom	Canada	8

As demonstrated by our bibliometric analysis, academic publications in the field of pediatric disability and health services are distinctly concentrated in specialized journals. (Figure 4) The data show that in autism spectrum disorders specifically, the journals *AUTISM* (n = 57) and the *Journal of Autism and Developmental Disorders* (n = 55) are the dominant publication platforms. In the literature on child health and development, *Child: Care, Health and Development* (n = 40) and *Pediatrics* (n = 30) were identified as prominent sources. In the area of intellectual disability and developmental disorders, journals such as BMJ Open (n = 22), the *Journal of Intellectual Disability Research* (n = 20), and *Research in Developmental Disabilities* (n = 20) are seen to have made significant contributions. Such findings indicate that research on this population is approached from a multidisciplinary perspective, but a more intensive accumulation of knowledge has occurred in journals specializing in autism and developmental disorders.

The Keywords Plus analysis presented in Figure 5 reveals the primary research trends and conceptual focus within the literature on children with disabilities and health services. The prominent terms in the analysis, "autism spectrum disorder" and "developmental disabilities," show that studies in the field are concentrated on neurodevelopmental disorders. Emphases such as "mental health services" and "psychiatric disorders" indicate that the mental health needs of children within the disability community play a central role in research.

Terms such as "young children," "health impact," "outcomes," "diagnosis," and "parents" highlight the importance of early intervention and family-centered approaches. The concepts of "health services access" and "disparities" draw attention to the systemic barriers encountered, particularly in vulnerable groups.

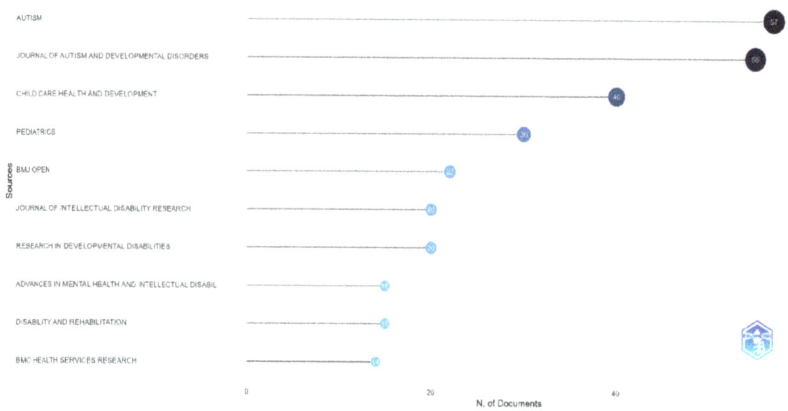

Figure 4. Distribution of the most prolific journals in the field of children with disabilities and health services.

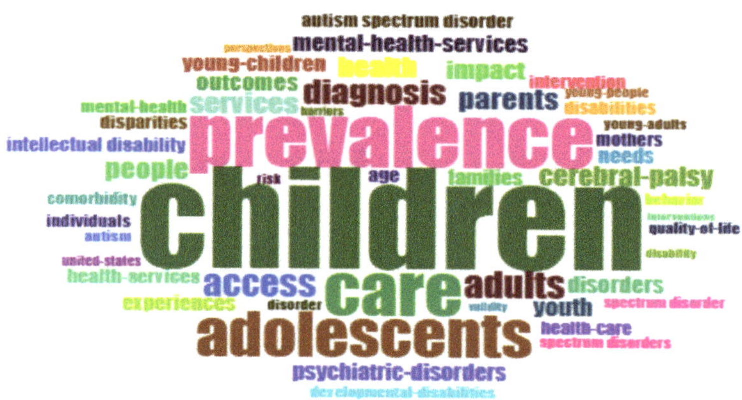

Figure 5. Word cloud based on keywords plus data.

The prominence of specific diagnostic groups like "intellectual disability" and "cerebral palsy", alongside demographic factors such as "families" and "age," shows that the research encompasses sociodemographic dimensions as well as clinical ones. Geographical references like "Mediterranean" and "United States" point to the existence of academic interest in regional health policies and practices.

This conceptual structure clarifies that research in the field of children experiencing disabilities and health services exhibits a multilayered structure. Studies are seen to be shaped across a wide spectrum, ranging from diagnostic classifications to mental health service access and from family dynamics to social inequalities. Our findings here are important, as they provide a conceptual framework for future research in the field.

The three-field analysis presented in Figure 6 depicts the intellectual architecture of the literature on pediatric disability populations and health services. The analysis reflects the dominant contributions of North America-based authors (Zuckerman, Brookman-Frazee, Mandell, etc.). Their work is seen to focus on themes such as autism spectrum disorder ("autism"), access issues ("access"), and family-centered interventions ("parents").

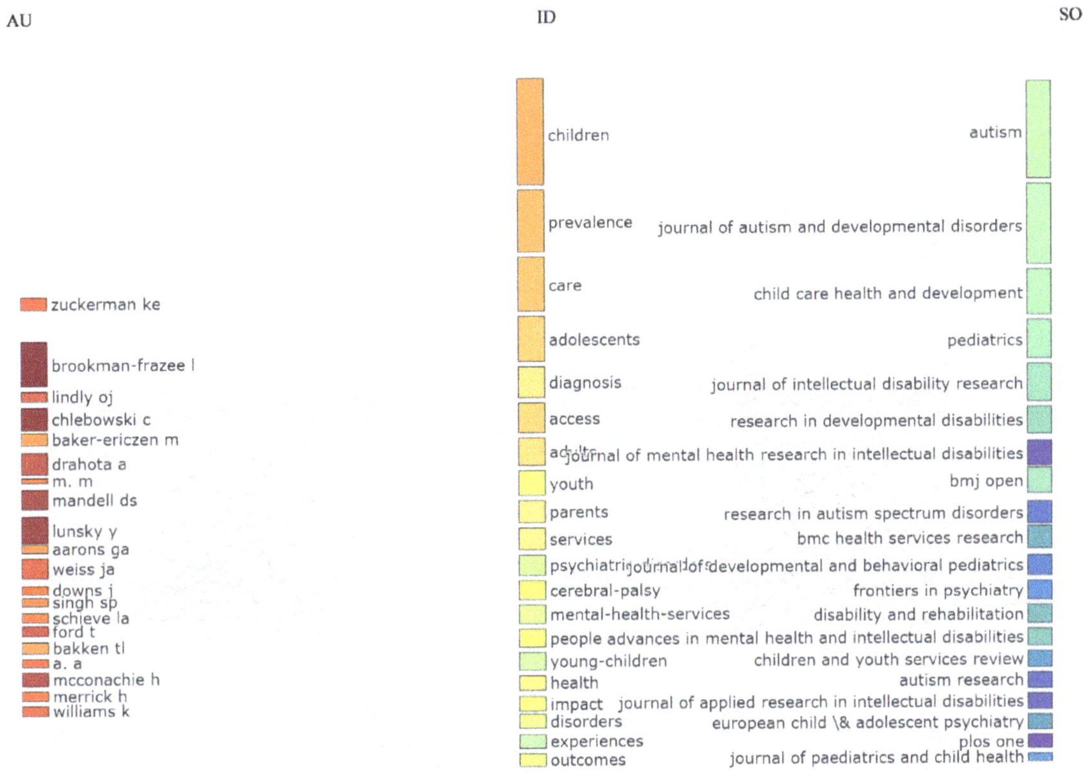

Figure 6. Structural dynamics of research on children with disabilities and health services: a three-fields analysis of authors, keywords, and journals.

Distribution of keywords illustrates that the clinical ("diagnosis," "mental-health-services") and social ("care," "services") dimensions of the research are intertwined. The prominence of terms like "prevalence" and "adolescents" reflects the importance given to age-specific epidemiological analyses in the field. The presence of specific diagnostic groups such as "cerebral palsy" and "developmental disabilities" establishes the heterogeneous structure of literature.

Consistency between authors' areas of expertise and their publication preferences (e.g., autism researchers gravitating toward developmental disability journals, mental health experts toward psychiatry publications) confirms that academic production is shaped within niche areas. Such findings offer significant clues that the literature on children in this demographic and health services develops at the intersection of clinical expertise and societal needs.

An examination of the most-cited publications in the field (Table 3) highlights the prominence of studies [20–22]. When evaluated in terms of total citations and normalized citation scores, one work stands out distinctly from other studies with both its total citation count and average annual citations [20]. Analysis of normalized citation scores identified that relatively recent studies also exhibited high citation performance [23,24].

Table 3. The 10 most-cited articles on health services for children with disabilities.

Cited Article (From the References List)	Total Citations	Citations per Year	Normalized Citations
[20]	774	110.57	22.42
[21]	743	67.55	16.92
[22]	607	40.47	10.95
[25]	583	34.29	10.80
[26]	540	33.75	6.21
[24]	505	56.11	14.14
[27]	457	25.39	8.68
[28]	362	51.71	10.48
[29]	334	17.58	3.76
[30]	307	43.86	8.89
[23]	304	50.67	15.04

Note. Data retrieved from Web of Science on 15 June 2025. Normalized citations refer to the total citations of an article normalized by the total citations of the journal in the same year.

The thematic mapping in Figure 7 was generated by keyword plus co-word analysis using the Bibliometrix package in R. The analysis is based on research articles from the WOS between 1984 and 2025. A total of 432 articles and 1712 keywords were analyzed. The thematic map was constructed according to the method of Callon et al. (1991), which positions themes on a two-dimensional plane according to their centrality (degree of relevance) and density (degree of development) [31]. Centrality measures the degree of interaction of a theme with other themes in the network, while density assesses a theme's internal strength and development. This scientific mapping approach consists of four theme categories: motor themes, niche themes, emerging/declining themes, and basic themes.

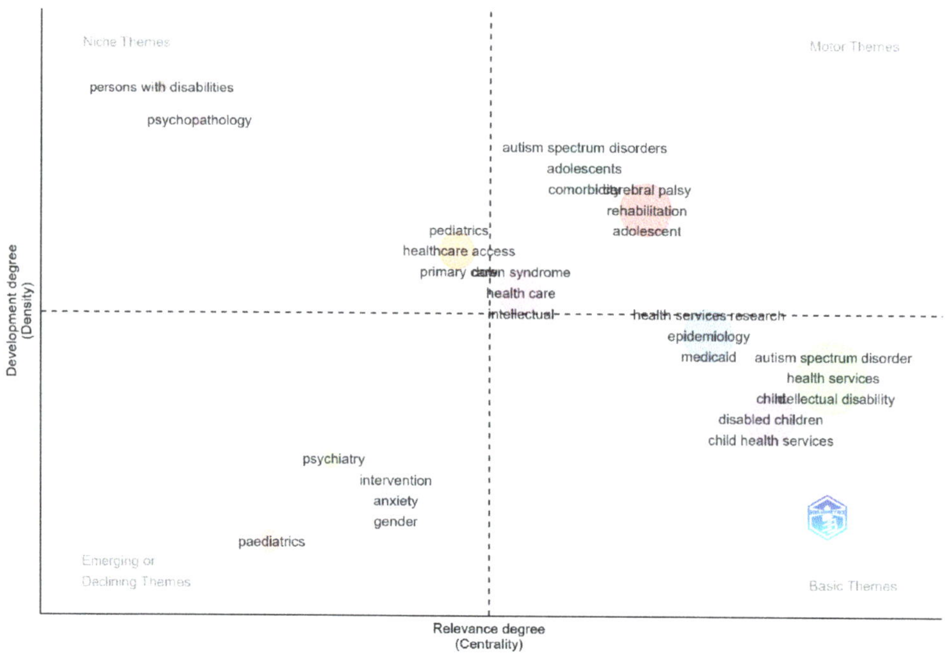

Figure 7. Thematic analysis.

Themes located in the Motor Themes (Developed Themes) category, such as "autism spectrum disorders," "adolescents," "comorbidity," "cerebral palsy," "rehabilitation," and "adolescent," are prominent for their high centrality and high-density values. This positioning substantiates that the themes in question are both well-developed within the literature and highly interactive with other themes. The themes of "autism spectrum disorders" and "cerebral palsy" are among the mature fields that are the subject of multidisciplinary studies.

The themes in the Niche Themes category, "persons with disabilities" and "psychopathology," are defined by high density but low centrality values. These themes represent sub-fields of study that are well-developed within specific areas of expertise but have limited interaction with other themes in the literature. The theme of "psychopathology," in particular, is an important area of specialization that, despite its high level of development, has a limited central contribution to the overall structure of literature.

Themes in the Emerging/Declining Themes category, such as "psychiatry," "intervention," "anxiety," "gender," and "pediatrics," have low values in terms of both density and centrality. This placement suggests that these themes are either newly entering the research area or are experiencing a decline in interest compared to previous years. Themes like "psychiatry" and "anxiety," despite their potential in the context of mental health and service access for children with disabilities, are considered underdeveloped areas in the current literature.

The themes located in the Basic Themes category—"health services research," "epidemiology," "Medicaid," "autism spectrum disorder," "health services," "child," "intellectual disability," "disabled children," and "child health services"—possess high centrality but relatively low-density values. These themes constitute the central topics of literature, forming the methodological and theoretical foundation for the field. The central position of the "disabled children" and "child health services" themes, in particular, demonstrates that these areas form a fundamental axis in health services research.

In summary, the positioning of themes like "autism spectrum disorders" and "cerebral palsy" as strong motor themes in the upper-right quadrant of the map pinpoints the areas where the literature is concentrated. On the other hand, the fact that themes like "psychopathology" and "persons with disabilities" remain in the niche quadrant suggests that these areas, while studied in-depth, have limited interaction within the general literature. The location of themes such as "psychiatry," "intervention," and "gender" in the emerging/declining themes category signals that mental health services and gender-based studies are not yet sufficiently mature or are seeing diminished interest in the context of children with disabilities. The relatively low density of basic themes, such as "health services research" and "child health services," despite their high centrality, attests to the fact that while these areas are methodologically and structurally important, they require more in-depth, content-focused research.

The results of the trend analysis presented in Figure 8 disclose that monitoring and case-focused data collection studies, such as those involving "patients," "disabilities monitoring networks," and "11 sites," have shown an increase, particularly after 2015. This development signals that large-sample, multi-center, and monitoring-based research is gaining importance in the field.

A marked rise in the terms "neurodevelopmental disorders" and "autism spectrum disorder" after 2010 reflects the rapid increase in clinical and service-oriented research centered on autism and neurodevelopmental disorders. This finding testifies to the deepening of clinical interest in neurodevelopmental diagnostic groups and the corresponding health services research.

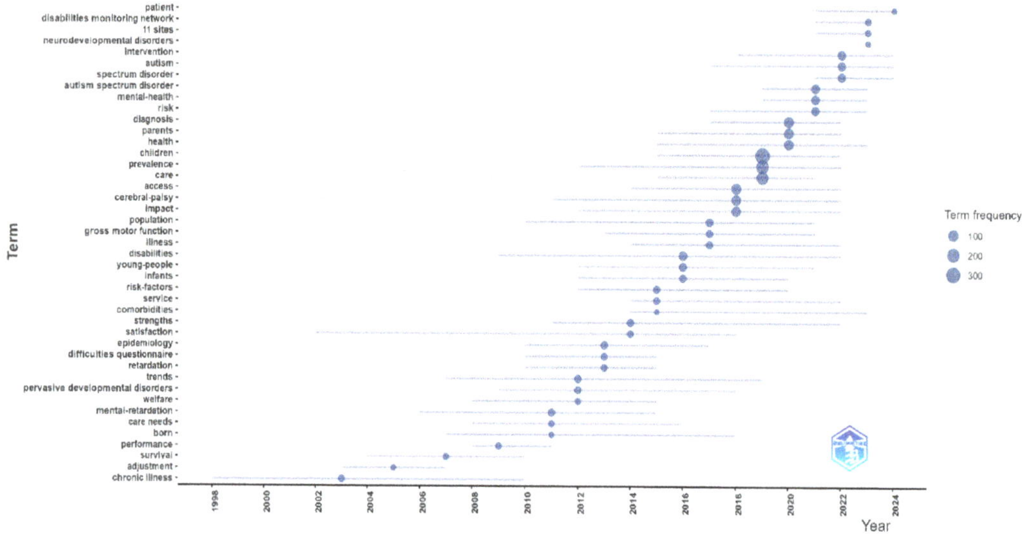

Figure 8. Topic trends.

A sharp increase observed in the terms "mental-health" and "comorbidities" after 2016 corroborates that mental health problems and psychiatric comorbidities in children with disabilities are being studied more frequently in the literature. This trend suggests a need for a multidisciplinary approach in health service planning and asserts that inequities in access to mental health services have gained priority in research.

Constant use of the terms "prevalence" and "epidemiology" over time affirms that the literature rests on a strong epidemiological foundation and that prevalence data are used as a fundamental reference point in service planning for the field. The increase in the terms "care," "access," and "services" over the last five years evidences a research trend concentrating on access to health services, service quality, and care models.

The term "mental-retardation" began to fall out of use from the 2010s onward, being replaced by more current and inclusive terminology. This change can be evaluated as a reflection of the terminological transformation in diagnostic classifications within the academic literature. The consistent study of terms like "gross motor function" and "cerebral-palsy" since the early 2000s upholds the view that the impact of neurological disorders on physical functionality has remained a permanent fixture on the research agenda for many years. By contrast, the relatively low frequency of terms focused on patient experience and quality of life, such as "welfare," "satisfaction," and "performance," points to the fact that topics like service quality and patient/parent satisfaction are still not adequately addressed in the literature, which can be construed to imply that quantitative service research in the field is open to development in terms of content richness.

Taken together, the findings indicate that in the field of pediatric disability populations and health services, there has been a research trend over the past 10–15 years concentrating on neurodevelopmental disorders, mental health, and access inequities. Terminological transformations and the increase in multi-center epidemiological studies have strengthened methodological diversification and monitoring-based data production processes in the field. However, the limited number of studies focused on patient experience, service satisfaction, and social welfare confirms that there is a literature gap in these topics, which points to potential areas for future research.

The thematic evolution analysis provided in Figure 9 visualizes how the subject headings in the literature on pediatric disability populations and health services have transformed between 1984 and 2025, and from which themes the research focus has evolved.

Figure 9. Thematic evolution analysis.

Between 1984 and 2014, the primary research axes of the literature were predominantly shaped around the themes of "access," "anxiety," "cerebral palsy," "children," and "gross motor function." During this period, clinical problems such as access inequities, the effects of neurological conditions like cerebral palsy on child health, and motor function disorders emerged as priority research areas. The inclusion of psychological factors like anxiety in previous work attests to the period's consideration of psychosocial dimensions, albeit to a limited extent.

In the period from 2015 to 2025, a significant transformation in research focus is observed. The prominence of themes such as "care," "diagnosis," "disorder," and "parents" illustrates that service delivery models, diagnostic processes, and family-centered approaches have increasingly gained priority. The appearance of "deficit-hyperactivity disorder" and "virus infection" on the research agenda can be interpreted as a reflection in the literature of health threats specific to the post-pandemic era and of neurodevelopmental disorders.

In general terms, the thematic analysis establishes that the literature on children experiencing disabilities and health services has undergone a significant transformation over approximately 40 years. It clarifies that while initially focusing on motor function disorders and access issues, the literature has now evolved into a more thorough and holistic structure that includes diagnostic processes, family support systems, and psychosocial factors. The recent prominence of research on attention deficit/hyperactivity disorder, viral infections, and parent-focused studies, in particular, reflects a broadening paradigm shift in health services, moving from the individual toward family- and community-based approaches.

The network graph provided in Figure 10 illustrates the relationships and clustering among the most frequently used keywords in the relevant publications.

The clusters, shown in different colors, represent the sub-thematic areas of the topic; they are observed to be concentrated around focal concepts such as "children," "care," and "prevalence." In the network, node size represents the frequency of the word's use, whereas the lines between nodes represent the frequency of co-occurrence. This analysis determined that themes such as access to health services, care processes, and mental health problems for children experiencing disabilities are the main areas of study highlighted in the literature. The relationships between clusters also serve as an indicator of interdisciplinary collaboration and the need for a holistic approach.

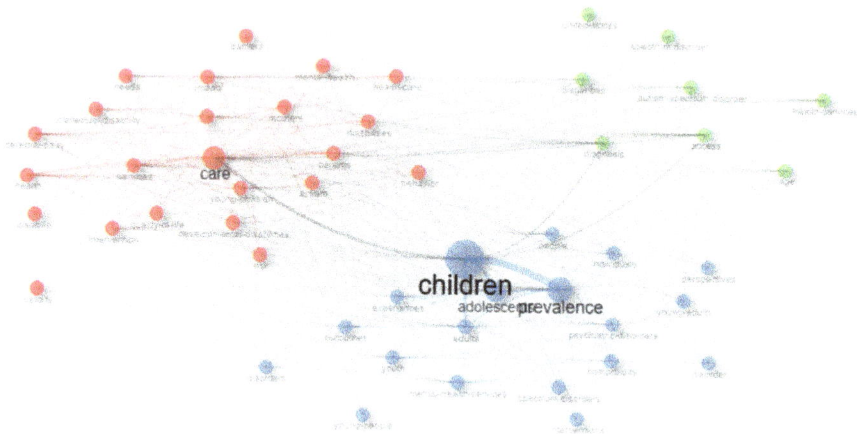

Figure 10. Keyword association network in publications on children with disabilities and health services.

4. Discussion

Our study presents a thorough bibliometric analysis that systematically examines research trends concerning access to health services for pediatric disability populations. The literature in the field has been documented to have undergone a significant quantitative and qualitative development during the 1984–2025 period. The calculated annual publication growth rate of 8.37% and the distinct upward trend observed, especially after 2015, seem to confirm that the topic has become a focus of academic interest.

According to our country-based analyses, high-income countries, such as the USA, the United Kingdom, and Australia, play a dominant role in research production, which means that the perspective of developed nations largely shapes research on healthcare access for minors with disabilities. On the other hand, the intensive collaborations among European countries attest to the strength of regional research networks.

Keyword co-occurrence network analysis demonstrates that publications on pediatric disability populations and health services are shaped around specific thematic clusters. The central placement of concepts such as "children" and "care" establishes that care processes for this population and prevalence studies are among the priority topics in the field. Other clusters developing around the "autism spectrum disorder" and "health services" axis substantiate that the processes of accessing health services for children with autism spectrum disorder have gained traction in the literature. This thematic distribution constitutes a valuable resource for health policy developers and clinicians in identifying priority research areas.

Our thematic map analysis revealed a research ecosystem shaped under four distinct categories, each featuring unique patterns of scholarly engagement within the field of childhood disability healthcare. The high density and centrality values of topics such as "autism spectrum disorders" and "cerebral palsy" in the motor themes category suggest that these areas hold a mature and influential position in the literature. The predominance of studies on autism spectrum disorders underscores that neurodevelopmental disorders are a priority research topic in the context of healthcare for pediatric disability populations. The fact that topics in the niche themes category, such as "psychopathology" and "persons with disabilities," have high density but low centrality implies that although specialized work is being performed in such areas, they have limited interaction with the broader scholarly discourse, thus suggesting intellectual fragmentation. This outcome alludes to the need for further psychopathology and disability studies equipped with a more constructive interdisciplinary approach. High centrality values of topics in the basic themes category, such as "health services research" and "child health services," indicate that such areas form the methodological backbone of the literature. However, the relatively low density of these themes suggests a need for more content-focused research.

Thematic evolution analysis also corroborates that the literature has undergone a significant transformation over time, with research focusing on motor function disorders and access issues in earlier periods having lately evolved into a more holistic structure that includes diagnostic processes, family-centered approaches, and psychosocial factors. The recent prominence of themes like "deficit-hyperactivity disorder" and "viral infection," in particular, demonstrates the field's responsiveness to contemporary health challenges—a research agenda that adapts dynamically to current priorities in response to pressing public health needs.

Limitations of the study are especially linked to the analyzed databases. We have scanned only the Web of Science database, and probably other important databases have published valuable studies on this topic. Future research should also include publications from PubMed, Scopus, etc., in this type of analysis, and it should be oriented to the evolution of studies concerning the topic of disabilities at different ages and in different countries. It will also be important to emphasize this evolution in relation to national and international statistics on the topic.

5. Conclusions

Our study has shed light on key research trends in healthcare access for children with disabilities, identifying the current state of the field and promising directions for future research. One of the most significant contributions of the study is its emphasis on addressing this complex issue from a multidimensional perspective. The integrated execution of clinical practices, policy development, and public awareness initiatives is crucial for pediatric disability populations to benefit equally from health services. Although high-income countries currently dominate research production, expanding international collaborations and achieving more equitable resource distribution will be essential for developing truly inclusive and globally applicable solutions.

Future research is recommended to prioritize more comprehensive and detailed analyses of the social, economic, and cultural barriers that confront this population in accessing healthcare. At the intersection of caregiving, child protection systems, and social services, adopting a socio-health perspective can offer valuable insights and contributions to the field. Broader deployment of qualitative and mixed methods should afford richer insights into patient and family experiences. Importantly, cross-country differences in resources, policies, and cultural perspectives on children with disabilities can point to identifiable patterns: for example, high-income settings generally offer more structured service systems, while low- and middle-income settings emphasize the roles of extended family and community networks in accessing healthcare. Such patterns are crucial, as they can guide policymakers in designing context-sensitive strategies that leverage existing strengths and address systemic gaps. In this context, comparative insights across contexts can inform international policy dialogues and support the development of adaptable, inclusive healthcare frameworks. Developing evidence-based guidelines for policymakers and healthcare providers can help address the challenges often encountered in practice. This study has the potential to serve as a foundational reference for researchers, clinicians, and policymakers committed to advancing equitable healthcare access for children with disabilities. Additionally, as much of the existing literature focuses primarily on the perspectives of parents, guardians, and healthcare professionals, future research should prioritize studies conducted directly with children with disabilities. Incorporating children's needs and lived experiences into research will help provide a more comprehensive and inclusive understanding of the needs and barriers they face in accessing healthcare.

Author Contributions: Conceptualization, E.G.; literature review, E.G., Y.O., A.C., M.Z., M.S., and R.S.; writing—original draft preparation, E.G., Y.O., A.C., M.Z., M.S., and R.S.; writing—review and editing, E.G., Y.O., A.C., M.Z., M.S., and R.S.; visualization, E.G.; supervision, Y.O. and M.S. All authors have an equal contribution. All authors have read and agreed to the published version of the manuscript.

Funding: This research was funded by EACEA, project ERASMUS-SPORT-2024-SCP, title Building Bridge to Accessible Fitness: Empowering Personal Trainers and Persons with Disabilities through Education, Community, and AI-Driven Coaching/Bridge4Fitness (project number 101181099) and the APC was funded by the budget of this project.

Conflicts of Interest: The authors declare no conflicts of interest.

References

1. World Health Organization. Global Report on Health Equity for Persons with Disabilities. 2022. Available online: https://www.who.int/publications/i/item/9789240063600 (accessed on 7 April 2025).
2. UNICEF. Seen, Counted, Included: Using Data to Shed Light on the Well-Being of Children with Disabilities. 2021. Available online: https://data.unicef.org/resources/children-with-disabilities-report-2021/ (accessed on 7 April 2025).
3. Gréaux, M.; Moro, M.F.; Kamenov, K.; Russell, A.M.; Barrett, D.; Cieza, A. Health equity for persons with disabilities: A global scoping review on barriers and interventions in healthcare services. *Int. J. Equity Health* **2023**, *22*, 236. [CrossRef]
4. Cieza, A.; Kamenov, K.; Sanchez, M.G.; Chatterji, S.; Balasegaram, M.; Lincetto, O.; Servili, C.; Bermejo, R.; Ross, D.A. Burden of disability in children and adolescents must be integrated into the global health agenda. *BMJ (Clin. Res. Ed.)* **2021**, *372*, n9. [CrossRef]
5. Levesque, J.F.; Harris, M.F.; Russell, G. Patient-centered access to health care: Conceptualizing access at the interface of health systems and populations. *Int. J. Equity Health* **2013**, *12*, 18. [CrossRef] [PubMed]
6. Ministry of Family and Social Services. 2023. Available online: https://www.sma.org.tr/en/announcement/342/disability-health-board-reports-and-information-about-special-needs-report-for-children-cozger (accessed on 9 April 2025).
7. UNICEF; European Disability Forum. Everybody Counts: A Situation Analysis of the Inclusion of Children with Disabilities in the Western Balkans and Turkey. 2018. Available online: https://www.unicef.org/eca/media/5361/file/Children%20with%20Disabilities%20in%20Western%20Balkans%20and%20Turkey%202018.pdf (accessed on 9 April 2025).
8. United Nations Human Rights, Office of the High Commissioner. Committee on the Rights of Persons with Disabilities Considers the Report of Turkey. 2019. Available online: https://www.ohchr.org/en/news/2019/03/committee-rights-persons-disabilities-considers-report-turkey (accessed on 9 April 2025).
9. UNICEF România. Incluziunea Copiilor cu Dizabilități în Școală și Comunitate. 2021. Available online: https://www.unicef.org/romania/media/10941/file/Ghid%20de%20practici:%20Incluziunea%20copiilor%20%C8%99i%20a%20tinerilor%20cu%20dizabilit%C4%83%C8%9Bi%20%C3%AEn%20asisten%C8%9Ba%20medical%C4%83%20general%C4%83.pdf (accessed on 10 April 2025).
10. Ministerul Muncii și Solidarității Sociale. Raport privind Incluziunea Socială în România în Anul. 2022. Available online: https://mmuncii.ro/j33/images/Documente/Familie/RaportariPrivindIncluziuneaSociala/Raport_incluziune_2022.pdf (accessed on 10 April 2025).
11. Donthu, N.; Kumar, S.; Mukherjee, D.; Pandey, N.; Lim, W.M. How to conduct a bibliometric analysis: An overview and guidelines. *J. Bus. Res.* **2021**, *133*, 285–296. [CrossRef]
12. Cu, A.; Meister, S.; Lefebvre, B.; Ridde, V. Assessing healthcare access using the Levesque's conceptual framework—a scoping review. *Int. J. Equity Health* **2021**, *20*, 116. [CrossRef] [PubMed]
13. Doherty, A.J.; Atherton, H.; Boland, P.; Hastings, R.; Hives, L.; Hood, K.; James-Jenkinson, L.; Leavey, R.; Randell, E.; Reed, J.; et al. Barriers and facilitators to primary health care for people with intellectual disabilities and/or autism: An integrative review. *BJGP Open* **2020**, *4*, bjgpopen20X101030. [CrossRef] [PubMed]
14. Ma, Y.; Liu, M.; Liu, Y.; Liu, D.; Hou, M. Exploring Physical Activity in Children and Adolescents with Disabilities: A Bibliometric Review of Current Status, Guidelines, Perceived Barriers, and Facilitators and Future Directions. *Healthcare* **2024**, *12*, 934. [CrossRef]

15. McBride-Henry, K.; Nazari Orakani, S.; Good, G.; Roguski, M.; Officer, T.N. Disabled people's experiences accessing healthcare services during the COVID-19 pandemic: A scoping review. *BMC Health Serv. Res.* **2023**, *23*, 346. [CrossRef]
16. Aria, M.; Cuccurullo, C. Bibliometrix: An R-tool for comprehensive science mapping analysis. *J. Informetr.* **2017**, *11*, 959–975. [CrossRef]
17. Moher, D.; Liberati, A.; Tetzlaff, J.; Altman, D.G.; the PRISMA Group. Preferred reporting items for systematic reviews and meta-analyses: The PRISMA statement. *PLoS Med.* **2009**, *6*, e1000097. [CrossRef]
18. Tricco, A.C.; Zarin, W.; Ghassemi, M.; Nincic, V.; Lillie, E.; Page, M.J.; Shamseer, L.; Antony, J.; Rios, P.; Hwee, J.; et al. Same family, different species: Methodological conduct and quality varies according to purpose for five types of knowledge synthesis. *J. Clin. Epidemiol.* **2018**, *96*, 133–142. [CrossRef]
19. Saaiq, M.; Ashraf, B. Modifying "Pico" question into "Picos" model for more robust and reproducible presentation of the methodology employed in a scientific study. *World J. Plast. Surg.* **2017**, *6*, 390–392.
20. Zablotsky, B.; Black, L.I.; Maenner, M.J.; Schieve, L.A.; Danielson, M.L.; Bitsko, R.H.; Blumberg, S.J. Prevalence and trends of developmental disabilities among children in the United States: 2009–2017. *Pediatrics* **2019**, *144*, e20190811. [CrossRef]
21. Croen, L.A.; Zerbo, O.; Qian, Y.; Massolo, M.L.; Rich, S.; Sidney, S.; Kripke, C. The health status of adults on the autism spectrum. *Autism* **2015**, *19*, 814–823. [CrossRef]
22. Brugha, T.S.; McManus, S.; Bankart, J.; Scott, F.; Purdon, S.; Smith, J.; Bebbington, P.; Jenkins, R.; Meltzer, H. Epidemiology of autism spectrum disorders in adults in the community in England. *Arch. Gen. Psychiatry* **2011**, *68*, 459–465. [CrossRef] [PubMed]
23. Dalsgaard, S.; Thorsteinsson, E.; Trabjerg, B.B.; Schullehner, J.; Plana-Ripoll, O.; Brikell, I.; Wimberley, T.; Thygesen, M.; Madsen, K.B.; Timmerman, A.; et al. Incidence rates and cumulative incidences of the full spectrum of diagnosed mental disorders in childhood and adolescence. *JAMA Psychiatry* **2020**, *77*, 155–164. [CrossRef] [PubMed]
24. Thapar, A.; Cooper, M.; Rutter, M. Neurodevelopmental disorders. *Lancet Psychiatry* **2017**, *4*, 339–346. [CrossRef] [PubMed]
25. Kogan, M.D.; Blumberg, S.J.; Schieve, L.A.; Boyle, C.A.; Perrin, J.M.; Ghandour, R.M.; Singh, G.K.; Strickland, B.B.; Trevathan, E.; van Dyck, P.C. Prevalence of parent-reported diagnosis of autism spectrum disorder among children in the US, 2007. *Pediatrics* **2009**, *124*, 1395–1403. [CrossRef]
26. Simon, T.D.; Berry, J.; Feudtner, C.; Stone, B.L.; Sheng, X.; Bratton, S.L.; Dean, J.M.; Srivastava, R. Children With Complex Chronic Conditions in Inpatient Hospital Settings in the United States. *Pediatrics* **2010**, *126*, 647–655. [CrossRef]
27. Kogan, M.D.; Strickland, B.B.; Blumberg, S.J.; Singh, G.K.; Perrin, J.M.; van Dyck, P.C. A National Profile of the Health Care Experiences and Family Impact of Autism Spectrum Disorder Among Children in the United States, 2005–2006. *Pediatrics* **2008**, *122*, e1149–e1158. [CrossRef]
28. Kooij, J.; Bijlenga, D.; Salerno, L.; Jaeschke, R.; Bitter, I.; Balázs, J.; Thome, J.; Dom, G.; Kasper, S.; Filipe, C.N.; et al. Updated European Consensus Statement on diagnosis and treatment of adult ADHD. Eur. *Psychiatry* **2018**, *56*, 14–34. [CrossRef]
29. Ford, T.; Vostanis, P.; Meltzer, H.; Goodman, R. Psychiatric disorder among British children looked after by local authorities: Comparison with children living in private households. *Br. J. Psychiatry* **2007**, *190*, 319–325. [CrossRef]
30. Fiske, A.; Henningsen, P.; Buyx, A. Your Robot Therapist Will See You Now: Ethical Implications of Embodied Artificial Intelligence in Psychiatry, Psychology, and Psychotherapy. *J. Med Internet Res.* **2019**, *21*, e13216. [CrossRef]
31. Callon, M.; Courtial, J.P.; Laville, F. Co-word analysis as a tool for describing the network of interactions between basic and technological research: The case of polymer chemistry. *Scientometrics* **1991**, *22*, 155–205. [CrossRef]

MDPI AG
Grosspeteranlage 5
4052 Basel
Switzerland
Tel.: +41 61 683 77 34

Healthcare Editorial Office
E-mail: healthcare@mdpi.com
www.mdpi.com/journal/healthcare

www.ingramcontent.com/pod-product-compliance
Lightning Source LLC
Chambersburg PA
CBHW061604210926
51850CB00009B/2206
* 9 7 8 3 7 2 5 8 7 8 8 7 1 *